T0254581

ICSA Book Series in Statistics

Series editors
Jiahua Chen, University of British Columbia, Vancouver, Canada
Ding-Geng (Din) Chen, University of North Carolina, Chapel Hill, NC, USA

More information about this series at http://www.springer.com/series/13402

Ding-Geng Chen • Zhezhen Jin • Gang Li • Yi Li
Aiyi Liu • Yichuan Zhao

Editors

New Advances in Statistics and Data Science

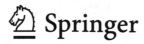 Springer

Editors
Ding-Geng Chen
University of North Carolina
Chapel Hill, NC, USA

Zhezhen Jin
Columbia University
New York, NY, USA

Gang Li
University of California
Los Angeles, CA, USA

Yi Li
University of Michigan-Ann Arbor
Ann Arbor, MI, USA

Aiyi Liu
National Institutes of Health
Bethesda, MD, USA

Yichuan Zhao
Georgia State University
Atlanta, GA, USA

ISSN 2199-0980   ISSN 2199-0999 (electronic)
ICSA Book Series in Statistics
ISBN 978-3-319-88776-0   ISBN 978-3-319-69416-0 (eBook)
https://doi.org/10.1007/978-3-319-69416-0

© Springer International Publishing AG 2017
Softcover re-print of the Hardcover 1st edition 2017
This work is subject to copyright. All rights are reserved by the Publisher, whether the whole or part of
the material is concerned, specifically the rights of translation, reprinting, reuse of illustrations, recitation,
broadcasting, reproduction on microfilms or in any other physical way, and transmission or information
storage and retrieval, electronic adaptation, computer software, or by similar or dissimilar methodology
now known or hereafter developed.
The use of general descriptive names, registered names, trademarks, service marks, etc. in this publication
does not imply, even in the absence of a specific statement, that such names are exempt from the relevant
protective laws and regulations and therefore free for general use.
The publisher, the authors and the editors are safe to assume that the advice and information in this book
are believed to be true and accurate at the date of publication. Neither the publisher nor the authors or
the editors give a warranty, express or implied, with respect to the material contained herein or for any
errors or omissions that may have been made. The publisher remains neutral with regard to jurisdictional
claims in published maps and institutional affiliations.

Printed on acid-free paper

This Springer imprint is published by Springer Nature
The registered company is Springer International Publishing AG
The registered company address is: Gewerbestrasse 11, 6330 Cham, Switzerland

Preface

This book is comprised of the most significant presentations at the 25th ICSA Applied Statistics Symposium held at Hyatt Regency Atlanta on June 12–15, 2016. This symposium attracted more than 700 statisticians and data scientists working in academia, government, and industry worldwide. The theme of this conference was "Challenges of Big Data and Applications of Statistics," which was in recognition of the advent of big data era. The symposium offered great opportunities for learning, receiving inspirations from old research ideas and developing new ones, and promoting research collaborations in data sciences. The invited and contributed talks in the symposium covered rich topics in big data analysis. From this very successful symposium, the six editors selected 19 high-quality presentations and invited the speakers to prepare full chapters for this book. All 19 chapters were thoroughly peer reviewed and consequently revised multiple times before final acceptance. We believe they provide invaluable contributions to statistics and data science.

The goal of this book is to disseminate the recent findings, showcase the scientific outputs of the symposium, and reflect new challenges and important advances in data science, statistics, business statistics, and biostatistics. The chapters in the book present the most recent developments in statistics, innovative methods in data science, and case applications from different fields of statistics, data sciences, and interdisciplinary research fields.

The 19 chapters are organized into four parts. Part I includes five chapters that present a review of the theoretical framework in data science. Part II consists of five chapters on complex and big data analysis. Part III is composed of four chapters that outline clinical trials, statistical shape analysis, and applications. Part IV presents statistical modeling and data analysis. The chapters are organized as self-contained units, and the references for each chapter are at the end of the chapter so that readers can refer to the cited sources for each chapter easily. To facilitate readers' understanding of the proposed methods and new procedures in the book, corresponding data and computing programs can be requested from the authors or the editors by email.

Part I: Review of Theoretical Framework in Data Science (Chapters 1–5)

The chapter "Statistical Distances and Their Role in Robustness" describes the statistical properties of some of the distance measures, which play a fundamental role in statistics, machine learning, and associated scientific disciplines. In this chapter, Markatou, Chen, and Lindsay illustrate the robust nature of Neyman's chi-squared and the non-robust nature of Pearson's chi-squared statistics and discuss the concept of discretization robustness.

In the chapter "The Out-of-Source Error in Multi-Source Cross Validation-Type Procedures," Afendras and Markatou propose the "out-of-source" error. The authors present an unbiased estimator of this error, discuss its variance, and derive natural assumptions under which the consistency of the estimator is guaranteed for a broad class of loss functions and data distributions.

In the following chapter "Meta-Analysis for Rare Events As Binary Outcomes," Dong provides a comprehensive review of the different methods of meta-analyses for rare events as binary outcomes. The methods covered in this chapter include nonparametric meta-analysis, parametric meta-analysis, and parametric bootstrap resampling meta-analysis. Several case studies using these methods are provided.

In the chapter "New Challenges and Strategies in Robust Optimal Design for Multicategory Logit Modelling," O'Brien provides key model-robust design strategies by deriving a larger unifying multi-category logit regression model and model nesting. These strategies are also extended to incorporate geometric and uniform designs. These designs are useful for both parameter estimation and model discrimination via checking for goodness of fit. Some examples are provided to illustrate these results.

The chapter "Testing of Multivariate Spline Growth Model" presents a new method, based on spline approximation and the F-test, for testing multivariate growth curves. Nummi, Möttönen, and Tuomisto show how the basic spline regression model can easily be extended to the multiple response case.

Part II: Complex and Big Data Analysis (Chapters 6–10)

In the chapter "Uncertainty Quantification Using the Nearest Neighbor Gaussian Process," Shi, Kang, Konomi, Vemaganti, and Madireddy demonstrate that the nearest-neighbor Gaussian process (NNGP) for analyzing a large dataset has the potential to be used for uncertainty quantification. The authors discover that when using NNGP to approximate a Gaussian process with strong smoothness, Bayesian inference needs to be carried out carefully with marginalizing over the random effects in the process. Using simulated and real data, the authors investigate the performance of NNGP to approximate the squared-exponential covariance function and its ability to handle change-of-support effects when only aggregated data over space are available.

In the following chapter "Tuning Parameter Selection in the LASSO with Unspecified Propensity," Zhao and Yang incorporate the missing data mechanism or the propensity in the penalized likelihood in order to correctly adopt the LASSO. Compared to the missing data methods with a concrete propensity, this assumption is relatively easier to satisfy in reality. The authors illustrate the proposed methods using real data from a melanoma study.

In the chapter "Adaptive Filtering Increases Power to Detect Differentially Expressed Genes," Nie and Liang propose a novel adaptive filtering procedure that improves power by filtering out genes that are unlikely to be differentially expressed. The authors show that the proposed procedure controls the false discovery rate asymptotically. Simulation study further demonstrates its advantage over state-of-the-art competitors.

In the chapter "Estimating Parameters in Complex Systems with Functional Outputs: A Wavelet-Based Approximate Bayesian Computation Approach," Zhu, Lu, Ming, Gupta, and Müller introduce a wavelet-based approximate Bayesian computation (wABC) approach that is likelihood-free and computationally scalable to functional data measured on a dense, high-dimensional grid. The method relies on near-lossless wavelet decomposition and compression to reduce the high correlation between measurement points and high dimensionality. The authors adopt a Markov chain Monte Carlo algorithm with a Metropolis-Hastings sampler to obtain posterior samples of the parameters for Bayesian inference. A Gaussian process surrogate for the simulator is proposed, and the uncertainty of the resulting sampler is controlled by calculating the expected error rate of the acceptance probability.

The chapter "A Maximum Likelihood Approach for Non-invasive Cancer Diagnosis Using Methylation Profiling of Cell-Free DNA from Blood" designs a maximum likelihood approach and a corresponding computational method to estimate the fraction of tumor-derived cell-free DNA in blood samples using methylation sequencing data. In this chapter, Sun and Li model the cell-free DNA in blood samples as a mixture of normal and tumor-derived cell-free DNA and assume the distributions of methylation levels for both normal and tumor-derived cell-free DNA follow different beta distributions. Through simulations, the authors study the effects of sequencing depth and fraction of tumor-derived cell-free DNA on the estimation accuracy.

Part III: Clinical Trials, Statistical Shape Analysis, and Applications (Chapters 11–14)

In the chapter "A Simple and Efficient Statistical Approach for Designing an Early Phase II Clinical Trial: Ordinal Linear Contrast Test," Zhang, Deng, Wang, and

Ting present an ordinal linear contrast test to design an efficient early Phase II trial. Although the performance of both MCP-Mod and ordinal linear contrast test is comparable, the ordinal linear contrast test is simpler, more robust, and more efficient from a practical perspective. For practitioners, the ordinal linear contrast test is a useful alternative.

The chapter "Landmark-Constrained Statistical Shape Analysis of Elastic Curves and Surfaces" presents a framework for landmark-constrained elastic shape analysis of curves and surfaces. In this chapter, Strait and Kurtek propose a new method, which has its roots in elastic shape analysis and uses the square-root velocity function representation for curves and square-root normal field representation for surfaces to greatly simplify the implementation of these methods. The authors provide complex examples from graphics and computer vision, wherein the landmark-constrained shape analysis framework is able to provide natural deformations between shapes and representative summaries.

In the chapter "Phylogeny-Based Kernels with Application to Microbiome Association Studies," Xiao and Chen provide a three-parameter phylogeny-based kernel, which allows modeling a wide range of nonlinear relationships between bacterial species and the environment for microbiome data. Each parameter has a nice biological interpretation, and by tuning the parameter, the authors can gain insights about how the microbiome interacts with the environment. The authors demonstrate that the test based on their new kernel outperforms those that are based on traditional distance-converted kernels, and apply the phylogeny-based kernel to real gut microbiome data from a diet-microbiome association study.

The chapter "Accounting for Differential Error in Time-to-Event Analyses Using Imperfect Electronic Health Record-Derived Endpoints" addresses the implications of using an imperfectly assessed outcome with differential measurement error in time-to-event analyses, motivated by identifying secondary breast cancer events using electronic health record data. Hubbard, Milton, Zhu, Wang, and Chubak use simulation studies to demonstrate the magnitude of bias induced by failure to account for error in the status or timing of recurrence and compare several methods for correcting this bias.

Part IV: Statistical Modeling and Data Analysis (Chapters 15–19)

In the chapter "Modeling Inter-Trade Durations in the Limit Order Market," Yang, Li, Chen, and Xing discuss the limitations of the Markov-switching multifractal intertrade duration models in the analysis of the ultrahigh-frequency limit order book (LOB) data and propose extensions which replace the exponential distributions on the errors by Weibull and Gamma distributions. Comparing the original and extended models, the authors find that the extended models fit data better.

The chapter "Assessment of Drug Interactions with Repeated Measurements" investigates the problem of assessing the joint effects of combined therapies for in vitro studies with repeated measurements. In this chapter, Zhou, Shen, and Lee use mixed-effects linear regression to estimate the dose-effect curve and propose a procedure to construct the point and interval estimates of the interaction index. Their approach improves the accuracy of the confidence intervals for the interaction indices at observed combination dose levels.

The chapter "Statistical Indices for Risk Tracking in Longitudinal Studies" centers on statistical indices to measure the tracking abilities of variables of interest over time. In this chapter, Tian and Wu propose a series of global statistical tracking indices based on the weighted means of the corresponding local tracking indices. The authors investigate the statistical properties of the new global tracking indices and demonstrate the usefulness of these tracking indices through their application to a longitudinal study of cardiovascular risk factors for children and adolescents.

The chapter "Statistical Analysis of Labor Market Integration: A Mixture Regression Approach" studies the labor market integration of young males in Finland using data from 2005 to 2013. In this chapter, Nummi, Salonen, and O'Brien apply a multivariate logistic mixture regression model for the longitudinal data. The authors suggest that the mixture regression approach can reveal new information that may remain hidden in more formal, census-based labor market statistics.

The chapter "Bias Correction in Age-Period-Cohort Models Using Eigen Analysis" develops a bias correction method using eigenanalysis in the age-period-cohort models. Fu corrects the bias in the parameter estimation using simple calculations without requiring original data and provides accurate standard error estimation. The proposed method is illustrated using two real examples.

The editors are deeply grateful to many people who helped publish this book with Springer. First, we would like to thank the authors of each chapter for their expertise, contributions, and dedications. Second, our sincere appreciations go to all the reviewers for their excellent reviews and valuable time, which greatly improved the presentations and the quality of the book. Third, our deep gratitude goes to the leadership of the executive committee, the organizing committee, the program committee, the program book committee, the local organizing committee, and the numerous volunteers of the 25th ICSA Applied Statistics Symposium because this book would not be possible without this successful symposium. Last but not least, we would like to acknowledge the great support and wonderful assistance of Nicholas Philipson (Springer/ICSA Book Series coordinator and editorial director, Business/Economics & Statistics) and Nitza Jones-Sepulveda (associate editor) from Springer New York throughout the publication process.

We look forward to receiving any comments and suggestions on typos, errors, and improvements about the book. If there is an exchange, please contact Dr. Yichuan Zhao (email: yichuan@gsu.edu) as the corresponding author and, if desired,

Drs. Ding-Geng Chen (email: dinchen@email.unc.edu), Zhezhen Jin (email: zj7@columbia.edu), Gang Li (email: vli@ucla.edu), Yi Li (email: yili@umich.edu), and Aiyi Liu (email: liua@mail.nih.gov) as well.

Chapel Hill, NC, USA	Ding-Geng Chen
New York, NY, USA	Zhezhen Jin
Los Angeles, CA, USA	Gang Li
Ann Arbor, MI, USA	Yi Li
Bethesda, MD, USA	Aiyi Liu
Atlanta, GA, USA	Yichuan Zhao

Contents

Contributors

Georgios Afendras Department of Biostatistics, SPHHP and Jacobs School of Medicine and Biomedical Sciences, University at Buffalo, Buffalo, NY, USA

Jun Chen Division of Biomedical Statistics and Informatics, Department of Health Science Research and Center for Individualized Medicine, Mayo Clinic, Rochester, MN, USA

Yang Chen Department of Biostatistics, University at Buffalo, Buffalo, NY, USA

Xinyun Chen Department of Finance, Economics and Management School, Wuhan University, Wuhan, China

Jessica Chubak Kaiser Permanente Washington Health Research Institute, Seattle, WA, USA

Qiqi Deng Boehringer-Ingelheim Pharmaceuticals, Inc., Ridgefield, CT, USA

Gaohong Dong iStats Inc., Long Island City, NY, USA

Martina Fu Research Lab of Dr. Yi Li, Department of Biostatistics, University of Michigan, Ann Arbor, MI, USA

Anupam K. Gupta Department of Mechanical Engineering, Virginia Tech, Blacksburg, VA, USA

Rebecca A. Hubbard Department of Biostatistics, Epidemiology & Informatics, University of Pennsylvania, Philadelphia, PA, USA

Emily L. Kang Department of Mathematical Sciences, University of Cincinnati, Cincinnati, OH, USA

Bledar A. Konomi Department of Mathematical Sciences, University of Cincinnati, Cincinnati, OH, USA

Sebastian Kurtek Department of Statistics, The Ohio State University, Columbus, OH, USA

J. Jack Lee Department of Biostatistics, The University of Texas MD Anderson Cancer Center, Houston, TX, USA

Wenyuan Li Department of Pathology and Laboratory Medicine, University of California at Los Angeles, Los Angeles, CA, USA

Zhicheng Li Department of Economics, State University of New York, Stony Brook, NY, USA

Kun Liang University of Waterloo, Waterloo, ON, Canada

Changwon Lim Department of Applied Statistics, Chung Ang University, Seoul, South Korea

Bruce G. Lindsay Department of Statistics, The Pennsylvania State University, University Park, PA, USA

Ruijin Lu Department of Statistics, Virginia Tech, Blacksburg, VA, USA

Marianthi Markatou Department of Biostatistics, SPHHP and Jacobs School of Medicine and Biomedical Sciences, University at Buffalo, Buffalo, NY, USA

Sandeep Madireddy Argonne National Laboratory, Lemont, IL, USA

Joanna Harton Department of Biostatistics, Epidemiology & Informatics, University of Pennsylvania, Philadelphia, PA, USA

Chen Ming Department of Mechanical Engineering, Virginia Tech, Blacksburg, VA, USA

Jyrki Möttönen Department of Mathematics and Statistics, University of Helsinki, Helsinki, Finland

Rolf Müller Department of Mechanical Engineering, Virginia Tech, Blacksburg, VA, USA

Zixin Nie University of Waterloo, Waterloo, ON, Canada

Tapio Nummi Faculty of Natural Sciences, University of Tampere, Tampere, Finland

Timothy E. O'Brien Department of Mathematics and Statistics and Institute of Environmental Sustainability, Loyola University of Chicago, Chicago, IL, USA

Janne Salonen Research Department, The Finnish Centre for Pensions, Helsinki, Finland,

Chan Shen Department of Health Services Research, Division of Cancer Prevention and Population Sciences, The University of Texas MD Anderson Cancer Center, Houston, TX, USA

Hongxiang Shi Department of Mathematical Sciences, University of Cincinnati, Cincinnati, OH, USA

Justin Strait Department of Statistics, The Ohio State University, Columbus, OH, USA

Carol K. Sun Oak Park High School, Oak Park, CA, USA

Xin Tian Office of Biostatistics Research, National Heart, Lung, and Blood Institute, Bethesda, MD, USA

Naitee Ting Boehringer-Ingelheim Pharmaceuticals, Inc., Ridgefield, CT, USA

Martti T. Tuomisto Faculty of Social Sciences (Psychology), University of Tampere, Tampere, Finland

Kumar Vemaganti Department of Mechanical and Materials Engineering, University of Cincinnati, Cincinnati, OH, USA

Le Wang Department of Biostatistics, Epidemiology & Informatics, University of Pennsylvania, Philadelphia, PA, USA

Susan Wang Boehringer-Ingelheim Pharmaceuticals, Inc., Ridgefield, CT, USA

Colin O. Wu Office of Biostatistics Research, National Heart, Lung, and Blood Institute, Bethesda, MD, USA

Jian Xiao Division of Biomedical Statistics and Informatics, Center for Individualized Medicine, Mayo Clinic, Rochester, MN, USA

Haipeng Xing Department of Applied Mathematics and Statistics, University of New York, Stony Brook, NY, USA

Jianzhao Yang Department of Applied Mathematics and Statistics, University of New York, Stony Brook, NY, USA

Yang Yang Department of Biostatistics, State University of New York at Buffalo, Buffalo, NY, USA

Jiwei Zhao Department of Biostatistics, State University of New York at Buffalo, Buffalo, NY, USA

Yaohua Zhang Department of Statistics, University of Connecticut, Storrs, CT, USA

Hongxiao Zhu Department of Statistics, Virginia Tech, Blacksburg, VA, USA

Weiwei Zhu Kaiser Permanente Washington Health Research Institute, Seattle, WA, USA

Shouhao Zhou Department of Biostatistics, The University of Texas MD Anderson Cancer Center, Houston, TX, USA

About the Editors

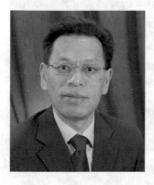

Professor Ding-Geng Chen is a fellow of the American Statistical Association and is currently the Wallace Kuralt distinguished professor at the University of North Carolina at Chapel Hill, USA, and an extraordinary professor at the University of Pretoria, South Africa. He was a biostatistics professor at the University of Rochester and the Karl E. Peace endowed eminent scholar chair in biostatistics at Georgia Southern University. He is also a senior statistics consultant for biopharmaceuticals and government agencies with extensive expertise in Monte Carlo simulations, clinical trial biostatistics, and public health statistics. Professor Chen has more than 150 referred professional publications; coauthored and coedited 15 books on clinical trial methodology, meta-analysis, and public health applications; and has been invited nationally and internationally to give presentations on his research. Professor Chen was honored with the "Award of Recognition" in 2014 by the Deming Conference Committee for creating highly successful advanced biostatistics workshop tutorials with his books.

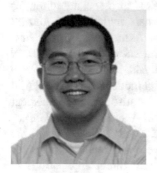

Professor Zhezhen Jin is a professor of biostatistics at Columbia University. His research interests in statistics include survival analysis, resampling methods, longitudinal data analysis, and nonparametric and semiparametric models. Dr. Jin has collaborated on research in the areas of cardiology, neurology, hematology, oncology, and epidemiology. He is a founding editor-in-chief of *Contemporary Clinical Trials Communications*; serves a associate editor for *Lifetime Data Analysis, Contemporary Clinical Trials*, and *Communications for Statistical Applications and Methods*; and is on the editorial board for *Kidney International*, the journal of the International Society of Nephrology. Dr. Jin has published over 150 peer-reviewed research papers in statistical and medical journals. He is a fellow of the American Statistical Association.

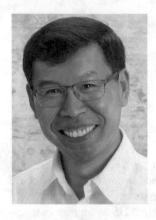

Professor Gang Li is a professor of biostatistics and biomathematics at the University of California at Los Angeles (UCLA) and the director of UCLA's Jonsson Comprehensive Cancer Center Biostatistics Shared Resource. His research interests include survival analysis, longitudinal data analysis, high-dimensional and omics data analysis, clinical trials, and evaluation and development of biomarkers. He has published over 100 papers in a wide variety of prestigious journals such as the *Annals of Statistics, the Journal of the American Statistical Association, the Journal of the Royal Statistical Society-B, Biometrika,* and *Biometrics.* He is an elected fellow of the Institute of Mathematics, the American Statistical Association, and the Royal Statistical Society, as well as an elected member of the International Statistical Institute. He has been serving on the editorial board of several statistical journals including *Biometrics.* Dr. Li has been active in collaborating with researchers in basic science, translational research, and clinical trials and has been a statistics principal investigator for multiple NIH-funded projects.

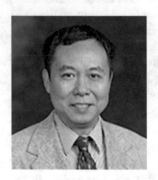

Professor Yi Li is a professor of biostatistics and global public health at the University of Michigan School of Public Health (UM-SPH). He is currently the director of China Initiatives at UM-SPH and served as the director of the Kidney Epidemiology and Cost Center at the University of Michigan from 2011 to 2016. Dr. Li is an elected fellow of the American Statistical Association and is serving as an associate editor for several major statistical journals, including the *Journal of the American Statistical Association, Biometrics, Scandinavian Journal of Statistics,* and *Lifetime Data Analysis.* His current research interests are survival analysis, longitudinal and correlated data analysis, measurement error problems, spatial models, and clinical trial designs. He has published more than 140 papers in major statistical and biomedical journals, including the *Journal of the American Statistical Association*, the *Journal of the Royal Statistical Society-B*, *Biometrika*, *Biometrics*, and *Proceedings of the National Academy of Sciences.* His group has been developing methodologies for analyzing large-scale and high-dimensional datasets, with direct applications in observational studies as well as in genetics/genomics. His methodologic research is funded by various NIH statistical grants starting from 2003. As the principal investigator, Dr. Li has been leading a multiyear national project to develop new measures to evaluate all dialysis facilities in the United States, with the goal of improving renal health care, saving lives, and reducing costs. Dr. Li is actively involved in collaborative research in clinical trials and observational studies with researchers from the University of Michigan and Harvard University. The applications have included chronic kidney disease surveillance, organ transplantation, cancer preventive studies, and cancer genomics.

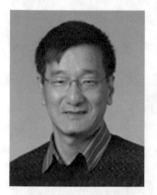

Dr. Aiyi Liu is a senior investigator in the Biostatistics and Bioinformatics Branch of the Division of Intramural Population Health Research at the Eunice Kennedy Shriver National Institute of Child Health and Human Development, National Institutes of Health. A fellow of the American Statistical Association, Dr. Liu has authored/coauthored about 90 statistical methodological publications covering various topics including general statistical estimation theory, sequential methodology and adaptive designs, and statistical methods for diagnostic biomarkers.

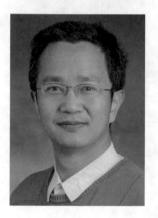

Professor Yichuan Zhao is a professor of statistics at Georgia State University in Atlanta. His current research interest focuses on survival analysis, empirical likelihood methods, nonparametric statistics, analysis of ROC curves, bioinformatics, Monte Carlo methods, and statistical modeling of fuzzy systems. He has published over 70 research articles in statistics and biostatistics research fields. Dr. Zhao initiated the Workshop Series on Biostatistics and Bioinformatics in 2012. He was a chair of the organizing committee for the 25th ICSA Applied Statistics Symposium in Atlanta, which was held to great success. He is currently serving as editor and is on the editorial board for several statistical journals. Dr. Zhao is an elected member of the International Statistical Institute.

List of Chapter Reviewers

Dr. Georgios Afendras Department of Biostatistics, SPHHP and Jacobs School of Medicine and Biomedical Sciences, University at Buffalo, Buffalo, NY, USA

Dr. Sounak Chakraborty Department of Statistics, University of Missouri-Columbia, Columbia, MO, USA

Dr. Ding-Geng Chen University of North Carolina, Chapel Hill, NC, USA

University of Pretoria, Pretoria, South Africa

Dr. Feng Chen School of Mathematics and Statistics, University of New South Wales, Sydney, Australia

Dr. Jian Chen Model Risk Management, Chicago, IL, USA

Jun Chen Division of Biomedical Statistics and Informatics, Department of Health Science Research and Center for Individualized Medicine, Mayo Clinic, Rochester, MN, USA

Dr. Guoqing Diao Department of Statistics, George Mason University, Fairfax, VA, USA

Dr. Ruzong Fan Department of Biostatistics, Bioinformatics, and Biomathematics, Georgetown University, Washington, DC, USA

Dr. Yixin Fang Department of Mathematical Sciences, New Jersey Institute of Technology, Newark, NJ, USA

Dr. Wenge Guo Department of Mathematical Sciences, New Jersey Institute of Technology, Newark, NJ, USA

Dr. Zhezhen Jin Department of Biostatistics, Columbia University, New York, NY, USA

Dr. Jian Kang Department of Biostatistics, University of Michigan, Ann Arbor, MI, USA

Dr. Linglong Kong Department of Mathematical and Statistical Sciences, University of Alberta, Edmonton, AB, Canada

Dr. Suprateek Kundu Department of Biostatistics and Bioinformatics, Emory University, Atlanta, GA, USA

Dr. Gang Li Department of Biostatistics, University of California, Los Angeles, CA, USA

Dr. Qizhai Li Academy of Mathematics and Systems Science, Chinese Academy of Sciences, Beijing, China

Dr. Yi Li Department of Biostatistics, University of Michigan, Ann Arbor, MI, USA

Dr. Chunfang (Devon) Lin Department of Mathematics and Statistics, Queen's University, Kingston, ON, Canada

Dr. Lizhen Lin Department of Applied and Computational Mathematics and Statistics, The University of Notre Dame, Notre Dame, IN, USA

Dr. Aiyi Liu Biostatistics and Bioinformatics Branch, Division of Intramural Population Health Research, National Institutes of Health, Bethesda, MD, USA

Dr. Anna Liu Department of Mathematics and Statistics, University of Massachusetts, Amherst, MA, USA

Dr. Rong Liu Department of Mathematics and Statistics, The University of Toledo, Toledo, OH, USA

Dr. Marianthi Markatou Department of Biostatistics, SPHHP and Jacobs School of Medicine and Biomedical Sciences, University at Buffalo, Buffalo, NY, USA

Dr. Yajun Mei H. Milton Stewart School of Industrial and Systems Engineering, Georgia Institute of Technology, Atlanta, GA, USA

Dr. Shuelei (Sherry) Ni Department of Statistics and Analytical Sciences, Kennesaw State University, Kennesaw, GA, USA

Dr. Jingyong Su Department of Mathematics & Statistics, Texas Tech University, Lubbock, TX, USA

Dr. Xin Tian Office of Biostatistics Research, National Heart, Lung, and Blood Institute, Bethesda, MD, USA

Dr. Naitee Ting Boehringer-Ingelheim Pharmaceuticals, Inc., Ridgefield, CT, USA

Dr. Antai Wang Department of Mathematical Sciences, New Jersey Institute of Technology, Newark, NJ, USA

Dr. Colin O. Wu Office of Biostatistics Research, National Heart, Lung, and Blood Institute, Bethesda, MD, USA

Dr. Xiaowei Wu Department of Statistics, Virginia Tech, Blacksburg, VA, USA

Dr. Weixin Yao Department of Statistics, University of California, Riverside, CA, USA

Dr. Xiang Zhang Eli Lilly and Company, Indianapolis, IN, USA

Dr. Jiwei Zhao Department of Biostatistics, State University of New York at Buffalo, Buffalo, NY, USA

Dr. Yichuan Zhao Department of Mathematics and Statistics, Georgia State University, Atlanta, GA, USA

Dr. Zhigen Zhao Department of Statistical Science, Temple University, Philadelphia, PA, USA

Dr. Shouhao Zhou Department of Biostatistics, The University of Texas MD Anderson Cancer Center, Houston, TX, USA

Dr. Hongxiao Zhu Department of Statistics, Virginia Tech, Blacksburg, VA, USA

Part I
Review of Theoretical Framework in Data Science

Statistical Distances and Their Role in Robustness

Marianthi Markatou, Yang Chen, Georgios Afendras, and Bruce G. Lindsay

1   Introduction

Distance measures play a ubiquitous role in statistical theory and thinking. However, within the statistical literature this extensive role has too often been played out behind the scenes, with other aspects of the statistical problems being viewed as more central, more interesting, or more important.

The behind the scenes role of statistical distances shows up in estimation, where we often use estimators based on minimizing a distance, explicitly or implicitly, but rarely studying how the properties of the distance determine the properties of the estimators. Distances are also prominent in goodness-of-fit (GOF) but the usual question we ask is how powerful is our method against a set of interesting alternatives not what aspects of the difference between the hypothetical model and the alternative are we measuring?

How can we interpret a numerical value of a distance? In goodness-of-fit we learn about Kolmogorov-Smirnov and Cramér-von Mises distances but how do these compare with each other? How can we improve their properties by looking at what statistical properties are they measuring?

Past interest in distance functions between statistical populations had a two-fold purpose. The first purpose was to prove existence theorems regarding some

M. Markatou (✉) • G. Afendras
Department of Biostatistics, SPHHP and Jacobs School of Medicine and Biomedical Sciences, University at Buffalo, Buffalo, NY, USA
e-mail: markatou@buffalo.edu; gafendra@buffalo.edu

Y. Chen
Department of Biostatistics, University at Buffalo, Buffalo, NY 14214, USA
e-mail: ychen57@buffalo.edu

B.G. Lindsay
Department of Statistics, The Pennsylvania State University, University Park, PA 16820, USA
e-mail: bgl@psu.edu

© Springer International Publishing AG 2017
D.-G. Chen et al. (eds.), *New Advances in Statistics and Data Science*,
ICSA Book Series in Statistics, https://doi.org/10.1007/978-3-319-69416-0_1

optimum solutions in the problem of statistical inference. Wald (1950) in his book on statistical decision functions gave numerous definitions of distance between two distributions which he primarily introduced for the purpose of creating decision functions. In this context, the choice of the distance function is not entirely arbitrary, but it is guided by the nature of the mathematical problem at hand.

Statistical distances are defined in a variety of ways, by comparing distribution functions, density functions or characteristic functions and moment generating functions. Further, there are discrete and continuous analogues of distances based on comparing density functions, where the word "density" is used to also indicate probability mass functions. Distances can also be constructed based on the divergence between a nonparametric probability density estimate and a parametric family of densities. Typical examples of distribution-based distances are the Kolmogorov-Smirnov and Cramér-von Mises distances. A separate class of distances is based upon comparing the empirical characteristic function with the theoretical characteristic function that corresponds, for example, to a family of models under study, or by comparing empirical and theoretical versions of moment generating functions.

In this paper we proceed to study in detail the properties of some statistical distances, and especially the properties of the class of chi-squared distances. We place emphasis on determining the sense in which we can offer meaningful interpretations of these distances as measures of statistical loss. Section 2 of the paper discusses the definition of a statistical distance in the discrete probability models context. Section 3 presents the class of chi-squared distances and their statistical interpretation again in the context of discrete probability models. Section 3.3 discusses metric and other properties of the symmetric chi-squared distance. One of the key issues in the construction of model misspecification measures is that allowance should be made for the scale difference between observed data and a hypothesized model continuous distribution. To account for this difference in scale we need the distance measure to exhibit discretization robustness, a concept that is discussed in Sect. 4.1. To achieve discretization robustness we need sensitive distances, and this requirement dictates a balance of sensitivity and statistical noise. Various strategies that deal with this issue are discussed in the literature and we briefly discuss them in Sect. 4.1. A flexible class of distances that allows the user to adjust the noise/sensitivity trade-off is the kernel smoothed distances upon which we briefly remark on in Sect. 4. Finally, Sect. 5 presents further discussion.

2 The Discrete Setting

Procedures based on minimizing the distance between two density functions express the idea that a fitted statistical model should summarize reasonably well the data and that assessment of the adequacy of the fitted model can be achieved by using the value of the distance between the data and the fitted model.

The essential idea of density-based minimum distance methods has been presented in the literature for quite some time as it is evidenced by the method of minimum chi-squared (Neyman 1949). An extensive list of minimum chi-squared methods can be found in Berkson (1980). Matusita (1955) and Rao (1963) studied minimum Hellinger distance estimation in discrete models while Beran (1977) was the first to use the idea of minimum Hellinger distance in continuous models.

We begin within the discrete distribution framework so as to provide the clearest possible focus for our interpretations. Thus, let $\mathscr{T} = \{0, 1, 2, \cdots, T\}$, where T is possibly infinite, be a discrete sample space. On this sample space we define a true probability density $\tau(t)$, as well as a family of densities $\mathscr{M} = \{m_\theta(t) : \theta \in \Theta\}$, where Θ is the parameter space. Assume we have independent and identically distributed random variables $X_1, X_2, \cdots, X_n$ producing the realizations $x_1, x_2, \cdots, x_n$ from $\tau(\cdot)$. We record the data as $d(t) = n(t)/n$, where $n(t)$ is the number of observations in the sample with value equal to t.

Definition 1 We will say that $\rho(\tau, m)$ is a statistical distance between two probability distributions with densities τ, m if $\rho(\tau, m) \geq 0$, with equality if and only if τ and m are the same for all statistical purposes.

Note that we do not require symmetry or the triangle inequality, so that $\rho(\tau, m)$ is not formally a metric. This is not a drawback as well known distances, such as Kullback-Leibler, are not symmetric and do not satisfy the triangle inequality.

We can extend the definition of a distance between two densities to that of a distance between a density and a class of densities as follows.

Definition 2 Let $\mathscr{M}$ be a given model class and τ be a probability density that does not belong in the model class $\mathscr{M}$. Then, the distance between τ and $\mathscr{M}$ is defined as

$$\rho(\tau, \mathscr{M}) = \inf_{m \in \mathscr{M}} \rho(\tau, m),$$

whenever the infimum exists. Let $m_{\text{best}} \in \mathscr{M}$ be the best fitting model, then

$$\rho(\tau, m_{\text{best}}) \triangleq \rho(\tau, \mathscr{M}).$$

We interpret $\rho(\tau, m)$ or $\rho(\tau, \mathscr{M})$ as measuring the "lack-of-fit" in the sense that larger values of $\rho(\tau, m)$ mean that the model element m is a worst fit to τ for our statistical purposes. Therefore, we will require $\rho(\tau, m)$ to indicate the worst mistake that we can make if we use m instead of τ. The precise meaning of this statement will be obvious in the case of the total variation distance, as we will see that the total variation distance measures the error, in probability, that is made when m is used instead of τ.

Lindsay (1994) studied the relationship between the concepts of efficiency and robustness for the class of f- or ϕ-divergences in the case of discrete probability models and defined the concept of Pearson residuals as follows.

Definition 3 For a pair of densities τ, m define the Pearson residual by

$$\delta(t) = \frac{\tau(t)}{m(t)} - 1, \tag{1}$$

with range the interval $[-1, \infty)$.

This residual has been used by Lindsay (1994), Basu and Lindsay (1994), Markatou (2000, 2001), and Markatou et al. (1997, 1998) in investigating the robustness of the minimum disparity and weighted likelihood estimators respectively. It also appears in the definition of the class of power divergence measures defined by

$$\rho(\tau, m) = \frac{1}{\lambda(\lambda + 1)} \sum \tau(t) \left\{ \left(\frac{\tau(t)}{m(t)} \right)^{\lambda} - 1 \right\}$$

$$= \frac{1}{\lambda(\lambda + 1)} \sum m(t) \{ (1 + \delta(t))^{\lambda+1} - 1 \}.$$

For $\lambda = -2, -1, -1/2, 0$ and 1 one obtains the well-known Neyman's chi-squared (divided by 2) distance, Kullback-Leibler divergence, twice-squared Hellinger distance, likelihood disparity and Pearson's chi-squared (divided by 2) distance respectively. For additional details see Lindsay (1994) and Basu and Lindsay (1994).

A special class of distance measures we are particularly interested in is the class of chi-squared measures. In what follows we discuss in detail this class.

3 Chi-Squared Distance Measures

We present the class of chi-squared disparities and discuss their properties. We offer loss function interpretations of the chi-squared measures and show that Pearson's chi-squared is the supremum of squared Z-statistics while Neyman's chi-squared is the supremum of squared t-statistics. We also show that the symmetric chi-squared is a metric and offer a testing interpretation for it.

We start with the definition of a generalized chi-squared distance between two densities τ, m.

Definition 4 Let $\tau(t)$, $m(t)$ be two discrete probability distributions. Then, define the class of generalized chi-squared distances as

$$\chi_a^2(\tau, m) = \sum \frac{[\tau(t) - m(t)]^2}{a(t)},$$

where $a(t)$ is a probability density function.

Notice that if we restrict ourselves to the multinomial setting and choose $\tau(t) = d(t)$ and $a(t) = m(t)$, the resulting chi-squared distance is Pearson's chi-squared statistic. Lindsay (1994) studied the robustness properties of a version of $\chi_a^2(\tau, m)$ by taking $a(t) = [\tau(t) + m(t)]/2$. The resulting distance is called *symmetric chi-squared*, and it is given as

$$S^2(\tau, m) = \sum \frac{2[\tau(t) - m(t)]^2}{\tau(t) + m(t)}.$$

The chi-squared distance is symmetric because $S^2(\tau, m) = S^2(m, \tau)$ and satisfies the triangle inequality. Thus, by definition it is a proper metric, and there is a strong dependence of the properties of the distance on the denominator $a(t)$. In general we can use as a denominator $a(t) = \alpha\tau(t) + \bar{\alpha}m(t)$, $\bar{\alpha} = 1 - \alpha$, $\alpha \in [0, 1]$. The so defined distance is called blended chi-squared (Lindsay 1994).

3.1 Loss Function Interpretation

We now discuss the loss function interpretation of the aforementioned class of distances.

Proposition 1 *Let τ, m be two discrete probabilities. Then*

$$\rho(\tau, m) = \sup_h \frac{\{\mathbb{E}_\tau(h(X)) - \mathbb{E}_m(h(X))\}^2}{\mathrm{Var}_a(h(X))},$$

where $a(t)$ is a density function, and $h(X)$ has finite second moment.

Proof Let h be a function defined on the sample space. We can prove the above statement by looking at the equivalent problem

$$\sup_h \{\mathbb{E}_\tau(h(X)) - \mathbb{E}_m(h(X))\}^2, \quad \text{subject to } \mathrm{Var}_a(h(X)) = 1.$$

Note that the transformation from the original problem to the simpler problem stated above is without loss of generality because the first problem is scale invariant, that is, the functions $\widehat{h}$ and $c\widehat{h}$ where c is a constant give exactly the same values. In addition, we have location invariance in that $h(X)$ and $h(X) + c$ give again the same values, and symmetry requires us to solve

$$\sup_h \{\mathbb{E}_\tau(h(X)) - \mathbb{E}_m(h(X))\}, \quad \text{subject to } \sum h^2(t)a(t) = 1.$$

To solve this linear problem with its quadratic constraint we use Lagrange multipliers. The Lagrangian is given as

$$L(t) = \sum h(t)(\tau(t) - m(t)) - \lambda \left\{ \sum h^2(t)a(t) - 1 \right\}.$$

Then

$$\frac{\partial}{\partial h}L(t) = 0, \text{ for each value of } t,$$

is equivalent to

$$\tau(t) - m(t) - 2\lambda h(t)a(t) = 0, \forall t,$$

or

$$\widehat{h}(t) = \frac{\tau(t) - m(t)}{2\lambda a(t)}.$$

Using the constraint we obtain

$$\sum \frac{[\tau(t) - m(t)]^2}{4\lambda^2 a(t)} = 1 \Rightarrow \widehat{\lambda} = \frac{1}{2} \left\{ \sum \frac{[\tau(t) - m(t)]^2}{a(t)} \right\}^{1/2}.$$

Therefore,

$$\widehat{h}(t) = \frac{\tau(t) - m(t)}{a(t)\sqrt{\sum \frac{[\tau(t) - m(t)]^2}{a(t)}}}.$$

If we substitute the above value of h in the original problem we obtain

$$\sup_{h}\{\mathbb{E}_\tau(h(X)) - \mathbb{E}_m(h(X))\}^2 = \sup_{h} \left\{ \sum h(t)[\tau(t) - m(t)]^2 \right\}$$

$$= \left\{ \sum \frac{[\tau(t) - m(t)]^2}{a(t)\sqrt{\sum \frac{[\tau(t) - m(t)]^2}{a(t)}}} \right\}^2$$

$$= \left\{ \frac{1}{\sqrt{\sum \frac{[\tau(t) - m(t)]^2}{a(t)}}} \left(\sum \frac{[\tau(t) - m(t)]^2}{a(t)} \right) \right\}^2 = \sum \frac{[\tau(t) - m(t)]^2}{a(t)},$$

as was claimed.   □

Remark 1 Note that $\widehat{h}(t)$ is the least favorable function for detecting differences between means of two distributions.

Corollary 1 *The standardized function which creates the largest difference in means is*

$$\widehat{h}(t) = \frac{\tau(t) - m(t)}{a(t)\sqrt{\chi_a^2}},$$

where $\chi_a^2 = \sum \frac{[\tau(t) - m(t)]^2}{a(t)}$, and the corresponding difference in means is

$$\mathbb{E}_\tau[\widehat{h}(t)] - \mathbb{E}_m[\widehat{h}(t)] = \sqrt{\chi_a^2}.$$

Remark 2 Are there any additional distances that can be obtained as solutions to an optimization problem? And what is the statistical interpretation of these optimization problems? To answer the aforementioned questions we first present the optimization problems associated with the Kullback-Leibler and Hellinger distances. In fact, the entire class of the blended weighted Hellinger distances can be obtained as a solution to an appropriately defined optimization problem. Secondly, we discuss the statistical interpretability of these problems by connecting them, by analogy, to the construction of confidence intervals via Scheffé's method.

Definition 5 The Kullback-Leibler divergence or distance between two discrete probability density functions is defined as

$$KL(\tau, m_\beta) = \sum_x m_\beta(x)[\log m_\beta(x) - \log \tau(x)].$$

Proposition 2 *The Kullback-Leibler distance is obtained as a solution of the optimization problem*

$$\sup_h \sum_x h(x) m_\beta(x), \quad \text{subject to } \sum_x e^{h(x)} \tau(x) \le 1,$$

where $h(\cdot)$ is a function defined on the same space as τ.

Proof It is straightforward if one writes the Lagrangian and differentiates with respect to h.   □

Definition 6 The class of squared blended weighted Hellinger distances ($BWHD_\alpha$) is defined as

$$(BWHD_\alpha)^2 = \sum_x \frac{[\tau(x) - m_\beta(x)]^2}{2\left[\alpha\sqrt{\tau(x)} + \overline{\alpha}\sqrt{m_\beta(x)}\right]^2},$$

where $0 < \alpha < 1, \overline{\alpha} = 1 - \alpha$ and $\tau(x), m_\beta(x)$ are two probability densities.

Proposition 3 *The class of $BWHD_\alpha$ arises as a solution to the optimization problem*

$$\sup_h \sum_x h(x)[\tau(x) - m_\beta(x)], \quad \text{subject to } \sum_x h^2(x)\left[\alpha\sqrt{\tau(x)} + \overline{\alpha}\sqrt{m_\beta(x)}\right]^2 \le 1.$$

When $\alpha = \overline{\alpha} = 1/2$, the $(BWHD_{1/2})^2$ gives twice the squared Hellinger distance.

Proof Straightforward.   □

Although both Kullback-Leibler and blended weighted Hellinger distances are solutions of appropriate optimization problems, they do not arise from optimization problems in which the constraints can be interpreted as variances. To exemplify and illustrate further this point we first need to discuss the connection with Scheffé's confidence intervals.

One of the methods of constructing confidence intervals is Scheffé's method. The method adjusts the significance levels of the confidence intervals for general contrasts to account for multiple comparisons. The procedure, therefore, controls the overall significance for any possible contrast or set of contrasts and can be stated as follows,

$$\sup_c \left| c^T(y - \mu) \right| < K\widehat{\sigma}, \quad \text{subject to } \|c\| = 1, \ c^T 1 = 0,$$

where $\widehat{\sigma}$ is an estimated contrast variance, $\|\cdot\|$ denotes the Euclidean distance and K is an appropriately defined constant.

The chi-squared distances extend this framework as follows. Assume that $\mathcal{H}$ is a class of functions which are taken, without loss of generality, to have zero expectation. Then, we construct the optimization problem $\sup_h \int h(x)[\tau(x) - m_\beta(x)]dx$, subject to a constraint that can possibly be interpreted as a constraint on the variance of $h(x)$ either under the hypothesized model distribution or under the distribution of the data.

The chi-squared distances arise as solutions of optimization problems subject to variance constrains. As such, they are interpretable as tools that allow the construction of "Scheffé-type" confidence intervals for models. On the other hand, distances such as the Kullback-Leibler or blended weighted Hellinger distance do not arise as solutions of optimization problems subject to interpretable variance constraints. As such they cannot be used to construct confidence intervals for models.

3.2 Loss Analysis of Pearson and Neyman Chi-Squared Distances

We next offer interpretations of the Pearson chi-squared and Neyman chi-squared statistics. These interpretations are not well known; furthermore, they are useful in illustrating the robustness character of the Neyman statistic and the non-robustness character of the Pearson statistic.

Recall that the Pearson statistic is

$$\sum \frac{[d(t) - m(t)]^2}{m(t)} = \sup_h \frac{[\mathbb{E}_d(h(X)) - \mathbb{E}_m(h(X))]^2}{\text{Var}_m(h(X))}$$

$$= \frac{1}{n} \sup_h \frac{[\frac{1}{n}\sum h(X_i) - \mathbb{E}_m(h(X))]^2}{\frac{1}{n}\text{Var}_m(h(X))} = \frac{1}{n} \sup_h Z_h^2,$$

that is, the Pearson statistic is the supremum of squared Z-statistics.

A similar argument shows that Neyman's chi-squared equals $\sup_h t_h^2$, the supremum of squared t-statistics.

This property shows that the chi-squared measures have a statistical interpretation in that a small chi-squared distance indicates that the means are close on the scale of standard deviation. Furthermore, an additional advantage of the above interpretations is that the robustness character of these statistics is exemplified. Neyman's chi-squared, being the supremum of squared t-statistics, is robust, whereas Pearson's chi-squared is non-robust, since it is the supremum of squared Z-statistics.

Signal-to-Noise There is an additional interpretation of the chi-squared statistic that rests on the definition of signal-to-noise ratio that comes from the engineering literature.

Consider the pair of hypotheses $H_0 : X_i \sim \tau$ versus the alternative $H_1 : X_i \sim m$, where X_i are independent and identically distributed random variables. If we consider the set of randomized test functions that depend on the "output" function h, the distance between H_0 and H_1 is

$$S^2(\tau, m) = \frac{[\mathbb{E}_m(h(X)) - \mathbb{E}_\tau(h(X))]^2}{\mathrm{Var}_\tau(h(X))}.$$

This quantity is a generalization of one of the more common definitions of signal-to-noise ratio. If, instead of working with a given output function h, we take supremum over the output functions h, we obtain Neyman's chi-squared distance, which has been used in the engineering literature for robust detection. Further, the quantity $S^2(\tau, m)$ has been used in the design of decision systems (Poor 1980).

3.3 Metric Properties of the Symmetric Chi-Squared Distance

The symmetric chi-squared distance, defined as

$$S^2(\tau, m) = \sum \frac{2[\tau(t) - m(t)]^2}{m(t) + \tau(t)},$$

can be viewed as a good compromise between the non-robust Pearson distance and the robust Neyman distance. In what follows, we prove that $S^2(\tau, m)$ is indeed a metric. The following series of lemmas will help us establish the triangle inequality for $S^2(\tau, m)$.

Lemma 1 *If a, b, c are numbers such that $0 \leq a \leq b \leq c$ then*

$$\frac{c-a}{\sqrt{c+a}} \leq \frac{b-a}{\sqrt{b+a}} + \frac{c-b}{\sqrt{c+b}}.$$

Proof First we work with the right-hand side of the above inequality. Write

$$\frac{b-a}{\sqrt{b+a}} + \frac{c-b}{\sqrt{c+b}} = (c-a)\{\frac{b-a}{c-a}\frac{1}{\sqrt{b+a}} + \frac{c-b}{c-a}\frac{1}{\sqrt{c+b}}\}$$

$$= (c-a)\{\frac{\alpha}{\sqrt{a+b}} + (1-\alpha)\frac{1}{\sqrt{c+b}}\},$$

where $\alpha = (b-a)/(c-a)$. Set $g(t) = 1/\sqrt{t}, t > 0$. Then $g''(t) = \frac{d^2}{dt^2}g(t) > 0$, hence the function $g(t)$ is convex. Therefore, the aforementioned relationship becomes

$$(c-a)\{\alpha g(a+b) + (1-\alpha)g(c+b)\}.$$

But

$$\alpha g(a+b) + (1-\alpha)g(c+b) \geq g(\alpha(a+b) + (1-\alpha)(c+b)),$$

where

$$\alpha(a+b) + (1-\alpha)(c+b) = \frac{b-a}{c-a}(a+b) + \frac{c-b}{c-a}(b+c) = c+a.$$

Thus

$$\alpha g(a+b) + (1-\alpha)g(c+b) \geq g(c+a),$$

and hence

$$\frac{b-a}{\sqrt{b+a}} + \frac{c-b}{\sqrt{c+b}} \geq \frac{c-a}{\sqrt{c+a}},$$

as was stated.   □

Note that because the function is strictly convex we do not obtain equality except when $a = b = c$.

Lemma 2 *If a, b, c are numbers such that $a \geq 0$, $b \geq 0$, $c \geq 0$ then*

$$\left|\frac{c-a}{\sqrt{c+a}}\right| \leq \left|\frac{b-a}{\sqrt{b+a}}\right| + \left|\frac{c-b}{\sqrt{c+b}}\right|.$$

Proof We will distinguish three different cases.

Case 1: $0 \leq a \leq b \leq c$ is already discussed in Lemma 1.
Case 2: $0 \leq c \leq b \leq a$ can be proved as in Lemma 1 by interchanging the role of
    a and c.
Case 3:   In this case b is not between a and c, thus either $a \leq c \leq b$ or $b \leq a \leq c$.

Assume first that $a \leq c \leq b$. Then we need to show that

$$\frac{c-a}{\sqrt{c+a}} \leq \frac{b-a}{\sqrt{b+a}}.$$

We will prove this by showing that the above expressions are the values of an increasing function at two different points. Thus, consider

$$f_1(t) = \frac{t-a}{\sqrt{t+a}}.$$

It follows that

$$f_1(b) = \frac{b-a}{\sqrt{b+a}} \quad \text{and} \quad f_1(c) = \frac{c-a}{\sqrt{c+a}}.$$

The function $f_1(t)$ is increasing because $f_1' > 0$ (recall $a \geq 0$) and since $c \leq b$ this implies $f_1(c) \leq f_1(b)$. Similarly we prove the inequality for $b \leq a \leq c$. $\quad\square$

Lemma 3 *The triangle inequality holds for the symmetric chi-squared distance* $S^2(\tau, m)$, *that is,*

$$\{S^2(\tau, m)\}^{1/2} \leq \{S^2(\tau, g)\}^{1/2} + \{S^2(g, m)\}^{1/2}.$$

Proof Set

$$\alpha_t = \frac{|\tau(t) - g(t)|}{\sqrt{\tau(t) + g(t)}}, \quad \beta_t = \frac{|g(t) - m(t)|}{\sqrt{g(t) + m(t)}}.$$

By Lemma 2

$$\left\{\sum \alpha_t^2\right\}^{1/2} \leq \left\{\sum (\alpha_t + \beta_t)^2\right\}^{1/2}.$$

But

$$\sum (\alpha_t + \beta_t)^2 = \sum \alpha_t^2 + \sum \beta_t^2 + 2 \sum \alpha_t \beta_t$$
$$\leq \sum \alpha_t^2 + \sum \beta_t^2 + 2 \left\{\sum \alpha_t^2\right\}^{1/2} \left\{\sum \beta_t^2\right\}^{1/2}.$$

Therefore

$$\sum (\alpha_t + \beta_t)^2 \leq \left\{\sqrt{\sum \alpha_t^2} + \sqrt{\sum \beta_t^2}\right\}^2,$$

and hence

$$\left\{\sum (\alpha_t + \beta_t)^2\right\}^{1/2} \leq \left\{\sum \alpha_t^2\right\}^{1/2} + \left\{\sum \beta_t^2\right\}^{1/2},$$

as was claimed. $\square$

Remark 3 The inequalities proved in Lemmas 1 and 2 imply that if $\tau \neq m$ there is no "straight line" connecting τ and m, in that there does not exist g between τ and m for which the triangle inequality is an equality.

Therefore, the following proposition holds.

Proposition 4 *The symmetric chi-squared distance $S^2(\tau, m)$ is indeed a metric.*

A testing interpretation of the symmetric chi-squared distance: let ϕ be a test function and consider the problem of testing the null hypothesis that the data come from a density f versus the alternative that the data come from g. Let θ be a random variable with value 1 if the alternative is true and 0 if the null hypothesis is true. Then

Proposition 5 *The solution ϕ_{opt} to the optimization problem*

$$\min_\phi \mathbb{E}_\pi[(\theta - \phi(x))^2],$$

where $\pi(\theta)$ is the prior probability on θ, given as

$$\pi(\theta) = \begin{cases} 1/2, & \text{if } \theta = 0 \\ 1/2, & \text{if } \theta = 1 \end{cases},$$

is not a $0 - 1$ decision, but equals the posterior expectation of θ given X. That is

$$\phi(t) = \mathbb{E}(\theta \mid X = t) = \mathbb{P}(\theta = 1 \mid X = t) = \frac{\frac{1}{2}g(t)}{\frac{1}{2}f(t) + \frac{1}{2}g(t)} = \frac{g(t)}{f(t) + g(t)},$$

the posterior probability that the alternative is correct.

Proof We have

$$\mathbb{E}(\theta \mid X) = \frac{1}{2}\mathbb{E}_{H_1}[(1 - \phi)^2] + \frac{1}{2}\mathbb{E}_{H_0}(\phi^2).$$

But

$$\mathbb{E}_{H_1}[(1 - \phi(X))^2] = \sum_t (1 - \phi(t))^2 g(t),$$

and

$$\mathbb{E}_{H_0}(\phi^2(X)) = \sum_t \phi^2(t)f(t),$$

hence

$$\phi_{\text{opt}}(t) = \frac{g(t)}{f(t) + g(t)},$$

as was claimed.   □

Corollary 2 *The minimum risk is given as*

$$\frac{1}{4}\left(1 - \frac{S^2}{4}\right),$$

where

$$S^2 = S^2(f, g) = \sum \frac{[f(t) - g(t)]^2}{\frac{1}{2}f(t) + \frac{1}{2}g(t)}.$$

Proof Substitute ϕ_{opt} in $\mathbb{E}_\pi[(\theta - \phi)^2]$ to obtain

$$\mathbb{E}_\pi[(\theta - \phi_{\text{opt}})^2] = \frac{1}{2}\sum_t \frac{f(t)g(t)}{f(t) + g(t)}.$$

Now set

$$A = \sum_t \frac{[f(t) + g(t)]^2}{f(t) + g(t)} = 2, \quad B = \sum_t \frac{[f(t) - g(t)]^2}{f(t) + g(t)} = \frac{1}{2}S^2.$$

Then

$$A - B = 4\sum_t \frac{f(t)g(t)}{f(t) + g(t)} = 2 - \frac{1}{2}S^2,$$

or, equivalently,

$$\sum_t \frac{f(t)g(t)}{f(t) + g(t)} = \frac{1}{4}\left(2 - \frac{1}{2}S^2\right).$$

Therefore

$$\mathbb{E}_\pi[(\theta - \phi_{\text{opt}})^2] = \frac{1}{2}\sum_t \frac{f(t)g(t)}{f(t) + g(t)} = \frac{1}{4}\left(1 - \frac{S^2}{4}\right),$$

as was claimed.   □

Remark 4 Note that $S^2(f, g)$ is bounded above by 4 and equals 4 when f, g are mutually singular.

The Kullback-Leibler and Hellinger distances are extensively used in the literature. Yet, we argue that, because they are obtained as solutions to optimization problems with non-interpretable (statistically) constraints, are not appropriate for our purposes. However, we note here that the Hellinger distance is closely related to the symmetric chi-squared distance, although this is not immediately obvious. We elaborate on this statement below.

Definition 7 Let τ, m be two probability densities. The squared Hellinger distance is defined as

$$H^2(\tau, m) = \frac{1}{2} \sum_x \left[\sqrt{\tau(x)} - \sqrt{m(x)} \right]^2.$$

We can more readily see the relationship between the Hellinger and chi-squared distances if we rewrite $H^2(\tau, m)$ as

$$H^2(\tau, m) = \frac{1}{2} \sum_x \frac{[\tau(x) - m(x)]^2}{[\sqrt{\tau(x)} + \sqrt{m(x)}]^2}.$$

Lemma 4 *The Hellinger distance is bounded by the symmetric chi-squared distance, that is,*

$$\frac{1}{8} S^2 \leq H^2 \leq \frac{1}{4} S^2,$$

where S^2 denotes the symmetric chi-squared distance.

Proof Note that

$$\left(\sqrt{\tau(x)} + \sqrt{m(x)} \right)^2 = \tau(x) + m(x) + 2\sqrt{\tau(x)m(x)} \geq \tau(x) + m(x).$$

Also

$$\left(\sqrt{\tau(x)} + \sqrt{m(x)} \right)^2 \leq 2[\tau(x) + m(x)],$$

and putting these relationships together we obtain

$$\tau(x) + m(x) \leq \left(\sqrt{\tau(x)} + \sqrt{m(x)} \right)^2 \leq 2[\tau(x) + m(x)].$$

Therefore

$$H^2(\tau, m) \leq \frac{1}{2} \sum \frac{[\tau(x) - m(x)]^2}{\tau(x) + m(x)} = \frac{1}{4} S^2,$$

and

$$H^2(\tau, m) \geq \frac{1}{2} \sum \frac{[\tau(x) - m(x)]^2}{2[\tau(x) + m(x)]} = \frac{1}{8} S^2,$$

and so

$$\frac{1}{8} S^2(\tau, m) \leq H^2(\tau, m) \leq \frac{1}{4} S^2(\tau, m),$$

as was claimed. □

3.4 Locally Quadratic Distances

A generalization of the chi-squared distances is offered by the locally quadratic distances. We have the following definition.

Definition 8 A locally quadratic distance between two densities τ, m has the form

$$\rho(\tau, m) = \sum K_m(x, y)[\tau(x) - m(x)][\tau(y) - m(y)],$$

where $K_m(x, y)$ is a nonnegative definite kernel, possibly dependent on m, and such that

$$\sum_{x,y} a(x) K_m(x, y) a(y) \geq 0,$$

for all functions $a(x)$.

Example 1 The Pearson distance can be written as

$$\sum \frac{(d(t) - m(t))^2}{m(t)} = \sum \frac{\mathbb{1}[s = t]}{\sqrt{m(s)m(t)}} [d(s) - m(s)][d(t) - m(t)]$$

$$= \sum K_m(s, t)[d(s) - m(s)][d(t) - m(t)],$$

where $\mathbb{1}(\cdot)$ is the indicator function. It is a quadratic distance with kernel

$$K_m(s, t) = \frac{\mathbb{1}[s = t]}{\sqrt{m(s)m(t)}}.$$

Sensitivity and Robustness In the classical robustness literature one of the attributes that a method should exhibit so as to be characterized as robust is the attribute of being resistant, that is insensitive, to the presence of a moderate number of outliers and to inadequacies in the assumed model.

Similarly here, to characterize a statistical distance as robust it should be insensitive to small changes in the true density, that is, the value of the distance should not be greatly affected by small changes that occur in τ. Lindsay (1994), Markatou (2000, 2001), and Markatou et al. (1997, 1998) based the discussion of robustness of the distances under study on a mechanism that allows the identification of distributional errors, that is, on the Pearson residual. A different system of residuals is the set of symmetrized residuals defined as follows.

Definition 9 If τ, m are two densities the symmetrized residual is defined as

$$r_{\text{sym}}(t) = \frac{\tau(t) - m(t)}{\tau(t) + m(t)}.$$

The symmetrized residuals have range $[-1, 1]$, with value -1 when $\tau(t) = 0$ and value 1 when $m(t) = 0$. Symmetrized residuals are important because they allow us to understand the way different distances treat different distributions.

The symmetric chi-squared distance can be written as a function of the symmetrized residuals as follows

$$S^2(\tau, m) = 4 \sum \left(\frac{1}{2}\tau(t) + \frac{1}{2}m(t) \right) \left\{ \frac{\tau(t) - m(t)}{\tau(t) + m(t)} \right\}^2 = 4 \sum b(t) r_{\text{sym}}^2(t),$$

where $b(t) = [\tau(t) + m(t)]/2$.

The aforementioned expression of the symmetric chi-squared distance allows us to obtain inequalities between $S^2(\tau, m)$ and other distances.

A third residual system is the set of logarithmic residuals, defined as follows.

Definition 10 Let τ, m be two probability density. Define the logarithmic residuals as

$$\delta(t) = \log \left(\frac{\tau(t)}{m(t)} \right),$$

with $\delta \in (-\infty, \infty)$.

A value of this residual close to 0 indicates agreement between τ and m. Large positive or negative values indicate disagreement between the two models τ and m.

In an analysis of a given data set, there are two types of observations that cause concern: outliers and influential observations. In the literature, the concept of an outlier is defined as follows.

Definition 11 We define an outlier to be an observation (or a set of observations) which appears to be inconsistent with the remaining observations of the data set.

Therefore, the concept of an outlier may be viewed in relative terms. Suppose we think a sample arises from a standard normal distribution. An observation from this sample is an outlier if it is somehow different in relation to the remaining observations that were generated from the postulated standard normal model. This means that, an observation with value 4 may be surprising in a sample of size 10, but is less so if the sample size is 10,000. In our framework therefore, the extent to which an observation is an outlier depends on both the sample size and the probability of occurrence of the observation under the specified model.

Remark 5 Davies and Gather (1993) state that although detection of outliers is a topic that has been extensively addressed in the literature, the word "outlier" was not given a precise definition. Davies and Gather (1993) formalized this concept by defining outliers in terms of their position relative to a central model, and in relationship to the sample size. Further details can be found in their paper.

On the other hand, the literature provides the following definition of an influential observation.

Definition 12 (Belsley 1980) An influential observation is one which, either individually or together with several other observations, has a demonstrably larger impact on the calculated values of various estimates than is the case for most of the other observations.

Chatterjee and Hadi (1986) use this definition to address questions about measuring influence and discuss the different measures of influence and their interrelationships.

The aforementioned definition is subjective, but it implies that one can order observations in a sensible way according to some measure of influence. Outliers need not be influential observations and influential observations need not be outliers. Large Pearson residuals correspond to observations that are *surprising*, in the sense that they occur in locations with small model probability. This is different from influential observations, that is from observations for which their presence or absence greatly affects the value of the maximum likelihood estimator.

Outliers can be surprising observations as well as influential observations. In a normal location-scale model, an outlying observation is both surprising and influential on the maximum likelihood estimator of location. But in the double exponential location model, an outlying observation is possible to be surprising but never influential on the maximum likelihood estimator of location as it equals the median.

Lindsay (1994) shows that the robustness of these distances is expressed via a key function called *residual adjustment function* (RAF). Further, he studied the characteristics of this function and showed that an important class of RAFs is given by $A_\lambda(\delta) = \frac{(1+\delta)^\lambda - 1}{\lambda + 1}$, where δ is the Pearson residual (defined by Eq. (1)). From this class we obtain many RAFs; in particular, when $\lambda = -2$ we obtain the RAF corresponding to Neyman's chi-squared distance. For details, see Lindsay (1994).

4   The Continuous Setting

Our goal is to use statistical distances to construct model misspecification measures. One of the key issues in the construction of misspecification measures in the case of data being realizations of a random variable that follows a continuous distribution is that allowances should be made for the scale difference between observed data and hypothesized model. That is, data distributions are discrete while the hypothesized model is continuous. Hence, we require the distance to exhibit discretization robustness, so it can account for the difference in scale.

To achieve discretization robustness, we need a sensitive distance, which implies a need to balance sensitivity and statistical noise. We will briefly review available strategies to deal with the problem of balancing sensitivity of the distance and statistical noise.

In what follows, we discuss desirable characteristics we require our distance measures to satisfy.

4.1 Desired Features

Discretization Robustness Every real data distribution is discrete, and therefore is different from every continuous distribution. Thus, a reasonable distance measure must allow for discretization, by saying that the discretized version of a continuous distribution must get closer to the continuous distribution as the discretization gets finer.

A second reason for requiring discretization robustness is that we will want to use the empirical distribution to estimate the true distribution, but without this robustness, there is no hope that the discrete empirical distribution will be closed to any model point.

The Problem of Too Many Questions Thus, to achieve discretization robustness, we need to construct a sensitive distance. This requirement dictates us to carry out a delicate balancing act between sensitivity and statistical noise.

Lindsay (2004) discusses in detail the problem of too many questions. Here we only note that to illustrate the issue Lindsay (2004) uses the chi-squared distance and notes that the statistical implications of a refinement in partition are the widening of the sensitivity to model departures in new "directions" but, at the same time, this act increases the statistical noise and therefore decreases the power of the chi-squared test in every existing direction.

There are a number of ways to address this problem, but they all seem to involve a loss of statistical information. This means we cannot ask all model fit questions with optimal accuracy. Two immediate solutions are as follows. First, limit the investigation only to a finite list of questions, essentially boiling down to prioritizing the questions asked of the sample. A number of classical goodness-of-fit tests create exactly such a balance. A second approach to the problem of answering infinitely many questions with only a finite number of data points is through the construction of kernel smoothed density measures. Those measures provide a flexible class of distances that allows for adjusting the sensitivity/noise trade-off. Before we briefly comment on this strategy, we discuss statistical distances between continuous probability distributions.

4.2 The L_2-Distance

The L_2 distance is very popular in density estimation. We show below that this distance is not invariant to one-to-one transformations.

Definition 13 The L_2 distance between two probability density functions τ, m is defined as

$$L_2^2(\tau, m) = \int [\tau(x) - m(x)]^2 dx.$$

Proposition 6 *The L_2 distance between two probability density functions is not invariant to one-to-one transformations.*

Proof Let $Y = a(X)$ be a transformation of X, which is one-to-one. Then $x = b(y)$, $b(\cdot)$ is the inverse transformation of $a(\cdot)$, and

$$
\begin{aligned}
L_2^2(\tau_Y, m_Y) &= \int [\tau_Y(y) - m_Y(y)]^2 dy \\
&= \int [\tau_X(b(y)) - m_X(b(y))]^2 (b'(y))^2 dy \\
&= \int [\tau_X(x) - m_X(x)]^2 (b'(a(x)))^2 a'(x) dx \\
&= \int [\tau_X(x) - m_X(x)]^2 b'(a(x)) dx \\
&\neq \int [\tau_X(x) - m_X(x)]^2 dx = L_2^2(\tau_X, m_X).
\end{aligned}
$$

Thus, the L_2 distance is not invariant under monotone transformations. □

Remark 6 It is easy to see that the L_2 distance is location invariant. Moreover, scale changes appear as a constant factor multiplying the L_2 distance.

4.3 The Kolmogorov-Smirnov Distance

We now discuss the Kolmogorov-Smirnov distance used extensively in goodness-of-fit problems, and present its properties.

Definition 14 The Kolmogorov-Smirnov distance between two cumulative distribution functions F, G is defined as

$$\rho_{KS}(F, G) = \sup_x |F(x) - G(x)|.$$

Proposition 7 (Testing Interpretation) *Let $H_0 : \tau = f$ versus $H_1 : \tau = g$ and that only test functions φ of the form $\mathbb{1}(x \le x_0)$ or $\mathbb{1}(x > x_0)$ for arbitrary x_0 are allowed. Then*

$$\rho_{KS}(F, G) = \sup |\mathbb{E}_{H_1}[\varphi(X)] - \mathbb{E}_{H_0}[\varphi(X)]|\,.$$

Proof The difference between power and size of the test is $G(x_0) - F(x_0)$. Therefore,

$$\sup_{x_0} |G(x_0) - F(x_0)| = \sup_{x_0} |F(x_0) - G(x_0)| = \rho_{KS}(F, G),$$

as was claimed.   □

Proposition 8 *The Kolmogorov-Smirnov distance is invariant under monotone transformations.*

Proof Write

$$F(x_0) - G(x_0) = \int \mathbb{1}(x \le x_0)[f(x) - g(x)]dx.$$

Let $Y = a(X)$ be a one-to-one transformation and $b(\cdot)$ be the corresponding inverse transformation. Then $x = b(y)$ and $dy = a'(x)dx$, so

$$\begin{aligned}
F_Y(y_0) - G_Y(y_0) &= \int \mathbb{1}(y \le y_0)[f_Y(y) - g_Y(y)]dy \\
&= \int \mathbb{1}(y \le y_0)[f_X(b(y))b'(y) - g_X(b(y))b'(y)]dy \\
&= \int \mathbb{1}(x \le b(y_0))[f_X(b(y))b'(y) - g_X(b(y))b'(y)]dy \\
&= \int \mathbb{1}(x \le x_0)[f_X(x) - g_X(x)]dx.
\end{aligned}$$

Therefore,

$$\sup_{y_0} |F_Y(y_0) - G_Y(y_0)| = \sup_{x_0} |F_X(x_0) - G_X(x_0)|\,,$$

and the Kolmogorov-Smirnov distance is invariant under one-to-one transformations.   □

Proposition 9 *The Kolmogorov-Smirnov distance is discretization robust.*

Proof Notice that we can write

$$|F(x_0) - G(x_0)| = \left| \int \mathbb{1}(x \le x_0)d[F(x) - G(x)] \right|,$$

with $\mathbb{1}(x \leq x_0)$ being thought of as a "smoothing kernel". Hence, comparisons between discrete and continuous distributions are allowed and the distance is discretization robust.   □

The Kolmogorov-Smirnov distance is a distance based on the probability integral transform. As such, it is invariant under monotone transformations (see Proposition 8). A drawback of distances based on probability integral transforms is the fact that there is no obvious extension in the multivariate case. Furthermore, there is not a direct loss function interpretation of these distances when the model used is incorrect. In what follows, we discuss chi-squared and quadratic distances that avoid the issues listed above.

4.4 Exactly Quadratic Distances

In this section we briefly discuss exactly quadratic distances. Rao (1982) introduced the concept of an exact quadratic distance for discrete population distributions and he called it *quadratic entropy*. Lindsay et al. (2008) gave the following definition of an exactly quadratic distance.

Definition 15 (Lindsay et al. 2008) Let F, G be two probability distributions, and K is a nonnegative definite kernel. A quadratic distance between F, G has the form

$$\rho_K(F, G) = \iint K_G(x, y)d(F - G)(x)d(F - G)(y).$$

Quadratic distances are of interest for a variety of reasons. These include the fact that the empirical distance $\rho_K(\widehat{F}, G)$ has a fairly simple asymptotic distribution theory when G identifies with the true model τ, and that several important distances are exactly quadratic (see, for example, Cramér-von Mises and Pearson's chi-squared distances). Furthermore, other distances are asymptotically locally quadratic around $G = \tau$. Quadratic distances can be thought of as extensions of the chi-squared distance class.

We can construct an exactly quadratic distance as follows. Let F, G be two probability measures that a random variable X may follow. Let ε be an independent error variable with known density $k_h(\varepsilon)$, where h is a parameter. Then, the random variable $Y = X + \varepsilon$ has an absolutely continuous distribution such that

$$f_h^*(y) = \int k_h(y - x)dF(x), \quad \text{if} \quad X \sim F,$$

or

$$g_h^*(y) = \int k_h(y - x)dG(x), \quad \text{if} \quad X \sim G.$$

Let

$$P^{*2}(F, G) = \int \frac{[f^*(y) - g^*(y)]^2}{g^*(y)} dy,$$

be the kernel-smoothed Pearson's chi-squared statistic. In what follows, we prove that $P^{*2}(F, G)$ is an exactly quadratic distance.

Proposition 10 *The distance $P^{*2}(F, G)$ is an exactly quadratic distance provided that $\iint K(s, t)d(F - G)(s)d(F - G)(t) < \infty$, where $K(s, t) = \int \frac{k_h(y-s)k_h(y-t)}{g^*(y)} dy$.*

Proof Write

$$P^{*2}(F, G) = \int \frac{[f^*(y) - g^*(y)]^2}{g^*(y)} dy$$

$$= \int \frac{[\int k_h(y - x)dF(x) - \int k_h(y - x)dG(x)]^2}{g^*(y)} dy$$

$$= \int \frac{[\int k_h(y - x)d(F - G)(x)]^2}{g^*(y)} dy$$

$$= \int \frac{[\int k_h(y - s)d(F - G)(s)][\int k_h(y - t)d(F - G)(t)]}{g^*(y)} dy.$$

Now using Fubini's theorem, the above relationship can be written as

$$\iint \left\{ \int \frac{k_h(y - s)k_h(y - t)}{g^*(y)} dy \right\} d(F - G)(s)d(F - G)(t)$$

$$= \iint K(s, t)d(F - G)(s)d(F - G)(t),$$

with $K(s, t)$ given above. $\square$

Remark 7

(a) The issue with many classical measures of goodness-of-fit is that the balance between sensitivity and statistical noise is fixed. On the other hand, one might wish to have a flexible class of distances that allows for adjusting the sensitivity/noise trade-off. Lindsay (1994) and Basu and Lindsay (1994) introduced the idea of smoothing and investigated numerically the blended weighted Hellinger distance, defined as

$$BWHD_\alpha(\tau^*, m_\theta^*) = \int \frac{(\tau^*(x) - m_\theta^*(x))^2}{\left(\alpha \sqrt{\tau^*(x)} + \overline{\alpha} \sqrt{m_\theta^*(x)} \right)^2} dx,$$

where $\overline{\alpha} = 1 - \alpha$, $\alpha \in [1/3, 1]$. When $\alpha = 1/2$, the $BWHD_{1/2}$ equals the Hellinger distance.

(b) Distances based on kernel smoothing are natural extensions of the discrete distances. These distances are not invariant under one-to-one transformations, but they can be easily generalized to higher dimensions. Furthermore, numerical integration is required for the practical implementation and use of these distances.

5 Discussion

In this paper we study statistical distances with a special emphasis on the chi-squared distance measures. We also introduce an extension of the chi-squared distance, the quadratic distance, introduced by Lindsay et al. (2008). We offered statistical interpretations of these distances and showed how they can be obtained as solutions of certain optimization problems. Of particular interest are distances with statistically interpretable constraints such as the class of chi-squared distances. These allow the construction of confidence intervals for models. We further discussed robustness properties of these distances, including discretization robustness, a property that allows discrete and continuous distributions to be arbitrarily close. Lindsay et al. (2014) study the use of quadratic distances in problems of goodness-of-fit with particular focus on creating tools for studying the power of distance-based tests. Lindsay et al. (2014) discuss one-sample testing and connect their methodology with the problem of kernel selection and the requirements that are appropriate in order to select optimal kernels. Here, we outlined the foundations that led to the aforementioned work and showed how these elucidate the performance of statistical distances as inferential functions.

Acknowledgements The first author dedicates this paper to the memory of Professor Bruce G. Lindsay, a long time collaborator and friend, with much respect and appreciation for his mentoring and friendship. She also acknowledges the Department of Biostatistics, School of Public Health and Health Professions and the Jacobs School of Medicine and Biomedical Sciences, University at Buffalo, for supporting this work. The second author acknowledges the Troup Fund, Kaleida Foundation for supporting this work.

References

Basu, A., & Lindsay, B. G. (1994). Minimum disparity estimation for continuous models: Efficiency, distributions and robustness. *Annals of the Institute of Statistical Mathematics, 46,* 683–705.

Belsley, D. A., Kuh, E., & Welsch, R. E. (1980). *Regression diagnostics: Identifying influential data and sources of collinearity*. New York: Wiley.

Beran, R. (1977). Minimum Hellinger distance estimates for parametric models. *Annals of Statistics, 5,* 445–463.

Berkson, J. (1980). Minimum chi-square, not maximum likelihood! *Annals of Statistics, 8,* 457–487.

Chatterjee, S., & Hadi, A. S. (1986). Influential observations, high leverage points, and outliers in linear regression. *Statistical Science, 1*, 379–393.

Davies, L., & Gather, U. (1993). The identification of multiple outliers. *Journal of the American Statistical Association, 88*, 782–792.

Lindsay, B. G. (1994). Efficiency versus robustness: The case for minimum Hellinger distance and related methods. *Annals of Statistics, 22*, 1081–1114.

Lindsay, B. G. (2004). Statistical distances as loss functions in assessing model adequacy. In *The nature of scientific evidence: Statistical, philosophical and empirical considerations* (pp. 439–488). Chicago: The University of Chicago Press.

Lindsay, B. G., Markatou, M., & Ray, S. (2014). Kernels, degrees of freedom, and power properties of quadratic distance goodness-of-fit tests. *Journal of the American Statistical Association, 109*, 395–410.

Lindsay, B. G., Markatou, M., Ray, S., Yang, K., & Chen, S. C. (2008). Quadratic distances on probabilities: A unified foundation. *Annals of Statistics, 36*, 983–1006.

Markatou, M. (2000). Mixture models, robustness, and the weighted likelihood methodology. *Biometrics, 56*, 483–486.

Markatou, M. (2001). A closer look at weighted likelihood in the context of mixture. In C. A. Charalambides, M. V. Koutras, & N. Balakrishnan (Eds.), *Probability and statistical models with applications* (pp. 447–468). Boca Raton: Chapman & Hall/CRC.

Markatou, M., Basu, A., & Lindsay, B. G. (1997). Weighted likelihood estimating equations: The discrete case with applications to logistic regression. *Journal of Statistical Planning and Inference, 57*, 215–232.

Markatou, M., Basu, A., & Lindsay, B. G. (1998). Weighted likelihood equations with bootstrap root search. *Journal of the American Statistical Association, 93*, 740–750.

Matusita, K. (1955). Decision rules, based on the distance, for problems of fit, two samples, and estimation. *Annals of Mathematical Statistics, 26*, 613–640.

Neyman, J. (1949). Contribution to the theory of the χ^2 test. In *Proceedings of the Berkeley Symposium on Mathematical Statistics and Probability* (pp. 239–273). Berkeley: The University of California Press.

Poor, H. (1980). Robust decision design using a distance criterion. *IEEE Transactions on Information Theory, 26*, 575–587.

Rao, C. R. (1963). Criteria of estimation in large samples. *Sankhya Series A, 25*, 189–206.

Rao, C. R. (1982). Diversity: Its measurement, decomposition, apportionment and analysis. *Sankhya Series A, 44*, 1–21.

Wald, A. (1950). *Statistical decision functions*. New York: Wiley.

The Out-of-Source Error in Multi-Source Cross Validation-Type Procedures

Georgios Afendras and Marianthi Markatou

1 Introduction

In many situations data arise not from a single source but from multiple sources, each of which may have a specific generating process. An example of such a situation is the monitoring and diagnosis of cardiac arrhythmias.

Monitoring devices in cardiac intensive care units use data from electrocardiogram (ECG) channels to automatically diagnose cardiac arrhythmias. However, data from other sources like arterial pressure, ventilation, etc. are often available, and each of these sources has a specific data generating process. Other potential data sources include nuclear medicine tests and echocardiograms. Other examples arise in natural language processing where labeled data for information extraction or parsing are obtained from a limited set of document types.

Cross validation is a fundamental statistical method used extensively in both, statistics and machine learning. A fundamental assumption in using cross validation is that the observations are realizations of exchangeable random variables, that is both, the training and test data come from the same source. However, this is not necessarily the case when data come from multiple sources. Geras and Sutton (2013) state that "for data of this nature, a common procedure is to arrange the cross validation procedure by source". In this article we are interested in estimating the generalization error of learning algorithms when multi-source data are present.

G. Afendras (✉) • M. Markatou
Department of Biostatistics, SPHHP and Jacobs School of Medicine and Biomedical Sciences, University at Buffalo, Buffalo, NY, USA
e-mail: gafendra@buffalo.edu; markatou@buffalo.edu

© Springer International Publishing AG 2017
D.-G. Chen et al. (eds.), *New Advances in Statistics and Data Science*,
ICSA Book Series in Statistics, https://doi.org/10.1007/978-3-319-69416-0_2

27

The generalization error is defined as the error an algorithm makes on cases that the algorithm has never seen before, and is important because it relates to the algorithm's prediction capabilities on independent data. The literature includes both, theoretical investigations of risk performance of machine learning algorithms as well as numerical comparisons.

Estimation of the generalization error can be achieved via the use of resampling techniques. The process consists of splitting the available data into a learning or training set and a test set a large number of times and averaging over these repetitions. A very popular resampling technique is cross validation. We are interested in investigating the use of cross validation in the case of multi-source data, where testing occurs on elements that may not have been part of the training set on which the learning algorithm was trained. We do not offer here a detailed overview of cross validation. The interested reader is referred to Stone (1974, 1977) for foundational aspects of cross validation, Breiman et al. (1984, Ch.s 3,8), Geisser (1975), and to Arlot and Celisse (2010) for a comprehensive survey.

A recent article by Geras and Sutton (2013) addresses a formulation of the *out-of-source* (OOS) error in a multi-source data setting. In Sect. 2 we provide Geras and Sutton's detailed definition of the OOS error. In their framework there are k sources. If the data size is n, the sample size of each source is n/k. The observations of each source are independent and identically distributed (iid) realizations of random variables/vectors from an unknown distribution. The elements that belong to a specific source constitute a test set, while the union of the elements of the remaining sources constitutes the corresponding training set. Geras and Sutton (2013) construct their cross validation-type decision rule using the elements of the aforementioned training set. In this sense, their procedure can be thought of as k-fold cross validation with the fundamental difference that the test set data does not necessarily follow the same distribution as the training data.

Recently, multi-source data analysis has received considerable attention in the literature. Ben-David et al. (2010) study the performance of classifiers trained on source data but tested on target data, that is data that do not necessarily follow the same distribution with the source data. Specifically, they study conditions under which a classifier performs well, as well as strategies to combine a small amount of labeled target data at the training step of the classifier to facilitate better performance.

This paper is organized as follows. Section 2 presents motivation, reviews the most relevant literature and establishes the notation used in this paper. Section 3 presents our framework and defines the OOS error. Section 4 defines our OOS error estimator and discusses its properties. Section 5 presents simulation results while Sect. 6 offers a discussion. Appendix 1 presents useful relationships needed for the proof of some results, while Appendix 2 shows some useful existing results. Finally, Appendix 3 contains the proofs of the obtained results.

2 Literature Review and Notation

First we present the Geras and Sutton's (2013) framework and give a list of definitions and notations.

Assume k sources, where k is a fixed number, and let $\mathscr{Z}$ be a data set $\mathscr{Z} = \{Z_1, \ldots, Z_n\}$ of size n. Assume all sources have the same number of observations, $m = n/k$, and the observations of the jth source constitute an iid collection of size m from an unknown distribution $F_j, j = 1, \ldots, k$. For each $j = 1, \ldots, k$ the observations of the jth source is the jth test set and its complement set, the union of the observations of the other sources, is the corresponding training set; furthermore, the decision rule is constructed based on all of the elements of the training set for all $j = 1, \ldots, k$.

To formalize the above procedure, first we give a list of definitions and notations. Let $N = \{1, \ldots, n\}$. For each $A \subseteq N$, we denote by $\mathscr{Z}_A$ the set $\mathscr{Z}_A \doteq \{Z_i \mid i \in A\}$. The set of the indices of the jth source is denoted by S_j and the set of observation of this source is $\mathscr{Z}_{S_j}$. The loss function L is a measurable nonnegative real function $L(T, \widehat{d})$, where $\widehat{d}$ is a decision rule and T is the target variable. The decision rule is constructed using the elements of a set $\mathscr{Z}_A$, i.e. $\widehat{d} = \widehat{d}(\mathscr{Z}_A)$, while the target variable is an element $Z_i \notin \mathscr{Z}_A$. Hereafter, we write $\widehat{d}_j \equiv \widehat{d}_{j,n} = \widehat{d}(\mathscr{Z}_{S_j}), j = 1, \ldots, k$, when the decision rule is constructed based on the elements of the jth source, and $\widehat{d}_{-j} \equiv \widehat{d}_{-j,n} = \widehat{d}(\mathscr{Z} \smallsetminus \mathscr{Z}_{S_j}), j = 1, \ldots, k$, when the decision rule is constructed based on the elements of the complement of the jth source, where n is the total sample size.

The Geras and Sutton's OOS is defined as

$$\mu_{\text{CVS}} = \frac{1}{k} \sum_{j=1}^{k} \mathbb{E}[L(Z^{(j)}, \widehat{d}_{-j})],$$

where $Z^{(j)} \sim F_j$ and are independent from the data set; and its estimator is

$$\widehat{\mu}_{\text{CVS}} = \frac{1}{n} \sum_{j=1}^{k} \sum_{i \in S_j} L(Z_i, \widehat{d}_{-j}).$$

Geras and Sutton's hypothesis that each source has exactly the same number of elements is too restrictive (and some times not realistic) in practice. Also, the construction of the decision rule based on all of the elements of the training set often leads to various pathologies, as we see in the following example.

Example 1 Consider a data set of observations that are realizations of independent variables and has size $n = 30$, say $\{Z_1, \ldots, Z_{30}\}$. Assume that the data set arises from three sources with $n_1 = n_2 = n_3 = 10$ observations each; in general, denote by n_j the sample size associated with the jth source. A variable of the first source follows $N(-\mu, 1)$, of the second source follows $N(0, 1)$ and of the third source follows $N(\mu, 1)$. Let the squared error loss be used and suppose that a new variable Z comes from the second source and is independent from the remaining variables in the data set. Additionally, assume that the decision rule is the sample mean. According to Geras and Sutton's (2013) formulation, Z has an OOS error which is $\mathbb{E}(Z-\overline{Z}_{1,3})^2$, where $\widehat{d}_{-2} = \overline{Z}_{1,3}$ is the average of the union of the elements of the first and third sources, that is $\overline{Z}_{1,3} = \frac{1}{20}\sum_{i \in S_1 \cup S_3} Z_i$, where S_j denotes the set of indices of the elements of the jth source. One can easily see that $Z - \overline{Z}_{1,3} \sim N(0, 1.05)$. Therefore, $\mathbb{E}(Z - \overline{Z}_{1,3})^2 = \text{Var}(Z - \overline{Z}_{1,3}) + \mathbb{E}^2(Z - \overline{Z}_{1,3}) = 1.05$. Observe that in this case Geras and Sutton's formulation has the pathology that the preceding error is independent of the value of μ. We see below, see Example 2, that the OOS error that is addressed by Geras and Sutton (2013) is significantly different than the actual OOS error.

In view of the above, it is clear that we need to re-formulate the definition of the OOS error in the context of multi-source data to take into account the fact that in practice, not all sources have the same number of observations.

3   Framework

Assume k sources, where k is a fixed number. Let a data set $\{Z_1, \ldots, Z_n\}$ of size n be observed when the generating process is as follows. The observations come from the sources that follow a distribution $\boldsymbol{p} = (p_1, \ldots, p_k)$. That is, the percentage of observations of the jth source is $p_j, j = 1, \ldots, k$ (the sample size of the jth source is $n_j = np_j$). The vector of the numbers of observations of the sources is denoted by $\boldsymbol{n} = n\boldsymbol{p} = (n_1, \ldots, n_k)$. Each Z_i is labeled by its source and it is independent from the remaining observations whether those come from the same or different sources. The observations of the jth source constitute an iid collection of size n_j from an unknown distribution F_j.

A new unobserved variable, say Z, comes from a source and is independent from $\{Z_1, \ldots, Z_n\}$. The probability of the event "the variable Z belongs to the jth source" is $p_j = n_j/n$, and follows the distribution $F_j, j = 1, \ldots, k$. The OOS error is the error that arises between the variable Z and the $k - 1$ foreign sources with respect to Z, when a loss function L is used for measuring this error.

Now we are in a position to present the algebraic form of the OOS error. Hereafter we assume that the loss function has finite moment of the first order; that is, $\mathbb{E}|L(Z_i, \widehat{d}_l)| < \infty$ for all $Z_i \in \mathscr{Z}_j$ and $l \neq j$. Given that the variable Z comes from the jth source and that the decision is constructed based on the elements of the lth source, the error committed is

$$\mathsf{e}_{j;l} \doteq \mathbb{E}[L(Z, \widehat{d}_l)] \text{ when } Z \sim F_j \text{ and } Z, \mathscr{Z}_{S_l} \text{ are independent,}$$

that is, $\mathsf{e}_{j;l}$ is the expected value of the loss function when the decision rule is constructed based on the elements of the lth source and the target variable belongs to the jth source and is independent of the elements of the lth source. Taking into account the distribution of the sources and using the conditional total probability theorem, given that the variable Z comes from the jth source the error is

$$\mathsf{e}_j \doteq \frac{1}{1 - p_j} \sum_{l \neq j} p_l \mathsf{e}_{j;l};$$

this is the error that is created from an observation from the jth source when compared against observations from the other sources. According to the total probability theorem, the total OOS error is defined by

$$\mu_{\mathrm{os}}^{(n)} \doteq \sum_{j=1}^{k} p_j \mathsf{e}_j = \sum_{j=1}^{k} od_j \sum_{l \neq j} p_l \mathsf{e}_{j;l}, \tag{1}$$

where $od_j \doteq p_j/(1 - p_j)$ is the odds of the jth source. This error can be thought of as a generalization-type error.

Our definition of the OOS error differs from the definition given by Geras and Sutton (2013) in two fundamental aspects. The first corresponds to the fact that our construction does not assume that the different sources have the same number of observations. The second is that, in our construction, if the test set corresponds to one of the sources the remaining sources serve as individual training sets, avoiding the usage of their union as a single training set.

4   The OOS Error Estimation

Here, we give an estimator of the OOS error defined in the previous section and investigate the properties of this estimator.

4.1   Estimating the OOS Error

We are interested in estimating the OOS error. To simplify notation we use $\ell_{i,j}$ to denote $L(Z_i, \widehat{d}_j)$. By definition, a natural estimator of $\mathsf{e}_{j;l}$ is $\frac{1}{n_j} \sum_{i \in S_j} \ell_{i,l}$, and thus, a natural estimator of $\mu_{\mathrm{os}}^{(n)}$ is

$$\widehat{\mu}_{\mathrm{os}}^{(n)} \doteq \frac{1}{n} \sum_{j=1}^{k} \frac{1}{n - n_j} \sum_{l \neq j} n_l \sum_{i \in S_j} \ell_{i,l}. \tag{2}$$

This estimator is a cross validation-type estimator of the OOS error. When k-fold cross validation is used to estimate generalization error the data are split in k equal parts. Each of these parts is a test set and its complement set is the corresponding training set. The target variable is a variable of the test set and the decision rule is constructed based on the elements of the corresponding training set (for more details see, for example, Afendras and Markatou 2016). Here, we have k test sets $(\mathscr{Z}_{S_1}, \ldots, \mathscr{Z}_{S_k})$, which are defined by the labeling of the data and are a partitioning of the data set. For each test set $\mathscr{Z}_{S_j}$ the corresponding training set $\mathscr{Z}_{S_j}^c = \bigcup_{l \neq j} \mathscr{Z}_{S_l}$ is partitioned into $k-1$ training sub-sets $\mathscr{Z}_{S_1}, \ldots, \mathscr{Z}_{S_{j-1}}, \mathscr{Z}_{S_{j+1}}, \ldots, \mathscr{Z}_{S_k}$. The target variable is a variable of the test set and for each $l \neq j$ the decision rule is constructed based on the elements of the training sub-set $\mathscr{Z}_{S_l}$.

Hereafter we write μ_{os} and $\widehat{\mu}_{os}$ instead $\mu_{os}^{(n)}$ and $\widehat{\mu}_{os}^{(n)}$ respectively. The following example illustrates the difference between the OOS error that introduced by Geras and Sutton and that we have defined in relationship (1).

Example 2 (Example 1 Continued) Let the data be as in Example 1 and the squared error loss is used. Let us consider $Z^{(1)} \sim N(-\mu, 1)$, $Z^{(2)} \sim N(0, 1)$, $Z^{(3)} \sim N(\mu, 1)$ and $Z^{(1)}, Z^{(2)}, Z^{(3)}, \{Z_1, \ldots, Z_n\}$ are independent. If $\widehat{d}_{-1} = \overline{Z}_{2,3}$, $\widehat{d}_{-2} = \overline{Z}_{1,3}$ and $\widehat{d}_{-3} = \overline{Z}_{1,2}$, then $Z^{(1)} - \overline{Z}_{2,3} \sim N(-3\mu/2, 1.05)$, $Z^{(2)} - \overline{Z}_{1,3} \sim N(0, 1.05)$ and $Z^{(3)} - \overline{Z}_{1,2} \sim N(3\mu/2, 1.05)$. Hence, the OOS error given by Geras and Sutton (2013) is

$$\mu_{CVS} = \frac{1}{3} \left\{ \mathbb{E}(Z^{(1)} - \overline{Z}_{2,3})^2 + \mathbb{E}(Z^{(2)} - \overline{Z}_{1,3})^2 + \mathbb{E}(Z^{(3)} - \overline{Z}_{1,2})^2 \right\} = 1.05 + \frac{3}{2}\mu^2.$$

Using the more general Example 4(a) below, relation (3) gives that the OOS error given by (1) is $\mu_{os} = 1.1 + 2\mu^2$.

4.2 Bias and Variance of $\widehat{\mu}_{os}$

In this section we investigate the bias and variance, and so the mean square error, of the OOS error estimator $\widehat{\mu}_{os}$. Using E.1–E.5, see Appendix 1, we state and prove the following theorem.

Theorem 1 *Assume that* $\mathbb{E}[L(Z, \widehat{d}_l)]^2 < \infty$ *when* $Z \sim F_j$ *and* Z, $\mathscr{Z}_{S_l}$ *are independent for all* $j \neq l$. *Then,*

(a) *the estimator* $\widehat{\mu}_{os}$ *given by (2) is an unbiased estimator of the OOS error;*
(b) *the variance of* $\widehat{\mu}_{os}$ *is*

$$\mathsf{Var}(\widehat{\mu}_{\mathrm{os}}) = \sum_{j=1}^{k} \frac{od_j^2}{np_j} \left(\sum_{l \neq j} p_l^2 (\mathsf{V}_{j;l} + n(p_j - 1/n)\mathsf{C}_{j;l}) + \sum_{l \neq l'} \sum_{:l,l' \neq j} p_l p_{l'} \mathsf{C}_{j;l,l'} \right)$$

$$+ \sum_{j \neq j'} od_j od_{j'} \left(\sum_{l \neq j,j'} p_l(p_l \mathsf{C}_{j,j';l} + 2p_j \mathsf{C}_{j,j';l,j}) \right),$$

where $\mathsf{V}_{j;l} = \mathsf{Var}\, L(Z, \widehat{d}_l)$ when $Z \sim F_j$ and is independent of $\mathscr{L}_{S_l}$; $\mathsf{C}_{j;l} = \mathsf{Cov}(L(Z, \widehat{d}_l), L(Z', \widehat{d}_l))$ when Z and Z' are iid from F_j and are independent of $\mathscr{L}_{S_l}$; $\mathsf{C}_{j;l,l'} = \mathsf{Cov}(L(Z, \widehat{d}_l), L(Z, \widehat{d}_{l'}))$ when $Z \sim F_j$ and is independent of $\mathscr{L}_{S_l} \cup \mathscr{L}_{S_{l'}}$; $\mathsf{C}_{j,j';l} = \mathsf{Cov}(L(Z, \widehat{d}_l), L(Z', \widehat{d}_l))$ when $Z \sim F_j$, $Z' \sim F_{j'}$ and Z, Z', $\mathscr{L}_{S_l}$ are independent; and $\mathsf{C}_{j,j';l,j} = \mathsf{Cov}(L(Z, \widehat{d}_l), L(Z', \widehat{d}_j))$ when $Z \in \mathscr{L}_{S_j}$, $Z' \sim F_{j'}$ and Z', $\mathscr{L}_{S_j}$, $\mathscr{L}_{S_l}$ are independent.

Now we investigate the consistency of the estimator $\widehat{\mu}_{\mathrm{os}}$. First, we are interested in finding simple and natural conditions that imply the desired result. Very often the sequence, with respect to n, of the decision rules $\widehat{d}_{j;n}$ converges in probability to a constant for each j. For example, if the decision rule is the sample mean of the elements of the jth source, say $\overline{Z}_j$, and F_j has mean μ_j, then $\overline{Z}_j \xrightarrow{\mathrm{P}} \mu_j$. Also, the finiteness of the variance of the OOS error estimator requires that $\mathbb{E}[L(Z_i, \widehat{d}_l)]^2 < \infty$ for all $Z_i \in \mathscr{L}_{S_j}$ and $j \neq l$. In view the above observations, we state the following conditions/assumptions:

C.1: $\widehat{d}_{j;n} \xrightarrow{\mathrm{P}} d_j$, as $n \to \infty$, for all $j = 1, \ldots, k$, where d_js are constants.

C.2: There exist positive numbers θ and M such that $\mathbb{E}[L(Z, \widehat{d}_{l,n})]^{2+\theta} \leq M$ when $Z \sim F_j$ and Z, $\mathscr{L}_{S_l}$ are independent, for all $j \neq l$ and n.

The condition $\theta > 0$ is needed because for Theorem 2 to hold the sequence $L(Z, \widehat{d}_{l,n})L(Z', \widehat{d}_{l,n})$ is not generally necessarily uniformly integrable. This in turn does not guarantee the convergence to 0 of $\mathsf{C}_{j;l}$ defined in Theorem 1(b); the same holds for the remaining quantities $\mathsf{C}_{j,j',l}$ and $\mathsf{C}_{j,j';l,j}$ again defined in Theorem 1(b), facts that affect the consistency of the OOS estimator.

Theorem 2 *Let L be a continuous loss function and suppose that C.1, C.2 hold. Then, $\mathsf{Var}(\widehat{\mu}_{\mathrm{os}}) \to 0$ as $n \to \infty$ and, thus, $\widehat{\mu}_{\mathrm{os}}$ is a consistent estimator of μ_{os}.*

The following Examples 3 and 4 show the usefulness of Theorem 2.

Example 3 Let $\mathscr{L}_{S_j}$ be an iid collection of random variables (rv's) from F_j, $j = 1, \ldots, k$, the decision rules are the usual averages of the elements of the sources, F_j does not depend on n and has mean μ_j and variance σ_j^2.

(a) Let the absolute error loss be used. Suppose that F_j has finite moments of order $2 + \theta_j$ for some $\theta_j > 0$, $j = 1, \ldots, k$. Then, $\widehat{d}_j = \overline{Z}_j = \frac{1}{n_j} \sum_{i \in S_j} Z_i \xrightarrow{\mathrm{P}} \mu_j$, that is, C.1 is satisfied. Set $\theta = \min_{j=1,\ldots,k} \{\theta_j\} > 0$, $\beta_{2+\theta} = \max_{j=1,\ldots,k} \{\mathbb{E}|Z|^{2+\theta}$ when $Z \sim F_j\} < \infty$ and $M = 2^{3+\theta} \beta_{2+\theta} < \infty$.

For each $j \neq l$ and $Z \sim F_j$ such that $Z, \mathscr{Z}_{S_l}$ are independent we have that $\mathbb{E}|L(Z, \widehat{d}_{l,n})|^{2+\theta} = \mathbb{E}|Z - \overline{Z}_l|^{2+\theta} \leq 2^{2+\theta} \left(\mathbb{E}|Z|^{2+\theta} + \mathbb{E}|\overline{Z}_l|^{2+\theta}\right) \leq 2^{2+\theta} \left(\mathbb{E}|Z|^{2+\theta} + \frac{1}{n_l}\sum_{i \in S_l} \mathbb{E}|Z_i|^{2+\theta}\right) \leq 2^{3+\theta} \beta_{2+\theta} = M$; and so C.2 is satisfied. Therefore, Theorems 1 and 2 show that $\mathsf{MSE}(\widehat{\mu}_{\mathrm{os}}) = \mathsf{bias}^2(\widehat{\mu}_{\mathrm{os}}) + \mathsf{Var}(\widehat{\mu}_{\mathrm{os}}) = \mathsf{Var}(\widehat{\mu}_{\mathrm{os}}) \to 0$ as $n \to \infty$.

(b) Let the squared error loss be used, that is $L(Z, \widehat{d}_{l,n}) = (Z - \overline{Z}_l)^2$, and suppose that F_j has finite moments of order $4 + \theta_j$ for some $\theta_j > 0, j = 1, \dots, k$. Using the same arguments as in (a), we obtain that $\mathsf{MSE}(\widehat{\mu}_{\mathrm{os}}) \to 0$ as $n \to \infty$.

Example 4 Suppose $F_j \sim N(\mu_j, \sigma_j^2)$ and $\widehat{d}_j = \overline{Z}_j = \frac{1}{n_j}\sum_{i \in S_j} Z_i$.

(a) Let the squared error loss be used. Then, we calculate (see in Appendix 3)

$$\mu_{\mathrm{os}} = \sum_{j=1}^{k} p_j \sigma_j^2 + \sum_{j=1}^{k} od_j \sum_{l \neq j} p_l (\mu_j - \mu_l)^2 + \frac{1}{n} \sum_{j=1}^{k} od_j \sum_{l \neq j} \sigma_j^2; \qquad (3)$$

and the quantities $\mathsf{V}_{j;l}, \mathsf{C}_{j;l}, \mathsf{C}_{j;l,l'}, \mathsf{C}_{j,j';l}$ and $\mathsf{C}_{j,j';l,j}$ that appear in the variance of $\widehat{\mu}_{\mathrm{os}}$ in Theorem 1(b) are

$$\mathsf{V}_{j;l} = 2\left(\sigma_j + \frac{\sigma_l^2}{np_l}\right)\left[\sigma_j + \frac{\sigma_l^2}{np_l} + 2(\mu_j - \mu_l)^2\right], \qquad (4a)$$

$$\left.\begin{aligned}
\mathsf{C}_{j;l} &= 2\frac{\sigma_l^2}{np_l}\left(\frac{\sigma_l^2}{np_l} + 2(\mu_j - \mu_l)^2\right), \\
\mathsf{C}_{j;l,l'} &= 2\sigma_j^2\left(\sigma_j^2 + 2(\mu_j - \mu_l)(\mu_j - \mu_{l'})\right), \\
\mathsf{C}_{j,j';l} &= 2\frac{\sigma_l^2}{np_l}\left(\frac{\sigma_l^2}{np_l} + 2(\mu_j - \mu_l)(\mu_{j'} - \mu_l)\right), \\
\mathsf{C}_{j;l,l'} &= 2\frac{\sigma_j^2}{np_j}\left(\frac{\sigma_j^2}{np_j} - 2(\mu_j - \mu_l)(\mu_{j'} - \mu_j)\right).
\end{aligned}\right\} \qquad (4b)$$

Observe that $\mathsf{C}_{j;l}, \mathsf{C}_{j,j';l}, \mathsf{C}_{j,j';l,j} \to 0$ as $n \to \infty$; specifically, these covariances are $O(1/n)$ functions as $n \to \infty$. It is obvious that $\mathsf{Var}(\widehat{\mu}_{\mathrm{os}}) = O(1/n)$ as $n \to \infty$. This example is a confirmation of Theorem 2 for this case.

(b) Let the absolute error loss be used. Then, see in Appendix 3,

$$\mu_{\mathrm{os}} = \sum_{j=1}^{k} od_j \sum_{l \neq j} p_l \left\{ \mu_{j;l}\left[1 - 2\Phi\left(-\frac{\mu_{j;l}}{\sigma_{j;l}}\right)\right] + \sigma_{j;l}\sqrt{\frac{2}{\pi}} \exp\left(-\frac{\mu_{j;l}^2}{2\sigma_{j;l}^2}\right)\right\}, \qquad (5)$$

where $\mu_{j;l} = \mu_j - \mu_l$, $\sigma_{j;l}^2 = \sigma_j^2 + \sigma_l^2/(np_l)$ and Φ denotes the cumulative distribution function of the standard normal distribution. The calculations of the covariances $\mathsf{C}_{j;l}, \mathsf{C}_{j;l,l'}, \mathsf{C}_{j,j';l}$ and $\mathsf{C}_{j;l,l'}$ in Theorem 1(b) are rather difficult.

In practice, the data distributions of the sources are unknown and, thus, the OOS error must be estimated. There are loss functions for which the calculation of the variance of $\widehat{\mu}_{os}$ is difficult, or impossible, even if the distribution of the data sources is known, cf. Example 4(b). Furthermore, in the formulation of Example 3 where the absolute error loss is used, if we consider $F_j \sim U(a_j, b_j), j = 1, 2, 3$, the calculation of OOS error in closed form is impossible.

4.3 On Variance Estimation

In this section we study the estimation of variance of the OOS error. Recall that in random cross validation one splits randomly the data into two sets of sizes n_1 and n_2 ($n_1 + n_2 = n$ is the total sample size) that serve as training/test sets and repeats this process J times.

First, we present a general result and some useful observations that arise from it. Nadeau and Bengio (2003) study the variance estimation of the random cross validation estimator of the generalization error of a computer algorithm when $L(Z_i, \widehat{d}_j)$ for all realizations $\mathscr{Z}_{S_j}$ and $Z_i \in \mathscr{Z}^c_{S_j}$ are exchangeable. They prove that "There is no general unbiased estimator of the variance of the random cross validation estimator that involves the $L(Z_i, \widehat{d}_j)$s in a quadratic and/or linear way." (see Nadeau and Bengio 2003, Proposition 3, p. 246). This result holds in a more general form.

Lemma 1 *Let $X_1, X_2, \ldots, X_n$ be a collection of random variables. If $\mathbb{E}(X_j) = \mu$, $\mathsf{Var}(X_j) = \sigma^2$ and $\mathsf{Cov}(X_j, X_{j'}) = \mathsf{C}, j \neq j'$, are unknown parameters, then we can find unbiased estimators of the second moments of X_js only for the cases of linear combinations of $\sigma^2 + \mu^2$, $\mathsf{C} + \mu^2$.*

The following corollary follows immediately from Lemma 1.

Corollary 1 *Let $X_1, X_2, \ldots, X_n$ be as in Lemma 1. Then, (a) there does not exist an unbiased estimator of $\mathsf{Var}(\overline{X})$, where $\overline{X}$ is the usual average of X_js, and (b) there do not exist unbiased estimators of μ^2, σ^2, C.*

Remark 1

(a) If one of the parameters μ^2, σ^2 and C is known, then we can provide unbiased estimators for each linear combination of the other two parameters.

(b) The statistic $s^2 = \frac{1}{n-1} \sum_{j=1}^{n} (X_j - \overline{X})^2$ is an unbiased estimator of $\sigma^2 - \mathsf{C}$. The variance of this estimator is

$$\mathsf{Var}(s^2) = \frac{1}{(n-1)^2} \left\{ \sum_{j=1}^{n} \mathsf{Var}(X_j - \overline{X})^2 + \sum \sum_{1 \leq j < j' \leq n} \mathsf{Cov}\left((X_j - \overline{X})^2, (X_{j'} - \overline{X})^2\right) \right\}.$$

It is possible $\mathsf{Var}(s^2) \nrightarrow 0$, as $n \to \infty$, see Example 5 below; and thus, s^2 is not a consistent estimator of $\sigma^2 - \mathsf{C}$.

(c) In both random and k-fold cross validation estimators of the generalization error of a computer algorithm, the sequence of the test set errors are as in Lemma 1 (see Afendras and Markatou 2016, Proposition 1). For both of these cases the cross validation estimator is the usual average of the test set errors. Thus, the unbiased estimation of the variance of the cross validation estimator is impossible. Let $\widehat{\mu}_j, j = 1, \dots, J$, denote the estimates of the test set errors and $\widehat{\mu}_{\mathrm{CV,J}} = \frac{1}{J} \sum_{j=1}^J \widehat{\mu}_j$ be the cross validation estimator of the generalization error in the random cross validation procedure. If $s_{\widehat{\mu}_j}^2 = \frac{1}{J-1} \sum_{j=1}^J \left(\widehat{\mu}_j - \widehat{\mu}_{\mathrm{CV,J}} \right)$ and $\rho = \mathrm{Corr}(\widehat{\mu}_j, \widehat{\mu}_{j'})$, Nadeau and Bengio (2003, p. 248) state that "$\dots \left(1 + \frac{\rho}{1-\rho} \right) s_{\widehat{\mu}_j}^2$ is an unbiased estimator of $\mathrm{Var}(\widehat{\mu}_{\mathrm{CV,J}})$";
this sentence is incorrect because the parameter ρ is unknown and, thus, $\left(1 + \frac{\rho}{1-\rho} \right) s_{\widehat{\mu}_j}^2$ is not an estimator (statistic). Of course, it is a random variable with $\mathbb{E}\left[\left(1 + \frac{\rho}{1-\rho} \right) s_{\widehat{\mu}_j}^2 \right] = \mathrm{Var}(\widehat{\mu}_{\mathrm{CV,J}})$. In general, the estimation of the correlation ρ is difficult. Nevertheless, even in the case in which we find an unbiased estimator of ρ, say $\widehat{\rho}$, then $\left(1 + \frac{\widehat{\rho}}{1-\widehat{\rho}} \right) s_{\widehat{\mu}_j}^2$ is not an unbiased estimator of $\mathrm{Var}(\widehat{\mu}_{\mathrm{CV,J}})$, except if $\left(1 + \frac{\widehat{\rho}}{1-\widehat{\rho}} \right)$ and $s_{\widehat{\mu}_j}^2$ are uncorrelated. Moreover, if $\widehat{\rho}$ is consistent estimator of ρ, then $\left(1 + \frac{\widehat{\rho}}{1-\widehat{\rho}} \right) s_{\widehat{\mu}_j}^2$ might is not a consistent estimator of $\mathrm{Var}(\widehat{\mu}_{\mathrm{CV,J}})$, cf. (b).

(d) Markatou et al. (2005) provide moment approximation estimators for the variance of the test set errors and for their covariance in a broad and often used class of cross validation procedures, in both random and k-fold cross validation cases. In view of (c), it is clear that their results are very important in practice.

Example 5 Let $0 < C < \sigma^2 < \infty$ and $\mu \in \mathbb{R}$. Assume that $Y_1, \dots, Y_n$ is an iid collection from the distribution with probability mass function $p_Y\left(-(\sigma^2 - C)^{1/2}/2 \right) = p_Y\left((\sigma^2 - C)^{1/2}/2 \right) = (n^2-1)/(2n^2-1/2), p_Y\left(-n(\sigma^2 - C) \right) = p_Y\left(n(\sigma^2 - C) \right) = 3/(8n^2 - 2)$; and $\epsilon \sim N(\mu, C)$ which is independent to Y_js. By straightforward calculations, $\mathbb{E}(Y) = 0$, $\mathrm{Var}(Y) = \sigma^2 - C$. Consider the rv's $X_j = Y_j + \epsilon$, $j = 1, \dots, n$. Then, one can easily see that the X_js are exchangeable with $\mathbb{E}(X_j) = \mu$, $\mathrm{Var}(X_j) = \sigma^2$ and $\mathrm{Cov}(X_j, X_{j'}) = C$ for all $j \neq j'$. By definition of the X_js, $s_X^2 = \frac{1}{n-1} \sum_{j=1}^n (X_j - \overline{X}) = \frac{1}{n-1} \sum_{j=1}^n (Y_j - \overline{Y}) = s_Y^2$. So, $\mathrm{Var}(s_X^2) = \mathrm{Var}(s_Y^2) = \frac{\mu_4^{(Y)}}{n} + \frac{(n-3)\mathrm{Var}(Y)}{n(n-1)} = \frac{12n^4 + n^2 - 1}{n(16n^2 - 4)} + \frac{(n-3)(\sigma^2 - C)}{n(n-1)} \to \infty$ as $n \to \infty$.

In view of Theorem 1(a), Lemma 1 and Corollary 1, the unbiased estimation of the variance of $\widehat{\mu}_{\mathrm{os}}$ is impossible because the quantities $\mathsf{V}_{j;l}, \mathsf{C}_{j;l}, \mathsf{C}_{j;l,l'}, \mathsf{C}_{j,j';l}$ and $\mathsf{C}_{j,j';l,j}$ are as in Lemma 1. For example, let the jth source and the lth source be two different sources. Then, $\{\ell_{i,l}, i \in S_j\}$ is a set of exchangeable rv's of size n_j with unknown mean, say $\mu_{j,l}$, variance $\mathsf{V}_{j,l}$ and covariance between two elements $\mathsf{C}_{j,l}$.

It is a fact that there does not exist a general unbiased estimator of the variance of the OOS error. If someone needs an estimator of the variance of the OOS error for some reason (for example, for statistical inference on the OOS error), one may resort to the bootstrap resampling technique or can follow the moment approximation method of Markatou et al. (2005) when it is possible. Notice that the bootstrap resampling technique in this formulation has a very large computational cost.

5 Simulation Study

Assume we have $k = 3$ sources with probability vector $\boldsymbol{p} = (0.2, 0.3, 0.5)$, and thus odds vector $\boldsymbol{od} = (1/4, 3/7, 1)$. Suppose that the elements of each source are iid rv's from a distribution and the squared or absolute error loss is used.

Table 1 presents the true value of the OOS error, the empirical mean, variance and squared bias of the OOS error estimator $\widehat{\mu}_{os}$, when $N = 10^4$ Monte Carlo (M-C) repetitions are used, for various values of the sample size n. The elements of each source are normally distributed and the squared and absolute error loss are used. In this case we have the explicit expressions of μ_{os} given by the relations (3) and (5) for both cases of squared and absolute error loss respectively. We observe that for both cases, squared and absolute error loss, the empirical mean square error of $\widehat{\mu}_{os}$ tends to zero as n tends to infinity, confirming the statements of Theorems 1(a) and 2.

Tables 2, 3, and 4 present the empirical mean and the empirical variance of the OOS error estimator $\widehat{\mu}_{os}$, for $N = 10^4$ M-C repetitions for various values of the sample size n, when the elements of each source are uniformly distributed (Table 2), Student distributed (Table 3) and gamma distributed (Table 4), and the squared and absolute error loss are used. For both cases of loss function, squared and absolute error loss, and for all cases of the sources' distributions the empirical variance of $\widehat{\mu}_{os}$ tends to zero as n tends to infinity, confirming empirically the statement of Theorem 2. Note that for these cases of the sources' distributions we do not have explicit forms of μ_{os} and thus, we cannot present the values $\widehat{\text{bias}}^2(\widehat{\mu}_{os})$ and $\widehat{\text{MSE}}(\widehat{\mu}_{os})$. On the other hand, since $\widehat{\mu}_{os}$ is an unbiased estimator of μ_{os}, for large values of n we have that $\widehat{\text{MSE}}(\widehat{\mu}_{os}) \approx \widehat{\text{Var}}(\widehat{\mu}_{os})$.

Tables 5, 6, 7, and 8 present the OOS error estimator and its associate empirical variance estimate in the case of a linear regression model with four covariates

Table 1 The OOS error, μ_{os}, the average of $\widehat{\mu}_{os}$ and its empirical variance and squared bias, for $N = 10^4$ M-C repetitions, when $k = 3$, $\boldsymbol{p} = (0.2, 0.3, 0.5)$, $F_1 \sim N(0, 9)$, $F_2 \sim N(2, 1)$, $F_3 \sim N(5, 5)$ and the squared/absolute error loss is used, for various values of n

	n	100	200	300	500	700	10^3	10^4
Squared	μ_{os}	18.171	18.084	18.055	18.031	18.021	18.014	17.998
	$\widehat{\mu}_{os}$	18.164	18.084	18.055	18.038	18.038	18.017	17.999
	$\widehat{\text{bias}}^2(\widehat{\mu}_{os})$	$<10^{-3}$	$<10^{-3}$	$<10^{-4}$	$<10^{-4}$	$<10^{-5}$	$<10^{-5}$	$<10^{-6}$
	$\widehat{\text{Var}}(\widehat{\mu}_{os})$	11.524	5.897	3.873	2.314	1.664	1.177	0.117
Absolute	μ_{os}	3.639	3.636	3.635	3.635	3.634	3.634	3.633
	$\widehat{\mu}_{os}$	3.635	3.634	3.638	3.635	3.633	3.634	3.633
	$\widehat{\text{bias}}^2(\widehat{\mu}_{os})$	$<10^{-5}$	$<10^{-5}$	$<10^{-5}$	$<10^{-5}$	$<10^{-6}$	$<10^{-7}$	$<10^{-8}$
	$\widehat{\text{Var}}(\widehat{\mu}_{os})$	0.148	0.074	0.050	0.030	0.021	0.014	0.001

Table 2 The average of $\widehat{\mu}_{os}$ and its empirical variance $\widehat{\text{Var}}(\widehat{\mu}_{os})$, for $N = 10^4$ M-C repetitions, when $k = 3$, $\boldsymbol{p} = (0.2, 0.3, 0.5)$, $F_1 \sim U(-1, 1)$, $F_2 \sim U(1/2, 3/2)$, $F_3 \sim U(3, 7)$ and the squared/absolute error loss is used, for various values of n

	n	100	200	300	500	700	10^3	10^4
Squared	$\widehat{\mu}_{os}$	17.294	17.266	17.277	17.271	17.273	17.278	17.275
	$\widehat{\text{Var}}(\widehat{\mu}_{os})$	1.699	0.871	0.568	0.332	0.243	0.173	0.017
Absolute	$\widehat{\mu}_{os}$	3.8435	3.8451	3.8425	3.8433	3.8433	3.8430	3.8428
	$\widehat{\text{Var}}(\widehat{\mu}_{os})$	0.0229	0.0113	0.0077	0.0047	0.0033	0.0022	0.0002

Table 3 The average of $\widehat{\mu}_{os}$ and its empirical variance $\widehat{\text{Var}}(\widehat{\mu}_{os})$, for $N = 10^4$ M-C repetitions, when $k = 3$, $\boldsymbol{p} = (0.2, 0.3, 0.5)$, $F_1 \sim t_7$, $F_2 \sim t_5(2)$, $F_3 \sim t_6(5)$ (where $t_v(\mu) \stackrel{d}{=} t_v + \mu$) and the squared/absolute error loss is used, for various values of n

	n	100	200	300	500	700	10^3	10^4
Squared	$\widehat{\mu}_{os}$	14.976	14.927	14.954	14.943	14.936	14.936	14.925
	$\widehat{\text{Var}}(\widehat{\mu}_{os})$	2.677	1.376	0.941	0.548	0.388	0.274	0.027
Absolute	$\widehat{\mu}_{os}$	3.5182	3.5142	3.5153	3.5152	3.5150	3.5153	3.5147
	$\widehat{\text{Var}}(\widehat{\mu}_{os})$	0.0417	0.0209	0.0141	0.0084	0.0061	0.0042	0.0004

Table 4 The average of $\widehat{\mu}_{os}$ and its empirical variance $\widehat{\text{Var}}(\widehat{\mu}_{os})$, for $N = 10^4$ M-C repetitions, when $k = 3$, $\boldsymbol{p} = (0.2, 0.3, 0.5)$, $F_1 \sim \exp(1)$, $F_2 \sim \Gamma(2, 1)$, $F_3 \sim \Gamma(10, 2)$ and the squared/absolute error loss is used, for various values of n

	n	100	200	300	500	700	10^3	10^4
Squared	$\widehat{\mu}_{os}$	12.095	12.068	12.067	12.060	12.038	12.048	12.043
	$\widehat{\text{Var}}(\widehat{\mu}_{os})$	2.763	1.326	0.863	0.537	0.385	0.265	0.027
Absolute	$\widehat{\mu}_{os}$	3.0669	3.0636	3.0655	3.0662	3.0657	3.0647	3.0652
	$\widehat{\text{Var}}(\widehat{\mu}_{os})$	0.0469	0.0240	0.0163	0.0095	0.0070	0.0048	0.0005

Table 5 The average of $\widehat{\mu}_{os}$ and its empirical variance $\widehat{\text{Var}}(\widehat{\mu}_{os})$ in linear regression case with four covariates, when $k = 3$, $\boldsymbol{p} = (0.2, 0.3, 0.5)$

n	100	200	300	500	700	10^3	10^4
$\widehat{\mu}_{os}$	83.06	71.46	79.36	70.88	72.73	75.04	74.32
$\widehat{\text{Var}}(\widehat{\mu}_{os})$	10.21	4.78	3.31	1.76	1.29	0.93	0.09

The model of the jth source is $y^{(j)} = \beta_0^{(j)} + \beta_1^{(j)} X_1 + \beta_2^{(j)} X_2 + \beta_3^{(j)} X_3 + \beta_4^{(j)} X_4 + \epsilon$, $j = 1, 2, 3$, where $X_1 \sim \text{binomial}(0.6)$, $X_2 \sim \text{Poisson}(2)$, $X_3 \sim N(3, 1)$, $X_4 \sim U(0, 3)$ with $\epsilon \sim N(0, 1)$, and $\boldsymbol{\beta}^{(1)} = (2, 1, -1, -3, 1)$, $\boldsymbol{\beta}^{(2)} = (1, 3, -1, 1, 1)$ and $\boldsymbol{\beta}^{(3)} = (-2, -2, 1, 1, -1)$. The number of M-C repetitions is $N = 10^3$

and three sources, for various sample sizes. Tables 5 and 6 present results for two different vectors of probabilities for the sources but the composition of the sources in terms of covariate distributions and vectors of parameters is the same in both tables. Furthermore, the distribution of covariates is the same in all sources but the associated parameter vectors are source-specific, i.e. they vary from source to source. We observe that the variance of the OOS error estimator, for large n

Table 6 The average of $\widehat{\mu}_{os}$ and its empirical variance $\widehat{\text{Var}}(\widehat{\mu}_{os})$ in linear regression case with four covariates, when $k = 3, \boldsymbol{p} = (0.1, 0.3, 0.6)$

n	100	200	300	500	700	10^3	10^4
$\widehat{\mu}_{os}$	67.74	66.50	60.06	62.86	63.37	61.25	61.08
$\widehat{\text{Var}}(\widehat{\mu}_{os})$	12.33	4.56	3.00	1.69	1.19	0.81	0.08

The models of the sources are as in Table 5, and the number of M-C repetitions is $N = 10^3$

Table 7 The average of $\widehat{\mu}_{os}$ and its empirical variance $\widehat{\text{Var}}(\widehat{\mu}_{os})$ in linear regression case with four covariates, when $k = 3, \boldsymbol{p} = (0.2, 0.3, 0.5)$

n	100	200	300	500	700	10^3	10^4
$\widehat{\mu}_{os}$	4.447	2.566	2.055	1.613	1.477	1.320	1.033
$\widehat{\text{Var}}(\widehat{\mu}_{os})$	8.870	1.795	0.786	0.294	0.175	0.087	0.001

The model of the jth source is $y^{(j)} = 2 + X_1^{(j)} - X_2^{(j)} + 3X_3^{(j)} + X_4 + \epsilon, j = 1, 2, 3$, where $X_1^{(1)} \sim \text{binomial}(0.6), X_2^{(1)} \sim \text{Poisson}(2), X_3^{(1)} \sim N(3, 1), X_4^{(1)} \sim U(0, 3), X_1^{(2)} \sim \text{binomial}(0.8),$ $X_2^{(2)} \sim \text{Poisson}(1), X_3^{(2)} \sim N(1, 1), X_4^{(2)} \sim U(5, 7), X_1^{(3)} \sim \text{binomial}(0.2), X_2^{(3)} \sim \text{Poisson}(3),$ $X_3^{(3)} \sim N(0, 1), X_4^{(3)} \sim U(0, 1)$ and $\epsilon \sim N(0, 1)$. The number of M-C repetitions is $N = 10^3$

Table 8 The average of $\widehat{\mu}_{os}$ and its empirical variance $\widehat{\text{Var}}(\widehat{\mu}_{os})$ in linear regression case with four covariates, when $k = 3, \boldsymbol{p} = (0.1, 0.3, 0.6)$

n	100	200	300	500	700	10^3	10^4
$\widehat{\mu}_{os}$	5.715	2.705	2.300	1.775	1.585	1.364	1.037
$\widehat{\text{Var}}(\widehat{\mu}_{os})$	12.27	2.041	1.202	0.479	0.254	0.102	0.001

The models of the sources are as in Table 7, and the number of M-C repetitions is $N = 10^3$

converges to 0. We draw similar observations from the results of Tables 7 and 8; these tables present results for various sample sizes when the parameter vector is the same for all sources but the distribution of covariates is different among the different sources, and the probability of the different sources is different in the two tables. The results show that as $n \to \infty$ the variance of the OOS error estimator converges to 0.

6 Discussion

In this paper we discuss the definition, estimation and properties of the proposed estimator of the out-of-source error in the context of multi-source data, when it is not assumed that all sources have exactly the same number of observations and do not necessarily follow the same distribution. We show that our proposed estimator is unbiased, and we offer natural and easy to verify in practice conditions under which the estimator we propose is consistent.

Most research, both theoretical and empirical, assumes that a learning algorithm is trained and tested using data that follow the same distribution. This setting has been extensively studied in the literature, and uniform convergence theory guarantees that a learning algorithm's empirical error is close to its true error under appropriate assumptions. However, in many practical situations we wish to train a learning algorithm under one or more source domains and then test it on a domain that is potentially different from the source domains. Our work, presented here, studies the out-of-source error in this setting. We further supplement the theoretical results we present here with a simulation that essentially verifies these results.

One setting where our results may be potentially useful is in meta-analysis. Meta-analysis methods combine and further analyze, quantitative evidence from related studies. As such meta-analysis is an evidence generation method in medicine (Riley et al. 2010). There are two approaches to carry out meta-analysis. Traditional approaches synthesize, at the study level, aggregated data, obtained from different publications. An alternative approach is meta-analysis based on individual partic- ipant data. Here, the individual raw, study specific data are used. In this setting, one can consider the different studies as corresponding to different sources. A large OOS error then indicates differences in the populations that are associated with the different studies. We conjecture that similar comments hold in the case of variable selection with respect to the OOS error and note that further study of OOS error in both, individual participant meta-analysis and variable selection and regularization, is needed.

Acknowledgements Dr. Markatou would like to thank the Jacobs School of Medicine and Biomedical Science for facilitating this work through institutional financial resources (to M. Markatou) that supported the work of the first author of this paper.

Appendix 1: Some Useful Relations

Since Z_is are independent and the elements of each source are identically distributed, the following are obvious.

E.1: $\left(L(Z_i, \widehat{d_l}), L(Z_{i'}, \widehat{d_l})\right)$, $i \in S_j$, $i' \in S_{j'}$ with $j \neq j' \neq l \neq j$, are exchangeable;

E.2: $\left(L(Z_i, \widehat{d_l}), L(Z_i, \widehat{d_{l'}})\right)$, $i \in S_j$ with $j \neq l \neq l' \neq j$, are exchangeable;

E.3: $\left(L(Z_i, \widehat{d_l}), L(Z_{i'}, \widehat{d_{l'}})\right)$, $i \neq i' \in S_j$ with $j \neq l \neq l' \neq j$, are exchangeable;

E.4: $\left(L(Z_i, \widehat{d_l}), L(Z_{i'}, \widehat{d_j})\right)$, $i \in S_j$, $i' \in S_{j'}$ with $j \neq j' \neq l \neq j$, are exchangeable.

E.5: $L(Z_i, \widehat{d_l})$ and $L(Z_{i'}, \widehat{d_{l'}})$, $i \in S_j$, $i' \in S_{j'}$, are independent for all indices j, j', l, l' such that $\{j, l\} \cap \{j', l'\} = \varnothing$.

Appendix 2: On Moments of Bivariate Normal Distribution

Theorem 3 (Isserlis 1918) *Let* $(Y_1, Y_2) \sim N_2 \left(0, \left(\begin{smallmatrix} \sigma_1^2 & \sigma_{12} \\ \sigma_{12} & \sigma_2^2 \end{smallmatrix}\right)\right)$. *Then,* $\mathbb{E}(Y_i^4) = 3\sigma_i^4$, $\mathbb{E}(Y_1^2 Y_2^2) = \sigma_1^2 \sigma_2^2 + 2\sigma_{12}^2$ *and* $\mathbb{E}(Y_1^2 Y_2) = \mathbb{E}(Y_1 Y_2^2) = 0$.

An application of Isserlis's Theorem 3 gives

Corollary 2 *Let* $(X_1, X_2) \sim N_2 \left(\left(\begin{smallmatrix} \mu_1 \\ \mu_2 \end{smallmatrix}\right), \left(\begin{smallmatrix} \sigma_1^2 & \sigma_{12} \\ \sigma_{12} & \sigma_2^2 \end{smallmatrix}\right)\right)$. *Then, the covariance of* X_1^2 *and* X_2^2 *is* $\mathsf{Cov}(X_1^2, X_2^2) = 2\sigma_{12}(\sigma_{12} + 2\mu_1 \mu_2)$.

Appendix 3: Proofs

Proof of Theorem 1

(a) By definition of $e_{j;l}$,

$$\mathbb{E}(\widehat{\mu}_{os}) = \frac{1}{n} \sum_{j=1}^k \frac{1}{n - n_j} \sum_{l \neq j} n_l \sum_{i \in S_j} \mathbb{E}(\ell_{i,l}) = \frac{1}{n} \sum_{j=1}^k \frac{n_j}{n - n_j} \sum_{l \neq j} n_l e_{j;l}.$$

The result arises by $n_j/n = p_j$ for all $j = 1, \ldots, k$.

(b) Write $\Sigma_j = \sum_{l \neq j} n_l \sum_{i \in S_j} \ell_{i,l}$ and $\Sigma_{j,l} = \sum_{i \in S_j} \ell_{i,l}$. Hence, $\widehat{\mu}_{os} = \frac{1}{n} \sum_{j=1}^k \frac{1}{n-n_j} \Sigma_j$ and $\Sigma_j = \sum_{l \neq j} n_l \Sigma_{j,l}$. By straightforward calculations

$$\mathsf{Var}(\widehat{\mu}_{os}) = \frac{1}{n^2} \left\{ \sum_{j=1}^k \frac{\mathsf{Var}(\Sigma_j)}{(n - n_j)^2} + \sum_{j \neq j'} \sum \frac{\mathsf{Cov}(\Sigma_j, \Sigma_{j'})}{(n - n_j)(n - n_{j'})} \right\}. \tag{6}$$

The variance of Σ_j is $\mathsf{Var}(\Sigma_j) = \sum_{l \neq j} n_l^2 \mathsf{Var}(\Sigma_{j,l}) + \sum \sum_{l \neq l': l, l' \neq j} n_l n_{l'} \mathsf{Cov}(\Sigma_{j,l}, \Sigma_{j,l'})$. We compute $\mathsf{Var}(\Sigma_{j,l}) = \sum_{i \in S_j} \mathsf{Var}(\ell_{i,l}) + \sum \sum_{i,i' \in S_j : i \neq i'} \mathsf{Cov}(\ell_{i,l}, \ell_{i',l}) = n_j V_{j;l} + n_j(n_j - 1) C_{j;l}$, see E.1 and E.2. Also, we compute the covariance of $\Sigma_{j,l}$ and $\Sigma_{j,l'}$, $\mathsf{Cov}(\Sigma_{j,l}, \Sigma_{j,l'}) = \sum_{i \in S_j} \mathsf{Cov}(\ell_{i,l}, \ell_{i,l'}) + \sum \sum_{i,i' \in S_j : i \neq i'} \mathsf{Cov}(\ell_{i,l}, \ell_{i',l'}) = n_j C_{j;l,l'}$, see E.3 and E.5. Thus,

$$\mathsf{Var}(\Sigma_j) = \sum_{l \neq j} n_l^2 \left(n_j V_{j;l} + n_j(n_j - 1) C_{j;l}\right) + \sum \sum_{l \neq l': l, l' \neq j} n_l n_{l'} C_{j;l,l'}. \tag{7}$$

The covariance of Σ_j and $\Sigma_{j'}$ is $\mathsf{Cov}(\Sigma_j, \Sigma_{j'}) = \sum_{l \neq j} \sum_{l' \neq j'} n_l n_{l'} \mathsf{Cov}(\Sigma_{j,l}, \Sigma_{j',l'}) = \sum_{l \neq j, j'} n_l^2 \mathsf{Cov}(\Sigma_{j,l}, \Sigma_{j',l}) + \sum \sum_{l \neq j, l' \neq j' : l \neq l'} n_l n_{l'} \mathsf{Cov}(\Sigma_{j,l}, \Sigma_{j',l'})$. Now we compute $\mathsf{Cov}(\Sigma_{j,l}, \Sigma_{j',l}) = \sum_{i \in S_j} \sum_{i' \in S_{j'}} \mathsf{Cov}(\ell_{i,l}, \ell_{i',l}) = n_j n_{j'} C_{j,j';l}$. For $\mathsf{Cov}(\Sigma_{j,l}, \Sigma_{j',l'})$ when $l \neq l'$ we distinguish the following cases: If $l \neq j'$ and $l' \neq j$, $\mathsf{Cov}(\Sigma_{j,l}, \Sigma_{j',l'}) = 0$, see E.5; if $l \neq j'$ and $l' = j$,

$\mathsf{Cov}(\Sigma_{j,l}, \Sigma_{j',j}) = \sum_{i\in S_j}\sum_{i'\in S_{j'}} \mathsf{Cov}(\ell_{i,l}, \ell_{i',j}) = n_j n_{j'} C_{jj';l,j}$, see E.4; and if $l = j'$ and $l' \neq j$, similarly, $\mathsf{Cov}(\Sigma_{j,j'}, \Sigma_{j',l'}) = n_j n_{j'} C_{jj';j',l'}$. Thus, for each $j \neq j'$

$$\mathsf{Cov}(\Sigma_j, \Sigma_{j'}) = \sum_{l \neq j,j'} n_l n_j n_{j'}(n_l C_{jj';l} + 2n_j C_{jj';l,j}) \tag{8}$$

Combining (6)–(8),

$$\mathsf{Var}(\widehat{\mu}_{\mathrm{os}}) = \frac{1}{n^2}\left\{\sum_{j=1}^{k} \frac{\sum_{l\neq j} n_l^2\left(n_j V_{j;l} + n_j(n_j-1)C_{j;l}\right) + \sum\sum_{l\neq l':l,l'\neq j} n_j n_l n_{l'} C_{j;l,l'}}{(n-n_j)^2} \right.$$

$$\left. + \sum\sum_{j\neq j'} \frac{\sum_{l\neq j,j'} n_l n_j n_{j'}(n_l C_{jj';l} + 2n_j C_{jj';l,j})}{(n-n_j)(n-n_{j'})} \right\}.$$

Using $n_j = np_j$ and $od_j = p_j/(1 - p_j)$ for all j, after some algebra, the proof is completed.

□

Proof of Lemma 1 Since the joint distribution function of X_js is unknown, the only information that we have is with respect to the moments of X_js. Therefore, the only forms of estimators that we know to have expected values equal to linear combinations of μ^2, σ^2 and C are the linear combination of X_j^2s and $X_j X_{j'}$s. Consider $\delta = \sum_{j=1}^{n} a_j X_j^2 + \sum\sum_{1\leq j<j'\leq n} b_{jj'} X_j X_{j'}$. Observe that $\mathbb{E}(X_j^2) = \sigma^2 + \mu^2$ and $\mathbb{E}(X_j X_{j'}) = C + \mu^2$. Thus, setting $a = \sum_{j=1}^{n} a_j$ and $b = \sum\sum_{1\leq j<j'\leq n} b_{jj'}$, we get

$$\mathbb{E}(\delta) = a(\sigma^2 + \mu^2) + b(C + \mu^2),$$

completing the proof.

□

Proof of Corollary 1

(a) We compute $\mathsf{Var}(\overline{X}) = \frac{1}{n}\sigma^2 + \frac{n-1}{n}C$. Let now δ be an unbiased estimator of the variance of $\overline{X}$, $\delta = \sum_{j=1}^{n} a_j X_j^2 + \sum\sum_{1\leq j<j'\leq n} b_{jj'} X_j X_{j'}$. Setting $a = \sum_{j=1}^{n} a_j$ and $b = \sum\sum_{1\leq j<j'\leq n} b_{jj'}$, we get

$$a(\sigma^2+\mu^2)+b(C+\mu^2) = \frac{1}{n}\sigma^2+\frac{n-1}{n}C \Rightarrow \left\{a = \frac{1}{n},\ b = 1 - \frac{1}{n},\ a+b = 0\right\},$$

a contradiction.

(b) Using the same arguments as in (a), the proof is completed.

□

Proof of Theorem 2 Let $Z \sim F_j$ be independent of the elements of the lth source. Using Hölder inequality and C.2, $\mathsf{V}_{j,l} \leq \mathbb{E}[L(Z, \widehat{d}_{l,n})]^2 \leq \mathbb{E}\{[L(Z, \widehat{d}_{l,n})]^{2+\theta}\}^{2/(2+\theta)} \leq M^{2/(2+\theta)} = M^*$ for all $j \neq l$. Thus, $\sum_{j=1}^{k} \frac{od_j^2}{np_j}$ $(\sum_{l \neq j} p_l^2 \mathsf{V}_{j;l}) \leq \frac{M^*}{n} \sum_{j=1}^{k} \frac{od_j^2}{p_j}(\sum_{l \neq j} p_l^2) = O(1/n)$. An application of Cauchy–Schwarz inequality gives $|\mathsf{C}_{j,l,l'}| \leq \mathsf{V}_{j,l} \leq M^*$. So, $\sum_{j=1}^{k} \frac{od_j^2}{np_j}(\sum \sum_{l \neq l':l,l' \neq j} p_l p_{l'} \mathsf{C}_{j;l,l'})$ $\leq \frac{M^*}{n} \sum_{j=1}^{k} \frac{od_j^2}{p_j}(\sum \sum_{l \neq l':l,l' \neq j} p_l p_{l'}) = O(1/n)$.

It is remains to prove that $\mathsf{C}_{j;l}, \mathsf{C}_{j,j',l}, \mathsf{C}_{j,j';l,j} \to 0$ as $n \to \infty$. Let Z, Z' are iid from F_j and are independent of the elements of the lth source. Consider the sequence of random vectors $(Z, Z', \widehat{d}_{l,n})$ with respect to n. Then, C.1 gives $(Z, Z', \widehat{d}_{l,n}) \rightsquigarrow (Z, Z', d_l)$ as $n \to \infty$. Since L is continuous, the maps $(Z, Z', \widehat{d}_{l,n}) \mapsto L(Z, \widehat{d}_{l,n})$ and $(Z, Z', \widehat{d}_{l,n}) \mapsto L(Z, \widehat{d}_{l,n})L(Z', \widehat{d}_{l,n})$ are continuous. Using the Continuous Mapping Theorem, $L(Z, \widehat{d}_{l,n}) \rightsquigarrow L(Z, d_l)$ and $L(Z, \widehat{d}_{l,n})L(Z', \widehat{d}_{l,n}) \rightsquigarrow L(Z, d_l)L(Z', d_l)$ as $n \to \infty$. Observe that $\mathbb{E}|L(Z, \widehat{d}_{l,n})|^{1+(1+\theta)} \leq M$, see C.2, so the sequence $L(Z, \widehat{d}_{l,n})$ is uniformly integrable. Hence, $\mathbb{E}|L(Z, d_l)| < \infty$ and $\mathbb{E}[L(Z, \widehat{d}_{l,n})] \to \mathbb{E}[L(Z, d_l)]$ as $n \to \infty$ (see, e.g., Billingsley 1995, p. 338). Similarly, $\mathbb{E}|L(Z', d_l)| < \infty$ and $\mathbb{E}[L(Z', \widehat{d}_{l,n})] \to \mathbb{E}[L(Z', d_l)]$ as $n \to \infty$. Using Cauchy–Schwarz inequality we obtain $\mathbb{E}|L(Z, \widehat{d}_{l,n})L(Z', \widehat{d}_{l,n})|^{1+\theta/2} \leq (\mathbb{E}|L(Z, \widehat{d}_{l,n})|^{2+\theta})^{1/2}(\mathbb{E}|L(Z', \widehat{d}_{l,n})|^{2+\theta})^{1/2} \leq M$. So, $L(Z, \widehat{d}_{l,n})L(Z', \widehat{d}_{l,n})$ is uniformly integrable. Therefore, $\mathbb{E}|L(Z, d_l)L(Z', d_l)| < \infty$ and $\mathbb{E}[L(Z, \widehat{d}_{l,n})L(Z', \widehat{d}_{l,n})] \to \mathbb{E}[L(Z, d_l)L(Z', d_l)]$ as $n \to \infty$. Moreover, $L(Z, d_l)$ and $L(Z', d_l)$ are independent. So, $\mathbb{E}[L(Z, \widehat{d}_{l,n})L(Z', \widehat{d}_{l,n})] \to \mathbb{E}[L(Z, d_l)]\mathbb{E}[L(Z', d_l)]$ as $n \to \infty$. From the preceding analysis we have that $\mathsf{C}_{j;l} \to 0$ as $n \to \infty$. Using the same arguments as above it follows that $\mathsf{C}_{j,j',l}$, $\mathsf{C}_{j,j';l,j} \to 0$ as $n \to \infty$, and the proof is completed. □

Proof of Equations (3)–(5) Let j, j', l, l' are four distinct indices. Assume that $Z_{(j)}, Z'_{(j)} \in \mathscr{Z}_{S_j}$ (with $Z_{(j)} \neq Z'_{(j)}$) and $Z_{(j')} \in \mathscr{Z}_{S_{j'}}$. Consider the following random

vectors $(X_1, X_2) = (Z_{(j)} - \overline{Z}_l, Z'_{(j)} - \overline{Z}_l) \sim N_2\left(\begin{pmatrix} \mu_j - \mu_l \\ \mu_j - \mu_l \end{pmatrix}, \begin{pmatrix} \sigma_j^2 + \sigma_l^2/n_l & \sigma_l^2/n_l \\ \sigma_l^2/n_l & \sigma_j^2 + \sigma_l^2/n_l \end{pmatrix}\right)$,

$(X_3, X_4) = (Z_{(j)} - \overline{Z}_l, Z_{(j)} - \overline{Z}_{l'}) \sim N_2\left(\begin{pmatrix} \mu_j - \mu_l \\ \mu_j - \mu_{l'} \end{pmatrix}, \begin{pmatrix} \sigma_j^2 + \sigma_l^2/n_l & \sigma_j^2 \\ \sigma_j^2 & \sigma_j^2 + \sigma_{l'}^2/n_{l'} \end{pmatrix}\right)$,

$(X_5, X_6) = (Z_{(j)} - \overline{Z}_l, Z_{(j')} - \overline{Z}_l) \sim N_2\left(\begin{pmatrix} \mu_j - \mu_l \\ \mu_{j'} - \mu_l \end{pmatrix}, \begin{pmatrix} \sigma_j^2 + \sigma_l^2/n_l & \sigma_l^2/n_l \\ \sigma_l^2/n_l & \sigma_{j'}^2 + \sigma_l^2/n_l \end{pmatrix}\right)$,

$(X_7, X_8) = (Z_{(j)} - \overline{Z}_l, Z_{(j')} - \overline{Z}_j) \sim N_2\left(\begin{pmatrix} \mu_j - \mu_l \\ \mu_{j'} - \mu_j \end{pmatrix}, \begin{pmatrix} \sigma_j^2 + \sigma_l^2/n_l & -\sigma_j^2/n_j \\ -\sigma_j^2/n_j & \sigma_{j'}^2 + \sigma_j^2/n_j \end{pmatrix}\right)$. If

$X \sim N(\mu, \sigma^2)$, then $\mathrm{Var}(X^2) = 2\sigma^2(\sigma^2 + 2\mu^2)$. Since $\mathsf{V}_{j,l} = \mathrm{Var}(X_1^2)$, (4a) follows. Observe that $\mathsf{C}_{j;l} = \mathrm{Cov}(X_1^2, X_2^2)$, $\mathsf{C}_{j;l,l'} = \mathrm{Cov}(X_3^2, X_4^2)$, $\mathsf{C}_{j,j';l} = \mathrm{Cov}(X_5^2, X_6^2)$ and $\mathsf{C}_{j,j';l,j} = \mathrm{Cov}(X_7^2, X_8^2)$. Hence, an application of Corollary 2 proves (4b). Finally, If $X \sim N(\mu, \sigma^2)$, then $\mathbb{E}|X| = \mu[1 - 2\Phi(-\mu/\sigma)] + \sigma(2/\pi)^{1/2} \exp\{-\mu^2/(2\sigma^2)\}$. Because $\mathsf{e}_{j;l} = \mathbb{E}|X_1| = \mu_{j;l}\left[1 - 2\Phi\left(-\mu_{j;l}/\sigma_{j;l}\right)\right] + \sigma_{j;l}\sqrt{2/\pi} \exp\left(-\mu_{j;l}^2/2\sigma_{j;l}^2\right)$, using (1), (5) follows, completing the proof. □

Proof of Corollary 2 Consider $Y_1 = X_1 - \mu_1$ and $Y_2 = X_2 - \mu_2$. Then, $(Y_1, Y_2) \sim N_2\left(0, \begin{pmatrix} \sigma_1^2 & \sigma_{12} \\ \sigma_{12} & \sigma_2^2 \end{pmatrix}\right)$. Thus, $\mathsf{Cov}(X_1^2, X_2^2) = \mathsf{Cov}(Y_1^2 + 2\mu_1 Y_1 + \mu_1^2, Y_2^2 + 2\mu_2 Y_2 + \mu_2^2) = \mathsf{Cov}(Y_1^2, Y_2^2) + 2\mu_2 \mathsf{Cov}(Y_1^2, Y_2) + 2\mu_1 \mathsf{Cov}(Y_1, Y_2^2) + 4\mu_1\mu_2 \mathsf{Cov}(Y_1, Y_2)$. A simple application of Isserlis's Theorem completes the proof. □

References

Afendras, G., & Markatou, M. (2016). Optimality of training/test size and resampling effectiveness of cross-validation estimators of the generalization error. arXiv:1511.02980v1 [math.ST].

Arlot, S., & Celisse, A. (2010). A survey of cross-validation procedures for model selection. *Statistics Surveys, 4*, 40–79.

Ben-David, S., Blitzer, J, Crammer, K., Kulesza, A., Pereira, F., & Vaughan, J. W. (2010). A theory of learning from different domains. *Machine Learning, 79*, 151–175.

Breiman, L., Friedman, J. H., Olshen, R. A., & Stone, C. J. (1984). *Classification and regression trees*. Belmont, CA: Wadsworth.

Billingsley, P. (1995). *Probability and measure*, 3rd ed. Wiley series in probability and mathematical statistics. New York: Wiley.

Geisser, S. (1975). The predictive sample reuse method with applications. *Journal of the American Statistical Association, 70*(350), 320–328.

Geras, K., & Sutton, C. (2013). Multiple-source cross-validation. In *Proceedings of the 30 th International Conference on Machine Learning*, Atlanta, GA (2013). *JMLR: W&CP, 28*(3), 1292–1300.

Isserlis, L. (1918). On a formula for the product-moment coefficient of any order of a normal frequency distribution in any number of variables. *Biometrika, 12*, 134–139.

Markatou, M., Tian, H, Biswas, S., & Hripcsak, G. (2005). Analysis of variance of cross-validation estimators of the generalization error. *Journal of Machine Learning Research, 6*, 1127–1168.

Nadeau, C., & Bengio, Y. (2003). Inference for the generalization error. *Machine Learning, 52*, 239–281.

Riley, R. D., Lambert, P. C., & Abo-Zaid, G. (2010). Meta-analysis of individual participant data: Rationale, conduct, and reporting. *British Medical Journal, 340*, c221. https://doi.org/doi:10.1136/bmj.c221

Stone, M. (1974). Cross-validatory choice and assessment of statistical predictions. *Journal of the Royal Statistical Society. Series B, 36*(2), 111–147.

Stone, M. (1977). Asymptotics for and against cross-validation. *Biometrika, 64*(1), 29–35.

Meta-Analysis for Rare Events As Binary Outcomes

Gaohong Dong

1 Introduction

While the use of meta-analyses can be traced back to nineteenth century studies of astronomy (Plackett 1958), Glass first introduced the term "meta-analysis" in 1976 from his paper "Primary, secondary, and meta-analysis of research". Meta-analysis is a systematic and quantitative review of the results of a set of individual studies, intended to integrate their findings (Glass 1976). Meta-analysis has been frequently and widely used in pharmaceutical industry to estimate treatment effects in terms of efficacy and/or safety outcomes, or to update the estimates of treatment effects by further including recent relevant clinical studies to date.

To estimate treatment effects from the pooled data, Simpson's paradox is a main reason for the use of a meta-analysis rather than a naïve data pooling. One of the best-known examples of Simpson's paradox is a study of gender bias among graduate school admissions to University of California, Berkeley (e.g. Wikipedia). In 1973, The UC Berkeley admission figures showed that men applying were more likely than women to be admitted. As shown in Table 1, overall 44% men vs. 35% women were admitted per a naïve data pooling analysis. Therefore men were more successful in admissions than women. Bickel et al. (1975) revealed that women tended to apply to competitive departments with low rates of admission even among qualified applicants (such as in the English department), whereas men tended to apply to less-competitive departments with high rates of admission among the qualified applicants (such as in the engineering and chemistry departments). Basically gender and the department were confounded. There are many real-life examples of Simpson's paradox in the medical field. Confounding is a main reason

G. Dong (✉)
iStats Inc., Long Island City, NY, USA
e-mail: gaohong_dong@istats.org

© Springer International Publishing AG 2017
D.-G. Chen et al. (eds.), *New Advances in Statistics and Data Science*,
ICSA Book Series in Statistics, https://doi.org/10.1007/978-3-319-69416-0_3

Table 1 UC Berkeley applications and admissions in 1973

Department	Men		Woman	
	Applicants	Admitted	Applicants	Admitted
A	825	62%	108	82%
B	560	63%	25	68%
C	325	37%	593	34%
D	417	33%	375	35%
E	191	28%	393	24%
F	373	6%	341	7%
Overall	8442	44%	4321	35%

to run randomized clinical trials. However, randomization itself does not guarantee the elimination of all confounding effects. From analysis perspective, a way to remove confounding effect is a stratified analysis or meta-analysis (e.g. Dmitrienko et al. 2005; Pourhoseingholi et al. 2012).

When the outcomes of interest are rare events, which are not uncommon for drug safety assessments, it is quite challenging to conduct a meta-analysis. As Cochrane Handbook (Higgins and Green 2011) pointed out that meta-analysis may be the only way to obtain reliable evidence of the treatment effects if the events are rare, as individual studies are usually underpowered to detect differences in rare outcomes. The conventional meta-analysis methods rely on large-sample approximations to the distributions of the combined point estimators. Such approximations may be inaccurate and lead to invalid conclusions when the individual study sample sizes are small, the number of studies is not large, or the event rates are low (e.g. Brown et al. 2001). The inverse-variance weighted method (Cochran 1954) is widely used in meta-analyses (fixed and random effects). However, this method is inappropriate for rare events (e.g. Higgins and Green 2011; Shuster and Walker 2016). The DerSimonian and Laird (1986) approach has a serious deficiency when event rate is low (e.g. Higgins and Green 2011; Shuster and Walker 2016). Hoaglin (2016) discussed the misunderstanding about Cochran's Q for heterogeneity test in meta-analyses. He pointed out that the use of the inverse-variance weights is problematic.

Since the events of interest are rare, some clinical studies that qualify the inclusion of the meta-analyses the sponsor pre-planned have zero events in one treatment group or in both treatments groups (so called single-zero-events or double-zero-events studies). Conventional methods either exclude such studies or add an arbitrary positive value (sometimes called continuity correction) to each cell of the corresponding 2 × 2 tables in the analysis, which is usually the case when the inverse-variance weighted approach is used. In the past decade, there are new methodological developments on the meta-analyses for rare events. Sweeting et al. (2004), Bradburn et al. (2007), Kuss (2015) and Böhning et al. (2015) extensively evaluated the performance of different meta-analysis methods for rare events with or without a continuity correction. Rücker et al. (2009) investigated the arcsine difference as a measure of treatment effect. Tian et al. (2009) developed an exact and efficient inference procedure for meta-analysis and provided an application of rosiglitazone studies with all available data included but without artificial continuity correction. Cai et al. (2010) proposed alternative approaches based on Poisson random-effect models to make an inference about the relative risk between two treatment groups. Brockhaus et al. (2016) compared the Peto odds ratio with the usual odds ratio.

This chapter reviews the meta-analyses with rare events as binary outcomes. The methods covered in this chapter include non-parametric meta-analysis (Mantel-Haenszel method, the Peto odds ratio, and the exact method of constructing confidence intervals for risk differences by Tian et al. (2009)), parametric meta-analysis (random-effects regression model, random-effects beta-binomial model and random-effects Poisson model) and parametric bootstrap resampling meta-analysis. Case studies using these methods are provided.

2 Methods

2.1 Non-Parametric Meta-Analysis

The non-parametric meta-analyses reviewed in this section are the methods under the framework of fixed-effects models, which assume that all studies have the same treatment effect (i.e. there is no between-study heterogeneity).

2.1.1 Mantel-Haenszel Method

The Mantel-Haenszel method (Mantel and Haenszel 1959) is often used for meta-analyses on binary outcomes. Let n_{ijm} denote the frequency count of the cell in the ith row and jth column of the 2×2 table (e.g. the first row vs. the second row is for the investigational treatment vs. control, and the first column vs. the second column is for with vs. without events, respectively) of the mth study included in the meta-analysis ($m = 1, 2, \ldots, M$), and n_m the total sample size for the mth study. The Mantel-Haenszel odds ratio is computed as follows:

$$OR_{MH} = \frac{\sum\limits_{m=1}^{M} n_{11m}n_{22m}/n_m}{\sum\limits_{m=1}^{M} n_{12m}n_{21m}/n_m}. \tag{1}$$

Since the Mantel-Haenszel method takes sums before ratios and adjusts the calculation with study sample sizes (i.e. more weight is applied to a larger study), the Mantel-Haenszel method provides a similar or robust estimate of the odds ratio compared to logit, maximum likelihood and other estimates, in particular when the data are sparse (e.g. Agresti 2002, 2013). It should be noted that Agresti (2002,

2013) pointed out that if the variability of the odds ratio across the studies is not substantial, the Mantel-Haenszel odds ratio is still useful. The calculation of the Mantel-Haenszel odds ratio can include the studies without an event of interest unless the denominator is zero. However, the double-zero-events studies do not have a contribution to the Mantel-Haenszel odds ratio, which is unappealing. Continuity correction (i.e. adding 0.5 to each cell of the 2×2 table) has been suggested when the Mantel-Haenszel method is used to analyze rare events. However, it has been reported that, a continuity correction may result in an unpleasant element of arbitrariness (e.g. Agresti and Hartzel 2000) or a bias (Bradburn et al. 2007), therefore it is not suggested (e.g. Kuss 2015).

The Mantel-Haenszel risk ratio (RR_{MH}) and the Mantel-Haenszel risk difference (δ_{MH}) are also used in meta-analyses for rare events, which are calculated as

$$RR_{MH} = \frac{\sum_{m=1}^{M} n_{11m} n_{2\bullet m} / n_m}{\sum_{m=1}^{M} n_{21m} n_{1\bullet m} / n_m}, \tag{2}$$

and

$$\delta_{MH} = \frac{\sum_{m=1}^{M} (n_{11m} n_{2\bullet m} - n_{21m} n_{1\bullet m}) / n_m}{\sum_{m=1}^{M} n_{1\bullet m} n_{2\bullet m} / n_m}, \tag{3}$$

where $n_{1\bullet m}$ and $n_{2\bullet m}$ are the number of subjects in the investigational treatment and the control group, respectively. Typically the variance of the logarithm of the Mantel-Haenszel odds ratio is estimated using Robins et al. (1986), and Greenland and Robins (1985) is used to estimate the variances of the Mantel-Haenszel risk difference and the logarithm of the Mantel-Haenszel risk ratio. One advantage to use the Mantel-Haenszel risk difference is that this method can include any zero-events studies.

2.1.2   Peto Odds Ratio

The Peto odds ratio (Peto et al. 1977; Yusuf et al. 1985) is used for meta-analyses for rare events as well. Same as the Mantel-Haenszel odds ratio, double-zero-events studies do not have a contribution to the Peto odds ratio. The Peto odds ratio is calculated as follows:

$$OR_{Peto} = \exp \left(\frac{\sum_{m=1}^{M} n_{11m} - E(n_{11m})}{\sum_{m=1}^{M} V_m} \right), \tag{4}$$

where $E\left(n_{11m}\right) = \frac{(n_{11m}+n_{21m})(n_{11m}+n_{12m})}{n_m}$ is the expectation of n_{11m} and $V_m = \frac{E(n_{11m})(n_{21m}+n_{22m})(n_{12m}+n_{22m})}{n_m(n_m-1)}$.

Brockhaus et al. (2014, 2016) recently studied the Peto odds ratio. They demonstrated that the Peto odds ratio performs better in terms of mean percentage error, but not the confidence interval width and mean square error when the treatment effect is small and the sample sizes are similar between treatment groups; however when the treatment effect is large and group sizes are unbalanced, the Peto odds ratio leads to biased estimates. The latter had been reported by other researchers, e.g. Greenland and Salvan (1990) and Sutton et al. (2000). And bias is also possible when the estimated odds ratio is far from unity (Fleiss 1993). Sweeting et al. (2004) and Cochrane Handbook (Higgins and Green 2011) indicated that the Peto odds ratio can be least biased when the event rate is very low (e.g. <1%) and two groups are balanced; in other scenarios, the Mantel-Haenszel method without a continuity correction performs better. However, Kuss (2015) pointed out that this recommendation ignored that both the Mantel-Haenszel method for the odds ratio and the risk ratio and the Peto odds ratio exclude double-zero-events studies unless continuity corrections are applied, and continuity corrections are not suggested.

2.1.3 Exact Method of Constructing Confidence Intervals for Risk Differences (Tian et al. 2009)

Tian et al. (2010) developed an exact and efficient inference procedure for meta-analysis. Their method can handle any zero-events studies without artificial continuity corrections. The parameter of interest is the risk difference Δ, say to construct a $100(1 - \alpha)\%$ 1-sided confidence interval (a, ∞) for Δ. For a given η, there are M study-specific 1-sided η-level confidence intervals for Δ. Now, for any fixed value of Δ, say 0, let's examine whether 0 is the true value of Δ. If yes, then on average, 0 should belong to at least $100\eta\%$ of the above M intervals. Let $y_m = 1$, if 0 belongs to the observed η interval from the mth study, and $y_m = 0$, otherwise. Then, 0 is included in (a, ∞) if

$$t\left(\eta\right) = \sum_{m=1}^{M} w_m\left(y_m - \eta\right) \geq c \tag{5}$$

where w_m is a study-specific positive weight (e.g. total sample size), c is chosen such that $Prob\{T\left(\eta\right) < c\} \leq \alpha$. Similarly, one can obtain combined $100(1 - \alpha)\%$ 1-sided confidence interval $(-\infty, b)$. It follows that (a, b) would be a $100(1 - 2\alpha)\%$ 2-sided confidence interval for Δ. A point estimator for Δ may be obtained as $\hat{\Delta}$ such that $\hat{\Delta}$ belongs to the intersection of all nonempty 2-sided confidence intervals for Δ. Tian et al. (2009) provided an application of rosiglitazone studies with all available data included but without artificial continuity correction. It was reported by Tian et al. (2009) that this method can be over conservative in some cases.

2.2   Parametric Meta-Analysis

One benefit of parametric meta-analyses is to include covariates on the individual subject (participant) level, whereas the non-parametric meta-analyses typically use the summary data at the study level, which could be only data that can be extracted from the literatures. The meta-analysis using individual participant data (IPD) is becoming an increasingly popular tool. Since Stewart and Tierney (2002), there is a tendency to consider the IPD meta-analysis as a 'gold standard' as it can improve the quality of the meta-analysis that can be done and produce more reliable results. There are two statistical approaches for conducting an IPD meta-analysis: one-stage and two-stage. The one-stage approach analyzes the IPD from all studies simultaneously, for example, in a hierarchical regression model with random effects. The two-stage approach derives aggregate data (such as effect estimates) in each study separately and then combines them in a traditional meta-analysis model. Many researchers have compared the one-stage and two-stage approaches. Recently Burke et al. (2017) pointed out that most differences arise because of different modelling assumptions, rather than the choice of one-stage or two-stage itself. However, individual participant data may not be always available for a meta-analysis.

   In this section, I review the three parametric meta-analysis models: random-effects regression model, random-effects beta-binomial model and random-effects Poisson model. Each of them can be reduced to the corresponding fixed-effects model by removing the random study effect. Due to the low event rates, some model parameters may not be identifiable. Therefore, these models may need to be implemented under the Bayesian framework. However, Stijnen et al. (2010) pointed out that Bayesian methods are not always suited for meta-analyses for rare events due to the fact that the study data could be easily dominated by the priors, which are even thought to be non-informative. This chapter only describes the frequentist version of the parametric meta-analyses. However, it should be noted that the advantages of the Bayesian models could be beyond to have the model parameters identified.

2.2.1   Random-Effects Regression Model

Logistic regression model is a natural way to analyze binary outcomes. Let Y_{im} denote the number of subjects with an event in the ith treatment of the mth study, N_{im} the number of subjects and π_{im} the event rate in the ith treatment of the mth study, then we have,

$$Y_{im} \sim \text{Binomial} \left(N_{im}, \pi_{im} \right), \tag{6a}$$

$$\log it \left(\pi_{im} \right) = \mu + \delta_m + X_{im}\beta, \tag{6b}$$

where μ is the intercept, $\delta_m \sim N(0, \sigma^2)$ is the random study effect, X_{im} is the covariate metrics and β is the effect of the covariates. This is a random-effects logistic regression model on the event rate with the logit link function to estimate the odds ratio. It is can be parameterized to estimate the risk ratio by using the log link function, and to estimate the risk difference by using the identity link function. When the random study effect δ_m is removed, the (6a) and (6b) are reduced to a fixed-effects model (e.g. a conventionally simple logistic regression), which assumes that the treatment effect is the same for all studies. A random-effects regression model can be implemented via the SAS GLIMMIX or NLMIXED procedure.

2.2.2 Random-Effects Beta-Binomial Model

Beta-binomial model assumes (1) the number of subjects with an event in the ith treatment of the mth study, Y_{im} follows a binomial distribution with the event rate π_{im}; and (2) π_{im} follows a beta distribution. Therefore, Y_{im} follows a beta-binomial distribution. This model and Poisson-gamma/Poisson-normal model (see Sect. 2.2.3) are typically implemented via a non-linear mixed-effect model, which is available in most commercial softwares such as SAS NLMIXED procedure. Kuss (2015) compared various meta-analysis models for rare events and concluded his recommendation of the beta-binominal model to estimate the odds ratio, the risk ratio or the risk difference, and he reported that this method is comparable or superior in terms of convergence, empirical power and empirical coverage.

2.2.3 Random-Effects Poisson Model

A Poisson model for meta-analyses to analyze rare events has been reported by many researchers. The recent work would be a Poisson-gamma model by Cai et al. (2010) and a Poisson-normal model by Böhning et al. (2015). The Poisson model considers that the number of subjects with an event in the ith treatment of the mth study, Y_{im} follows a Poisson distribution. Further the random study effect is assumed to follow a gamma distribution (so called Poisson-gamma model) or a normal distribution (so called Poisson-normal model). Advantages of the Poisson model include (a) zero-events studies are naturally addressed; (b) the varying exposure or follow-up time can be considered. The random-effects Poisson model can be implemented via the SAS NLMIXED procedure.

2.3 Parametric Bootstrap Resampling Meta-Analysis

Parametric meta-analyses are typically implemented via the maximum likelihood approach with interferences based on the large sample theory. In practice, some model assumptions may not hold for some studies included in the analyses and the data may not be large enough to apply the large sample theory, which possibly result in biased estimates and inappropriate standard errors (Van Den Noortgate and Onghena 2005). As computing intensity is not a major concern nowadays, there have been discussions for the use of resampling for meta-analyses. Resampling methods used for meta-analyses include bootstrap, Jacknife procedure and randomization test.

A comprehensive view of bootstrap in a general setting can be found from Carpenter and Bithell (2000). The use of bootstrap in meta-analyses has been suggested by many researchers. Per my knowledge, a recent methodological work was by Van Den Noortgate and Onghena (2005). Dong et al. (2016) presented an application with rare events in transplant studies to address implausible estimated event rates (e.g. negative lower limits of 95% confidence intervals of event rates) provided from SAS NLMIXED per delta method (see more details from Sect. 3.2).

When the parametric bootstrap is applied to meta-analyses, a parametric model is assumed known up to unknown parameters. For example, the random-effects logistic regression model given in (6a) and (6b) is assumed known for the parameter of interest—the event rates π_{im} with unknown parameters μ (intercept), β (effect vector for the covariates) and δ_m (random study effect). The bootstrap to construct confidence intervals for event rates can be carried out as follows:

(a) Estimate the model parameters and their distributions, e.g. based on the maximum likelihood method;
(b) Draw a random sample for the parameters based on their estimated distributions;
(c) Estimate event rate $\hat{\pi}_i$ ($i = 1, 2, \ldots$, for treatment regimens), as well as $\hat{d}(\pi_i, \pi_j)$, a function of π_i and π_j ($i \neq j$) of interest if applicable, e.g. $\hat{d}(\pi_i, \pi_j) = \hat{\pi}_i - \hat{\pi}_j$ for the event rate difference between the treatment regimens i and j.
(d) Obtain bootstrap samples by repeating (b) and (c) B times (e.g. B=100,000);
(e) Construct confidence intervals for π_i and $d(\pi_i, \pi_j)$ based on the B bootstrap samples.

3 Case Studies

3.1 A Rosiglitazone Meta-Analysis Study

Nissen and Wolski (2007) performed a meta-analysis comparing rosiglitazone (a drug for treating type 2 diabetes mellitus) with placebo or active comparators to assess the effect of rosiglitazone on cardiovascular outcomes of myocardial infarction (MI) and cardiovascular disease related death (CVD). They screened 116 phase II, III and IV clinical trials. Of these, 48 trials met the predefined inclusion criteria of having a randomized comparator group, a similar duration of treatment in all groups, and more than 24 weeks of drug exposure (see Appendix). Six of the 48 trials did not report any MI or CVD and therefore were not included in their analysis. Of the remaining 42 studies, 38 with at least one MI reported and 23 with at least one CVD reported were included in their MI and CVD analysis, respectively.

Nissen and Wolski analyzed the rosiglitazone studies with the Peto odds ratio and concluded that rosiglitazone was associated with a significant increase in the risk of MI (odds ratio: 1.43; 95% CI: 1.03, 1.98; p-value $= 0.03$) and with an increase in the risk of CVD that had borderline significance (odds ratio: 1.64; 95% CI: 0.98, 2.74; p-value $= 0.06$). This analysis was criticized by many researchers primarily due to the exclusion of the clinical studies that did not have an event reported. The immediate criticism was from Shuster et al. (2007) who argued that the rosiglitazone studies had differing doses, differing follow-up, differing control medications, differing eligibility, and differing concomitant medications, therefore, performed a random-effects analysis with zero-events studies included. Subsequently, a number of further re-analyses were conducted to assess rosiglitazone effect on MI and CVD. Table 2 presents the meta-analysis by Nissen and Wolski and some re-analyses by other researchers. The latter showed inconsistent results compared to what Nissen and Wolski reported. Shuster et al. (2007) revealed the opposite significant results (e.g. insignificant for MI, but significant for CVD). Cai et al. (2010) reported a slightly lower significant p-value for MI than Shuster et al. (2007) (p-value $= 0.087$ vs. 0.110). However the odds ratio estimated by Cai et al. (2010) was also slightly lower than that per Shuster et al. (2007) (odds ratio $= 1.33$ vs. 1.51 for MI). It should be noted that the inverse-variance weighted approach, the Mantel-Haenszel method and Tian et al. (2009) showed a very similar point estimate of the risk difference (0.18% $\sim 0.19\%$). However, the statistical significances are very different: a very significant risk difference (p-value $= 0.001$ and 0.009 for MI and VCD, respectively) vs. a moderately significant risk difference (e.g. p-value $= 0.034$ and 0.048) vs. very insignificant risk difference (e.g. p-value $= 0.27$ and 0.83).

Nissen and Wolski (2010) re-analyzed rosiglitazone studies with additional eight recent studies included (in total of 56 studies) and re-stated their findings made in 2007. Subsequently, there are some re-analyses of these updated rosiglitazone study data (e.g. Böhning et al. 2015).

3.2 A Transplant Extrapolation Study with Everolimus

Ballerstedt et al. (2015) and Dong et al. (2016) reported a pediatric investigational plan (PIP) to assess the efficacy and safety of everolimus combined with reduced exposure calcineurin inhibitors (CNIs) in the pediatric kidney and liver transplant indications. This PIP commitment consisted of one new study in each of two indications. However, the very slow enrollment made it impossible to recruit patients in a timely manner. Following the recent EMA concept paper on extrapolation (EMA 2013) and with consultations with EMA, an extrapolation methodology was developed to bridge adult and pediatric data via meta-analyses, which included 57 adult studies with a total of 19,720 patients and seven pediatric studies with a total of 652 children. In the two pediatric studies, zero events were observed.

Table 2 Rosiglitazone meta-analysis results

Method	Treatment effect measure	MI			CVD		
		Point estimate	95% confidence interval	p-value	Point estimate	95% confidence interval	p-value
Peto odds ratio—Nissen and Wolski (2007)[a]	Odds ratio	1.43	1.03, 1.98	0.03	1.64	0.98, 2.74	0.06
Logistic regression[a, d]	Odds ratio	1.43	1.03, 1.98	0.033	1.66	0.98, 2.84	0.062
Mantel-Haenszel[b, d]	Odds ratio	1.43	1.05, 1.93	0.022	1.70	1.04, 2.77	0.034
DerSimonian and Laird (1986)—Random effect model[d]	Odds ratio	1.29	0.94, 1.76	0.12			
Random effect approach (Shuster et al. 2007)	Risk ratio	1.51	0.91, 2.48	0.110	2.37	1.38, 4.07	0.002
Poisson random-effects model by Cai et al. (2010)	Risk ratio	1.33	0.96, 1.84	0.087			
Inverse-variance weighted approach[c, d]	Risk difference	0.18%	0.07%, 0.28%	0.001	0.13%	0.03%, 0.22%	0.009
Mantel-Haenszel[d]	Risk difference	0.19%	0.01%, 0.37%	0.034	0.11%	0.00%, 0.21%	0.048
Exact approach for fixed effect model by Tian et al. (2009)	Risk difference	0.183%	−0.08%, 0.38%	0.27	0.063%	−0.13%, 0.23%	0.83

[a] Zero-events studies were excluded
[b] No contributions from the double-zero-events studies
[c] Double-zero-events studies had to be excluded in order to perform the calculation
[d] Analyzed by Shuster et al. (2007), Tian et al. (2009) and/or Lane (2011)

The meta-analysis model used for this extrapolation study was a random-effects logistic regression model as described in (6a) and (6b). The efficacy analyses considered the primary composite endpoint of biopsy-proven acute rejection (BPAR), graft loss or death and its main component of BPAR because most of the studies were from literature without the composite endpoint reported. Due to the same reason, the two timepoints Month 12 (primary) and Month 6 were considered. The covariates included population (adult vs. children) and various immunosuppressant drugs. This model assumed that the drug effects in combination therapies were additive in the log-odds scale.

The model was implemented via the SAS PROC NLMIXED. For the estimated event rates and differences in event rates, the confidence intervals (CIs) initially obtained were based on the delta method directly from the SAS NLMIXED procedure. However these intervals were deemed unsatisfactory, since the coverages were poor and especially the CI limits were nonsensical (i.e. negative lower limits for event rates). Therefore, appropriate CIs were constructed via a parametric bootstrap approach (Dong et al. 2016) as described in Sect. 2.3. However, the parameters of interest here for this bootstrap resampling were the average composite efficacy failure rates at Month 12 of the treatment regimens used in the pediatric studies for adults and children populations $\hat{\pi}_{ip}$ ($i = 1, 2, \ldots$, for treatment regimens, and p = 1 for children vs. 0 for adults) and the event rate differences between the two populations $d(\pi_{i1}, \pi_{i0}) = \pi_{i1} - \pi_{i0}$.

4   Summary

There are methodological challenges to perform meta-analyses for rare events, particularly for the analyses with zero-events studies included. The conventional analyses like the inverse-variance weighted approach and the DerSimonian and Laird random-effects method mostly provide biased results, or even could not be mathematically calculated. Excluding zero-events studies is not a reasonable approach at all as these studies do provide information, thus should not be ignored. The Peto odds ratio performs well in terms of mean percentage error (but not the confidence interval width and mean square error) when the treatment effect is small and the sample sizes are similar between the two treatment groups; the Mantel-Haenszel method without a continuity correction performs better in other scenarios. The Mantel-Haenszel method for the odds ratio and the risk ratio and the Peto odds ratio ignore the double-zero-events studies unless continuity corrections are applied. However, the recent research does not suggest continuity corrections.

Parametric meta-analyses have an advantage to include covariates on the individual subject level into the analysis models. However, conventional parametric approaches deriving the variances of parameters of interest based on the large sample theory or delta method may result in unsatisfactory results. Specific models such as beta-binomial model and Poisson model should be considered. Bootstrap may provide a reasonable tool to construct confidence intervals for the parameters of interest.

Acknowledgements The author would like to thank the anonymous reviewers for their comments and suggestions, and editors for their editorial support.

Appendix: Data for the rosiglitazone meta-analysis study from Nissen and Wolski (2007)

	Rosiglitazone			Control		
Study	Number of subjects	Number of subjects with MI	Number of subject with CVD	Number of subjects	Number of subjects with MI	Number of subject with CVD
1	357	0	1	176	0	1
2	391	1	0	207	0	2
3	774	1	0	185	0	3
4	213	1	0	109	0	4
5	232	0	1	116	0	5
6	43	1	0	47	0	6
7	121	0	0	124	0	7
8	110	2	3	114	2	8
9	382	0	0	384	0	9
10	284	0	0	135	0	10
11	294	1	2	302	1	11
12	563	0	0	142	0	12
13	278	1	0	279	1	13
14	418	0	0	212	0	14
15	395	1	2	198	0	15
16	203	1	1	106	1	16
17	104	2	0	99	0	17
18	212	0	1	107	0	18
19	138	1	1	139	0	19
20	196	0	1	96	0	20
21	122	1	0	120	0	21
22	175	1	0	173	0	22
23	56	0	0	58	0	23
24	39	0	0	38	0	24
25	561	2	1	276	0	25
26	116	3	2	111	1	26
27	148	0	2	143	0	27
28	231	0	1	242	0	28
29	89	0	0	88	0	29
30	168	0	1	172	0	30
31	116	0	0	61	0	31
32	1172	0	1	377	0	32

(continued)

33	706	0	1	325	0	33
34	204	2	0	185	1	34
35	288	0	1	280	0	35
36	254	0	0	272	0	36
37	314	0	0	154	0	37
38	162	0	0	160	0	38
39	442	0	1	112	0	39
40	394	0	1	124	0	40
41	2635	9	12	2634	10	41
42	1456	41	2	2895	5	42
43	101	0	0	51	0	43
44	232	0	0	115	0	44
45	70	0	0	75	0	45
46	25	0	0	24	0	46
47	196	0	0	195	0	47
48	676	0	0	225	0	48

References

Agresti, A. (2002). *Categorical data analysis* (2nd ed.). New York: John Wiley & Sons.

Agresti, A. (2013). *Categorical data analysis* (3rd ed.). New York: John Wiley & Sons.

Agresti, A., & Hartzel, J. (2000). Strategies for comparing treatments on a binary response with multi-centre data. *Statistics in Medicine, 19*(8), 1115–1139.

Ballerstedt, S., Fisch, R., Dumortier, T., Dong, G., & Ng, J. *Supporting a pediatric investigational plan using extrapolation from adults.* 36th annual conference of the International Society for Clinical Biostatistics (ISCB). Utrecht, Netherlands, August 23–27, 2015. http://www.iscb2015.info/documenten/documents/presentations/C20.2.pdf

Bickel, P. J., Hammel, E. A., & O'Connell, J. W. (1975). Sex bias in graduate admissions: Data from Berkeley. *Science, 187*(4175), 398–404.

Böhning, D., Mylona, K., & Kimber, A. (2015). Meta-analysis of clinical trials with rare events. *Biometrical Journal, 57,* 633–648.

Bradburn, M. J., Deeks, J. J., Berlin, J. A., & Russell, L. A. (2007). Much ado about nothing: A comparison of the performance of meta-analytical methods with rare events. *Statistics in Medicine, 26*(1), 53–77.

Brockhaus, A. C., Bender, R., & Skipka, G. (2014). The Peto odds ratio viewed as a new effect measure. *Statistics in Medicine, 33*(28), 4861–4874.

Brockhaus, A. C., Grouven, U., & Bender, R. (2016). Performance of the Peto odds ratio compared to the usual odds ratio estimator in the case of rare events. *Biometrical Journal, 58,* 1428–1444.

Brown, L., Cai, T., & Dasgupta, A. (2001). Interval estimation for a binomial proportion. *Statistical Science, 16,* 101–103.

Burke, D. L., Ensor, J., & Riley, R. D. (2017). Meta-analysis using individual participant data: One-stage and two-stage approaches, and why they may differ. *Statistics in Medicine, 36*(5), 855–875.

Cai, T., Parast, L., & Ryan, L. (2010). Meta-analysis for rare events. *Statistics in Medicine, 29*(20), 2078–2089.

Carpenter, J., & Bithell, J. (2000). Bootstrap confidence intervals: when, which, what? A practical guide for medical statisticians. *Statistics in Medicine, 19*(9), 1141–1164.

Cochran, W. G. (1954). The combination of estimates from different experiments. *Biometrics, 10,* 101–129.

DerSimonian, R., & Laird, N. (1986). Meta-analysis in clinical trials. *Controlled Clinical Trials, 7,* 177–188.

Dmitrienko, A., Molenberghs, G., Chuang-Stein, C., & Offen, W. (2005). *Analysis of clinical trials using SAS® : A practical guide.* Cary: SAS Institute.

Dong, G., Ng, J., Ballerstedt, S., & Vandemeulebroecke, M. *Parametric bootstrap in meta-analyses to construct CIs for event rates and differences in event rate.* 25th Annual ICSA Applied Statistics Symposium, Atlanta, GA, June 12–15, 2016.

European Medicines Agency (EMA). *Concept paper on extrapolation of efficacy and safety in medicine development.* http://www.sftox.com/actualites/WC500142358.pdf. 19 March 2013.

Fleiss, J. L. (1993). *Statistical methods for rates and proportions* (2nd ed.). New York: Wiley.

Glass, G. V. (1976). Primary, secondary, and meta-analysis of research. *Educational Researcher, 5*(10), 3–8.

Greenland, S., & Robins, J. M. (1985). Estimation of common effect parameter from sparse follow up data. *Biometrics, 41,* 55–68.

Greenland, S., & Salvan, A. (1990). The statistical bias of meta-analysis. *Statistical Methods in Medical Research, 2,* 121–145.

Higgins, J. P. T., & Green, S. (Eds.). (2011). *Cochrane handbook for systematic reviews of interventions* version 5.1.0 [updated March 2011]. The Cochrane Collaboration. Available from www.handbook.cochrane.org

Hoaglin, D. C. (2016). Misunderstandings about Q and 'Cochran's Q test' in meta-analysis (with discussions). *Statistics in Medicine, 35*(4), 485–495.

Kuss, O. (2015). Statistical methods for meta-analyses including information from studies without any events add nothing to nothing and succeed nevertheless. *Statistics in Medicine, 34,* 1097–1116.

Lane, P. (2011). Meta-analysis of incidence of rare events. *Statistical Method in Medical Research, 22*(2), 117–132.

Mantel, N., & Haenszel, W. (1959). Statistical aspects of analysis of data from retrospective studies of disease. *Journal of the National Cancer Institute, 22,* 719–748.

Nissen, S., & Wolski, K. (2007). Effect of rosiglitazone on the risk of myocardial infarction and death from cardiovascular causes. *New England Journal of Medicine, 356*(24), 2457–2471.

Nissen, S., & Wolski, K. (2010). Rosiglitazone revisited: An updated meta-analysis of risk for myocardial infarction and cardiovascular mortality. *Archives of Internal Medicine, 170,* 1191–1201.

Peto, R., Pike, M. C., Armitage, P., Breslow, N. E., Cox, D. R., Mantel, N., et al. (1977). Design and analysis of randomized clinical trials requiring prolonged observation of each patient. II. Analysis and examples. *British Journal of Cancer, 35*(1), 1–39.

Plackett, R. L. (1958). Studies in the history of probability and statistics: vii. The principle of the arithmetic mean. *Biometrika, 45*(1–2), 133.

Pourhoseingholi, M. A., Baghestani, A. R., & Vahedi, M. (2012). How to control confounding effects by statistical analysis. *Gastroenterology and Hepatology from Bed to Bench, 5*(2, Spring), 79–83.

Robins, J. M., Breslow, N., & Greenland, S. (1986). Estimators of the Mantel-Haenszel variance consistent in both sparse data and large-strata limiting models. *Biometrics, 42,* 311–323.

Rücker, G., Schwarzer, G., Carpenter, J., & Olkin, I. (2009). Why add anything to nothing? The arcsine difference as a measure of treatment effect in meta-analysis with zero cells. *Statistics in Medicine, 28*(5), 721–738.

Shuster, J. J., Jones, L. S., & Salmon, D. A. (2007). Fixed vs random effects meta-analysis in rare event studies: The rosiglitazone link with myocardial infarction and cardiac death. *Statistics in Medicine, 26*(24), 4375–4385.

Shuster, J. J., & Walker, M. A. (2016). Low-event-rate meta-analyses of clinical trials: Implementing good practices. *Statistics in Medicine, 35*(14), 2467–2478.

Stewart, L. A., & Tierney, J. F. (2002). To IPD or not to IPD? Advantages and disadvantages of systematic reviews using individual patient data. *Evaluation & the Health Professions, 25*(1), 76–97.

Stijnen, T., Hamza, T. H., & Ozdemir, P. (2010). Random effects meta-analysis of event outcome in the framework of the generalized linear mixed in sparse data model with applications. *Statistics in Medicine, 29*(29), 3046–3067.

Sutton, A., Abrams, K., Jones, D., Sheldon, T., & Song, F. (2000). *Methods for meta-analysis in medical research*. West Sussex: Wiley.

Sweeting, M. J., Sutton, A. J., & Lambert, P. C. (2004). What to add to nothing? Use and avoidance of continuity corrections in meta-analysis of sparse data. *Statistics in Medicine, 23*(9), 1351–1375.

Tian, L., Cai, T., Pfeffer, M., Piankov, N., Cremieux, P.-Y., & Wei, L. J. (2009). Exact and efficient inference procedure for meta-analysis and its application to the analysis of independent 2×2 tables with all available data but without artificial continuity correction. *Biostatistics, 10*, 275–281.

Van Den Noortgate, W., & Onghena, P. (2005). Parametric and nonparametric bootstrap methods for meta-analysis. *Behavior Research Methods, 37*(1), 11–22.

Wikipedia contributors. *Simpson's paradox*. Wikipedia, The Free Encyclopedia. Available at: https://en.wikipedia.org/w/index.php?title=Simpson%27s_paradox&oldid=759399357. Accessed 15 October 2017.

Yusuf, S., Peto, R., Lewis, J., Collins, R., & Sleight, P. (1985). Beta blockade during and after myocardial infarction: An overview of the randomized trials. *Progress in Cardiovascular Diseases, 27*(5), 335–371.

New Challenges and Strategies in Robust Optimal Design for Multicategory Logit Modelling

Timothy E. O'Brien and Changwon Lim

1 Introduction

Binary logistic and multi-category logit (MCL) regression models are amongst the most popular techniques in applied research where a goal is to determine relationships between attributes and/or adjusting for covariates. As such, introductory statistics texts cover these methods, and many applications-focused students note their usefulness in basic statistical methods courses. Aside from choosing from probit-based or logit-based link functions, modelling in the logistic case is relatively straightforward. But the situation is complicated in the multi-category case since several reasonable rival models have been suggested to handle these data. In these MCL cases, the practitioner is thus faced with choosing one of these models over the others, and, more importantly, deciding which experimental design to use. As in all cases of modelling, it is desired that this design should then allow for efficient model-parameter estimation and provide for a test of goodness-of-fit of the chosen model.

Important background to quantal, logistic and multicategory modelling is given in McCullagh and Nelder (1989), Agresti (2007, 2013), and Dobson and Barnett (2008), and extensions and applications are provided in Finney (1978). Optimal design strategies are introduced and illustrated in Silvey (1980), O'Brien and Funk (2003) and Atkinson et al. (2007), and geometric and uniform designs are explored in O'Brien et al. (2009).

T.E. O'Brien (✉)
Department of Mathematics and Statistics and Institute of Environmental Sustainability, Loyola University of Chicago, Chicago, IL, USA
e-mail: tobrie1@luc.edu

C. Lim
Department of Applied Statistics, Chung Ang University, Seoul, South Korea
e-mail: changwon77@gmail.com

© Springer International Publishing AG 2017
D.-G. Chen et al. (eds.), *New Advances in Statistics and Data Science*,
ICSA Book Series in Statistics, https://doi.org/10.1007/978-3-319-69416-0_4

In the context of typical MCL modelling situations, in what follows we provide needed background and introduce and demonstrate the usefulness of model-robust near optimal designs, highlighting extensions that allow for geometric and uniform design strategies. Thus, these results provide practitioners with useful guidelines in situations where potentially several MCL models can be chosen for a given dataset. Note that although the illustrations provided in this paper concern only three-level outcomes with a single explanatory variable, the results have been applied to numerous illustrations involving several independent variables and as many as five outcome categories.

2 Quantal Dose-Response Modelling

For the binary logistic model, where the x variable corresponds to dose or concentration, it is common that the researcher wishes to select the k dose points to run the experiment. This dose selection as well as the number of replicates at each of these points is the experimental design problem addressed here in a larger context. For n_i experimental units receiving dose x_i, the logistic model holds that the number of "successes" y_i has a binomial distribution with success probability π_i; under the assumed logit link, we obtain the generalized linear model equation, $\log\left(\frac{\pi_i}{1-\pi_i}\right) = \alpha + \beta x_i$. Also, when this model function is reparameterized so that the ED_{50} parameter $\gamma = \frac{-\alpha}{\beta}$ is a model parameter—so that the right-hand side in this expression is $\beta(x - \gamma)$—the model then becomes generalized nonlinear model. Important references for generalized linear and nonlinear models include McCullagh and Nelder (1989), Agresti (2007, 2013), and Dobson and Barnett (2008).

In contrast with binary logistic situation—where experiments result in "successes" or "failures"—often the number of outcomes is three or more. Commonly-used models for these data include the adjacent category logit (ACL), baseline category logit (BCL), continuation ratio (CR), and proportional odds (PO). For example, in the case of $K = 3$ outcomes and single predictor x, the ACL model is given by the simultaneous equations

$$\begin{cases} (i)\ \log\left(\frac{\pi_1}{\pi_2}\right) = \alpha_1 + \beta_1 x \\ (ii)\ \log\left(\frac{\pi_2}{\pi_3}\right) = \alpha_2 + \beta_2 x \end{cases} \tag{1}$$

Denoting $ex_1 = e^{\alpha_1 + \beta_1 x}, ex_2 = e^{\alpha_2 + \beta_2 x}, den = 1 + ex_1 + (ex_1)(ex_2)$, this expression is equivalent to $\pi_1 = (ex_1)(ex_2)/den, \pi_2 = ex_2/den, \pi_3 = 1/den$. To obtain parameter estimates, confidence regions/intervals and experimental designs, these expressions can be substituted into the log-likelihood expression. The BCL model amends the left-hand sides of the expressions in (1) with $(i)\log(\pi_1/\pi_3)$ and $(ii)\log(\pi_2/\pi_3)$. It is therefore observed that the BCL model is equivalent to the ACL model through a simple reparameterization, and it is therefore subsumed by

Table 1 Multicategory logit models for $K = 3$ outcomes

Continuation ratio A (CRA) model	Un-proportional odds (UPO) logit model
$\begin{cases} (i) \log\left(\frac{\pi_1}{\pi_2}\right) = \alpha_1 + \beta_1 x \\ (ii) \log\left(\frac{\pi_1+\pi_2}{\pi_3}\right) = \alpha_2 + \beta_2 x \end{cases}$	$\begin{cases} (i) \log\left(\frac{\pi_1}{\pi_2+\pi_3}\right) = \alpha_1 + \beta_1 x \\ (ii) \log\left(\frac{\pi_1+\pi_2}{\pi_3}\right) = \alpha_2 + \beta_2 x \end{cases}$
Adjacent category logit (ACL) model	Continuation ratio B (CRB) model
$\begin{cases} (i) \log\left(\frac{\pi_1}{\pi_2}\right) = \alpha_1 + \beta_1 x \\ (ii) \log\left(\frac{\pi_2}{\pi_3}\right) = \alpha_2 + \beta_2 x \end{cases}$	$\begin{cases} (i) \log\left(\frac{\pi_1}{\pi_2+\pi_3}\right) = \alpha_1 + \beta_1 x \\ (ii) \log\left(\frac{\pi_2}{\pi_3}\right) = \alpha_2 + \beta_2 x \end{cases}$

results for the ACL model. Additional details regarding multicategory logit models are given below as well as in Agresti (2007, 2013).

In addition to the ACL model, a listing of useful multicategory logit models is given in Table 1. For $K = 3$ outcomes, each of these models entails two equations. These expressions are easily extended to $K > 3$ outcomes where each model would then contain $(K - 1)$ equations.

As specified in Table 1, in addition to the ACL model, commonly-used models include the two variants of the Continuation Ratio model (denoted CRA and CRB here) as well as the Proportional Odds (PO) model. The PO model is derived from the UPO model imposing the equal-slope restriction, viz., $\beta_1 = \beta_2(=\beta)$. In addition to noting similarities and differences in models, an important goal in listing these models here is to unify them under one umbrella in order to provide the researcher with near-optimal robust designs (see Sect. 5).

Example 1 Price et al. (1987) provides toxicity data involving pregnant mice in which the predictor variable is the concentration of a certain ether. The chosen concentration levels in the study were $x_i = 0, 62.5, 125, 250, 500$ mg/kg per day. With respective sample sizes of $n_i = 297, 242, 312, 299, 285$, the total sample size is $n = 1435$ mice. The response variable here encompassed the three levels relating to the status of the offspring: death, malformed, or normal. Among the model functions given in Table 1, the model with the highest log-likelihood value (and thus AIC) here is the CRB model, with maximum likelihood estimates: $\widehat{\alpha}_1 = -3.2479, \widehat{\beta}_1 = 0.0064, \widehat{\alpha}_2 = -5.7019, \widehat{\beta}_2 = 0.0174$. In terms of interpretation of these estimates, since equation (i) in the CRB model contrasts dead with alive offspring and equation (ii) contrasts malformed with normal offspring, these results are best interpreted in terms of odds ratios: as the concentration level increases by an additional 100 mg/kg/day, the odds of a dead pup (versus alive) increases by a multiplicative factor of $e^{100\widehat{\beta}_1} = 1.89$ and the odds of a malformed pup (versus normal) increases by a multiplicative factor of $e^{100\widehat{\beta}_2} = 5.68$.

We return to this illustration below to demonstrate ways to improve upon the chosen experimental design.

3   Confidence Regions and Intervals

As noted in Seber and Wild (1989), in the case of normal linear and nonlinear models involving the p-vector $\boldsymbol{\theta}$ of model parameters, $(1-\alpha)100\%$ Wald confidence regions for $\boldsymbol{\theta}$ are of the form: $\left\{ \boldsymbol{\theta} \in \Theta : \left(\boldsymbol{\theta} - \widehat{\boldsymbol{\theta}}\right)^T \widehat{\boldsymbol{V}}^T \widehat{\boldsymbol{V}} \left(\boldsymbol{\theta} - \widehat{\boldsymbol{\theta}}\right) \leq ps^2 F_\alpha \right\}$.
In this expression, $\widehat{\boldsymbol{\theta}}$ is the least-squares (i.e., maximum likelihood) estimate of $\boldsymbol{\theta}$, $\widehat{\boldsymbol{V}}$ is the $n \times p$ Jacobian matrix of first derivatives evaluated at $\widehat{\boldsymbol{\theta}}$, s^2 is the mean square error (estimator of σ^2), and F_α is a tabled F percentile with p and $n-p$ degrees of freedom with tail probability of α. The $(1-\alpha)100\%$ likelihood-based confidence region in this situation is $\left\{ \boldsymbol{\theta} \in \Theta : S(\boldsymbol{\theta}) - S\left(\widehat{\boldsymbol{\theta}}\right) \leq ps^2 F_\alpha \right\}$.
Here, $S(\boldsymbol{\theta}) = (\boldsymbol{y} - \boldsymbol{\eta}(x, \boldsymbol{\theta}))^T (\boldsymbol{y} - \boldsymbol{\eta}(x, \boldsymbol{\theta})) = \boldsymbol{\varepsilon}^T \boldsymbol{\varepsilon}$. These two regions will be nearly equivalent depending upon the degree to which the (vector) model function, $\boldsymbol{\eta}(x, \boldsymbol{\theta})$, is well-approximated by the planar expression, $\boldsymbol{\eta}\left(x, \widehat{\boldsymbol{\theta}}\right) + \widehat{\boldsymbol{V}}\left(\boldsymbol{\theta} - \widehat{\boldsymbol{\theta}}\right)$. In normal linear models, this result is exactly met, and only approximately so for normal nonlinear, generalized linear, and generalized nonlinear models.

In non-normal situations, such as those considered here, approximate $(1-\alpha)100\%$ likelihood-based confidence regions are of the form $\left\{ \boldsymbol{\theta} \in \Theta : 2\left[LL(\boldsymbol{\theta}) - LL\left(\widehat{\boldsymbol{\theta}}\right) \right] \leq \chi_\alpha^2 \right\}$, where $LL(\boldsymbol{\theta})$ is the model log-likelihood and χ_α^2 is a tabled χ^2 percentile with p degrees of freedom and tail probability equal to α. Wald and likelihood confidence intervals can be obtained from these regions by conditioning or profiling; further details are given in Seber and Wild (1989) and Pawitan (2013). Notably, often the researcher wishes to choose an experimental design to reduce the length of the resulting confidence interval or the volume of the resulting confidence region.

4   Optimal Design Theory

An n-point design, denoted ξ, is written

$$\xi = \left\{ \begin{matrix} x_1 & x_2 & \ldots & x_n \\ \omega_1 & \omega_2 & \ldots & \omega_n \end{matrix} \right\} \tag{2}$$

The ω_i are non-negative design weights which sum to one, and the x_i are design points (or vectors) that belong to the design space, and which are not necessarily distinct. For the constant-variance normal setting with linear or nonlinear normal model function $\eta(x, \boldsymbol{\theta})$, the $n \times p$ Jacobian matrix is $V = \frac{\partial \eta}{\partial \theta}$. Denoting $\boldsymbol{\Omega} = \text{diag} \{\omega_1, \omega_2, \ldots, \omega_n\}$, the $p \times p$ (Fisher) information matrix is then written

$$M(\xi, \boldsymbol{\theta}) = V^T \boldsymbol{\Omega} V \tag{3}$$

In the more general case of either non-constant variance or non-normality, the corresponding information matrix is given by

$$M(\xi, \theta) = -E\left(\frac{\partial^2 LL}{\partial \theta \, \partial \theta^T}\right) \tag{4}$$

As underscored in Atkinson et al. (2007), the information matrix for the binary logistic model has the same form as in (3) with an appropriate modification of the weight matrix Ω. Since the (asymptotic) variance of $\widehat{\theta}_{MLE}$ is proportional to $M^{-1}(\xi, \theta)$, in many regression settings designs are often chosen to minimize some (convex) function of $M^{-1}(\xi, \theta)$. For example, designs which minimize its determinant are called D-optimal. As noted in Seber and Wild (1989), these designs minimize the volume of the confidence region given in the previous section. Since for nonlinear/logistic models, M depends upon θ, so-called local (or Bayesian) designs are typically obtained.

The (approximate) variance of the predicted response at the value x is

$$d(x, \xi, \theta) = \frac{\partial \eta(x, \theta)}{\partial \theta^T} M^{-1}(\xi) \frac{\partial \eta(x, \theta)}{\partial \theta} = tr\left\{M^{-1}(\xi) M(x)\right\} \tag{5}$$

Here, $M(x) = \frac{\partial \eta(x,\theta)}{\partial \theta} \frac{\partial \eta(x,\theta)}{\partial \theta^T}$ is the information matrix evaluated at the arbitrary value x; note that in contrasting with Eq. (4) where it is highlighted that for nonlinear models the information matrix depends upon the design and parameter values, occasionally one or both of these symbols are drop in what follows merely for typographic simplicity. Designs that minimize (over ξ) the maximum (over x) of $d(x, \xi, \theta)$ in (5) are called G-optimal. As stated above, since this predicted variance depends upon θ for logistic and nonlinear models, researchers often seek optimal designs either using a "best guess" for θ (called a local optimal design) or by assuming a plausible prior distribution on θ (called a Bayesian optimal design).

The General Equivalence Theorem (GET) of Kiefer and Wolfowitz (1960) establishes that D- and G-optimal designs are equivalent. This theorem also demonstrates that the variance function (5) evaluated using the D–/G-optimal design does not exceed the line $y = p$ (where p is the number of model function parameters)—but that it will exceed this line for all other designs. A corollary of the GET establishes that the maximum of the variance function is achieved for the D–/G-optimal design at the support points of this design. This result is very useful in demonstrating optimality of a given design, by substituting it into (5) and plotting the resulting variance function. Results and additional references for optimal design in binary logistic settings are given in Abdelbasit and Plackett (1983) and Minkin (1987), and in the general setting in Silvey (1980).

Example 1 Continued For the pregnant mice illustration and CRB model with the (MLE) parameter estimates given above and design points in the range [0, 2000], the local D-optimal design associates the respective weights $w = 0.4058, 0.3805, 0.2136$ with design support points (concentrations) $x = 222.59, 401.35, 767.91$. The

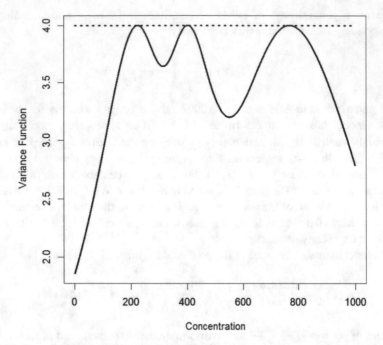

Fig. 1 Variance function for CRB model using D-optimal design—pregnant mice example

corresponding variance-function plot is shown in Fig. 1 along with the cut line, $y = 4$, since this model contains $p = 4$ parameters. D-optimality is established here by noting that the variance function does not exceed the cut-line.

Mindful that for the models considered here we are typically more interested in efficient estimation of only a subset of the model parameters, we partition the Fisher information matrix as

$$M = \begin{bmatrix} M_{11} & M_{12} \\ M_{21} & M_{22} \end{bmatrix} \qquad (6)$$

In this expression, each sub-matrix M_{ij} is of dimension $p_i \times p_j$ for $i, j = 1, 2$, and $p_1 + p_2 = p$. In the current situation, the parameter vector is similarly partitioned, $\theta = \begin{pmatrix} \theta_1 \\ \theta_2 \end{pmatrix}$ with θ_1 of dimension $p_1 \times 1$, θ_2 of dimension $p_2 \times 1$, and θ_1 is the parameter vector of interest and θ_2 are the nuisance parameters. Subset D-optimal designs for θ_2 in the joint model, as discussed in Atkinson et al. (2007), are obtained by maximizing

$$\left| M_{22} - M_{21} M_{11}^{-1} M_{12} \right| = \frac{|M|}{|M_{11}|} \qquad (7)$$

Noting problems associated with subset designs, O'Brien (2005) and Atkinson et al. (2007) instead combine the subset and full-parameter criteria and suggest that designs be chosen to maximize the objective function

$$\Phi_\phi\left(\xi, \boldsymbol{\theta}\right) = \frac{1 - \phi}{p_1}\log|\boldsymbol{M}_{11}| + \frac{\phi}{p_2}\log\left|\boldsymbol{M}_{22} - \boldsymbol{M}_{21}\boldsymbol{M}_{11}^{-1}\boldsymbol{M}_{12}\right| \qquad (8)$$

For ϕ chosen in the interval $\left[0, \frac{p_2}{p}\right]$, we call designs that maximize (8) D_ϕ-optimal. The resulting designs range from D-optimal designs for the $\boldsymbol{\theta}_1$ parameters in the smaller model containing only the $\boldsymbol{\theta}_1$ parameters for the choice $\phi = 0$ to D-optimal designs for the full $\boldsymbol{\theta}$ parameter vector in the larger model for the choice $\phi = \frac{p_2}{p}$. The corresponding variance function associated with (8) and an extension of the General Equivalence Theorem are then used to ensure D_ϕ-optimality of the resulting design by plotting the variance function, with the note that this normalized variance function has cut line $y = 1$ instead of $y = p$. To illustrate using the first example given in O'Brien (2005), the subset design for the two-parameter intermediate product model comprises only a single design support point and so is a singular design, whereas the D_ϕ-optimal design has two support points for ϕ in $\left(0, \frac{p_2}{p}\right]$.

A measure of the distance or discrepancy between an arbitrary design ξ_C and the D-optimal design ξ_D^* is the D-efficiency discussed in O'Brien and Funk (2003) and Atkinson et al. (2007), and given by the expression

$$\left(\frac{|\boldsymbol{M}\left(\xi_C\right)|}{|\boldsymbol{M}\left(\xi_D^*\right)|}\right)^{1/p} \qquad (9)$$

To illustrate, for an arbitrary design ξ_C with a D-efficiency of 66.7%, the researcher would need 50% more (1/0.667) experimental units to obtain the same information as the D-optimal design. Thus, in this setting, the same information would thus be achieved using the D-optimal design and only 120 experimental units as with the chosen (arbitrary) design using 180 experimental units.

The above advantage (i.e., optimality) notwithstanding, optimal designs can often only be used as a starting point in realistic situations since they often have some associated shortcomings. One important shortcoming is that often in practice, optimal designs for p-parameter model functions comprise only p support points, and so they provide little or no ability to test for lack of fit of the assumed model. Indeed, for the pregnant mice example discussed above, although the model contains $p = 4$ model parameters, the D-optimal design contains only three support points, so this design gives little or no means to check model adequacy. Further, in spite of the important theoretical optimal design results given in Zocchi and Atkinson (1999), Fan and Chaloner (2001), and Perevozskaya et al. (2003) for the CRB, CRA and PO models respectively, these works do not directly deal with the model-robustness issues raised and addressed here.

Table 2 Local D-optimal designs for pregnant mice example

Continuation ratio A (CRA) model	Un-proportional odds (UPO) logit model
$\xi_{CRA}^* = \left\{ \begin{array}{ccc} 194.5 & 428.1 & 1682.0 \\ 0.3023 & 0.4531 & 0.2445 \end{array} \right\}$	$\xi_{UPO}^* = \left\{ \begin{array}{ccc} 0 & 353.2 & 678.2 \\ 0.3575 & 0.4066 & 0.2359 \end{array} \right\}$
Adjacent category logit (ACL) model	Continuation ratio B (CRB) model
$\xi_{AC}^* = \left\{ \begin{array}{ccc} 193.5 & 425.5 & 1554.8 \\ 0.3037 & 0.4527 & 0.2435 \end{array} \right\}$	$\xi_{CRB}^* = \left\{ \begin{array}{ccc} 222.6 & 401.3 & 767.9 \\ 0.4058 & 0.3805 & 0.2136 \end{array} \right\}$

Importantly, optimal designs can also vary substantially—including the ACL, CRA, CRB and UPO models considered here. To illustrate, for the pregnant mice example and the concentration-range [0, 2000] as used in Price et al. (1987), the local D-optimal designs are given in Table 2 (obtained using the respective best fitting model parameter estimates). Note that whereas one such optimal design includes a concentration level as low as 0 mg/kg (i.e., for the UPO model), the highest concentration in another design is almost 1700 mg/kg (i.e., for the CRA model). This underscores the fact that optimal designs for one model may be very inefficient for another model.

As noted above, the designs and design strategies considered to date have focused primarily on efficiently estimating parameters in the assumed model, and not focused on allowing for—or discriminating amongst—other MCL models. Since in general rival models exist, clearly designs should also highlight which model best fits the data. That is, researchers often desire near-optimal so-called "robust" designs which have extra support points that can then be used to test for model adequacy. We next give very useful means to obtain these robust near-optimal designs.

5   Near-Optimal Robust Design Strategies

The structure of the four multicategory logit models considered in Table 1 suggest the following model function, which we refer to as the generalized ordinal logit (GOL) model function:

$$\left\{ \begin{array}{l} (i)\ \log\left(\frac{\pi_1}{\pi_2+\theta_1\pi_3}\right) = \alpha_1 + \beta_1 x \\ (ii)\ \log\left(\frac{\theta_2\pi_1+\pi_2}{\pi_3}\right) = \alpha_2 + \beta_2 x \end{array} \right. \tag{10}$$

In this expression, θ_1 and θ_2 are additional (or "hyper") parameters introduced to connect the above models. The ACL, CRA, CRB, and UPO models result by choosing $(\theta_1, \theta_2) = (0, 0), (0, 1), (1, 0), (1, 1)$, respectively. As a result, for the GOL model, we impose the constraints $0 \le \theta_1 \le 1, 0 \le \theta_2 \le 1$; numerically this is achieved by imposing for example for $i = 1, 2, \theta_i = \frac{e^{\psi_i}}{1+e^{\psi_i}}$ so when ψ_i varies between $-\infty$ and ∞, (θ_1, θ_2) is bounded in the unit square. Estimation of the six model parameters (including the hyper-parameters) can easily be achieved using maximum likelihood estimation algorithms. Although none of the ACL, CRA, CRB, or UPO models are special cases of another, since each of these models is nested in the larger GOL model, differences between each of these models and the best-fitting GOL model can be evaluated using the asymptotic χ^2 test statistic (i.e., two times the change in log-likelihood) with associated 2 degrees of freedom. Further, subsets of this larger family can also be connected: an important such special case of the GOL model is the UPOCRB model, obtain for $\theta_1 = 1$. This latter model connects UPO and CRB models, and is demonstrated in the illustration below.

The key goal of our introducing the GOL model here is to facilitate our obtaining model-robust near-optimal designs. This is achieved by viewing the assumed model function chosen from one of the constituents (viz, ACL, CRA, CRB, and UPO) as an element of the GOL family and using the modified subset design procedure given in (8) to obtain D_ϕ-optimal designs. For example, if the ACL is the assume model function with given *a priori* parameter estimates for this ACL model, it is suggested to use design criterion (8) with $\boldsymbol{\theta}_2^T = (\theta_1, \theta_2) = (0, 0)$ and $\boldsymbol{\theta}_1^T = (\alpha_1, \beta_1, \alpha_2, \beta_2)$ fixed at the *a priori* parameter estimates. We choose the tuning parameter ϕ in (8) so that the D-efficiency given in (9) for the ACL model exceeds some lower bound such as 90%. We thereby obtain an efficient model-robust D_ϕ-optimal design. This is illustrated in the following example.

Example 1 Continued For the pregnant mice illustration, the best fitting model is the CRB model and second best fitting model is the UPO model. As highlighted in Table 2, the (local) optimal designs for these two models differ substantially, with one design containing a lowest concentration of 0 and the other containing a lower bound in excess of 200. Further, since the fit of these two models to these data is far superior to the other two models, we view the chosen CRB model as embedded in the UPOCRB model. As noted above, we envision the frequently-encountered situation in which the researcher has the CRB model in mind (with *a priori* parameter estimates), and desires a near-optimal design which satisfies the dual objectives of: (1) efficiently estimating the CRB model parameters, and (2) providing for some ability to test for lack-of-fit in the direction of the UPO model. Taking $\phi = 0.05$, the local D_ϕ-optimal design assigns the weights $w = 0.0856, 0.3635, 0.3572, 0.1937$ to the design points (concentrations) $x = 0, 230.5, 405.8, 760.9$. We underscore that the additional design support point reflects the multi-objective nature of this design. Indeed, D_ϕ-optimality of this design is established by noting that the corresponding variance function, plotted in Fig. 2, lies below the cut line $y = 1$. The associated D-efficiency for this design for the CRB model is 95.3% and for the UPO model exceeds 80%, and so it is therefore quite efficient for both models. Certainly, if the researcher was concerned with departures from the assumed CRB model in the direction of the ACL and/or CRA models in addition to the UPO model, we would easily embed the CRB model in the larger GOL model and find the associated D_ϕ-optimal design.

The structure of the design chosen in Price et al. (1987), as well as several additional examples given in O'Brien et al. (2009), underscores the popularity of

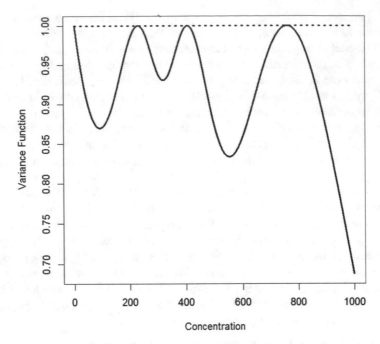

Fig. 2 Variance function for UPOCRB model using D_ϕ-optimal design—pregnant mice example

geometric and uniform designs in practical settings. Thus, we also examine here robust geometric designs of the form $x = a, ab, ab^2 \ldots ab^K$ for multicategory logit models, checking to see whether addition of the point $x = 0$ improves this geometric design. Here, K is specified by the researcher, and computer maximization algorithms are used to obtain optimal values of a and b as well as any associated information loss (as measured by the D-efficiency). We have also obtained optimal uniform designs of the form $A, A + B, A + 2B \ldots A + KB$, letting the final choice of the design structure (geometric or uniform) be the one with the higher D-efficiency or up to the researcher's discretion. So that the final design is robust to the assumed model function choice, we recommend obtaining local D_ϕ-optimal designs using the modified subset design procedure given in (8) and with ϕ chosen to yield a sufficiently-high final D-efficiency for the assumed sub-model.

Example 1 Continued For the pregnant mice illustration and now embedding the CRB model in the GOL model, we have noted somewhat higher D-efficiencies for geometric designs over uniform designs, so we highlight only geometric designs here. As such, we have sought designs which associate weights of the form $\omega^*, \frac{1-\omega^*}{4}, \frac{1-\omega^*}{4}, \frac{1-\omega^*}{4}, \frac{1-\omega^*}{4}$ respectively with support points $x = 0, a, ab, ab^2, ab^3$. Hence, robust geometric designs have been obtained here by optimizing over ω^*, a, b. Choosing $\phi = 0.10$ yields the optimal values $\omega^* = 0.054, a = 160.2, b = 1.65$, and produces a robust optimal design with D-efficiency (for the CRB model) of 90.6%. For the total sample size used by the authors ($n = 1435$), this design assigns $79, 339, 339, 339, 339$ mice to the respective concentrations $x = 0, 169.2, 264.2, 435.8, 718.9$. We emphasize that the original design used in Price et al. (1987) given above—with nearly uniform weights and geometric support points $x = 0, 62.5, 125, 250, 500$—has D-efficiency (for the CRB model) of only 62.8%. Therefore, with a D-efficiency in excess of 90%, the robust optimal geometric design strategy and design suggested here is strongly favored.

Some additional extensions—further demonstrating the breadth of our multiple-objective design strategy—are provided in the following illustration.

Example 2 Zocchi and Atkinson (1999) presents a dataset in which seven sets of 500 housefly pupae were exposed to one of seven doses of gamma radiation. The response variable for this study encompassed the three classes: death, opened but died before complete emergence, and complete emergence. The chosen radiation levels in the study were $x = 80, 100, 120, 140, 160, 180, 200$ Gy, and with equal replicates of $n_i = 500$ fly pupae per level, the total sample size was therefore $n = 3500$. Due to nonlinearities involved with these data, the authors suggest quadratic fits, and for the ACL, CRA, CRB and UPO models considered here, the best-fitting is the quadratic CRA model,

$$
\begin{cases}
(i)\ \log\left(\frac{\pi_1}{\pi_2}\right) = \alpha_1 + \beta_1 x + \gamma_1 x^2 \\
(ii)\ \log\left(\frac{\pi_1 + \pi_2}{\pi_3}\right) = \alpha_2 + \beta_2 x + \gamma_2 x^2
\end{cases}
\tag{11}
$$

We underscore that, with design points constrained to lie in the design space $[80, 200]$, the (local) D-optimal design for this model places equal weights at only three design points: $x = 80, 125.2, 163.6$. With only three support points, this design is thus of limited use to detect lack of fit of the assumed model. This model is easily embedded in the corresponding quadratic GOL model (which then contains eight parameters), and local D_ϕ-optimal designs using the modified subset design procedure given in (8) can then be easily obtained. Here, with $\phi = 0.25$, the local D_ϕ-optimal design associates the weights $w = 0.2423, 0.0456, 0.2272, 0.2454, 0.2395$ with the five design points $x = 80, 97.8, 116.1, 147.4, 182.1$. With a D-efficiency of 93.5%, this design represents only a minor information loss but a vast improvement in terms of additional design support points and thus the ability to test for model adequacy. To justify the claim of optimality, the corresponding scaled variance function is given in Fig. 3, and D_ϕ-optimality is established by noting that this function lies below the cut-line $y = 1$. Also, among designs of the form $A, A + B, A + 2B, \ldots, A + 6B$, using $\phi = 0.10$, the local D_ϕ-optimal uniform design has the support points, $x = 80, 96.6, 113.2, 129.8, 146.4, 163.0, 179.6$. Our final recommendation would be to allocate 500 fly pupae to each of these seven radiation levels. Whereas the original (uniform) seven-point design given in Zocchi and Atkinson (1999) has a D-efficiency (viz-a-viz the CRA model) of 84.1%, this proposed design increases the D-efficiency to 92.1%, and represents a modest improvement.

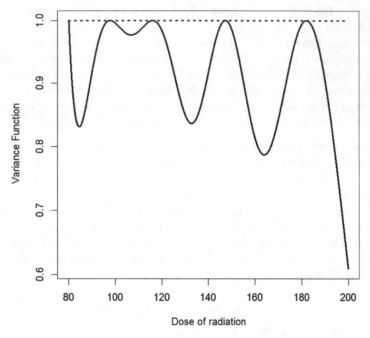

Fig. 3 Variance function for GOL model using D_ϕ-optimal design—house flies example

6 Discussion

In addition to linear and logistic regression models, researchers often find that multi-category logit models—including the adjacent category logit, baseline category logit, continuation ratio and proportional odds models considered here—are useful for modelling their data. The resulting parameter estimates then aid these researchers to make predictions or comparisons under different settings, for example using estimated odds ratios across strata. As such, practical experimental design methodologies are needed to gather the data to estimate these values and make needed predictions, and these researchers often consider using optimal designs.

But important theoretical optimal design results that are applicable only to the assumed model function are of only limited use to the practitioner. As noted, most optimal designs for models containing only p support points comprise no more than p support points, and this is certainly the case for the MCL models considered here. Underscoring this fact, Govaerts (1996) comments that this limitation prevents the use of optimal designs in most industrial settings. Therefore, the multiple-objective design strategies introduced and illustrated here for multi-category logit models—as well as in Hyun and Wong (2015) for normal nonlinear models—are paramount in applied research. Additionally, the extension of our GOL nesting strategy to incorporate geometric- and uniform-type designs gives practitioners clear suggestions as to how these designs in situations where they are desired. The suggested designs suggested here are indeed very "near" to the optimal designs in the sense that often the resulting D-efficiency is above 90%. As such, practitioners typically find that an information loss of less than 10% is relatively small compared to the practical nature of geometric and uniform robust designs and the resulting ability to assess model goodness-of-fit.

We conclude by pointing out that beyond the MCL models considered here— viz, the PO, UPO, ACL, CRA and CRB—authors such as Agresti (2010) and others have introduced yet more models for ordinal response data, and extensions of our methods provided here to these additional cases are now under study.

Acknowledgements The first author expresses his appreciation to the J. William Fulbright Foreign Scholarship Board for ongoing grant support and to Vietnam National University (Hanoi), Kathmandu University (Nepal) and Gadjah Mada University and Islamic University of Indonesia for kind hospitality and assistance during research visits.

References

Abdelbasit, K. M., & Plackett, R. L. (1983). Experimental design for binary data. *Journal of the American Statistical Association, 78*, 90–98.

Agresti, A. (2007). *An introduction to categorical data analysis* (2nd ed.). Hoboken, NJ: Wiley.

Agresti, A. (2010). *Analysis of ordinal categorical data* (2nd ed.). Hoboken, NJ: Wiley.

Agresti, A. (2013). *Categorical data analysis* (3rd ed.). Hoboken, NJ: Wiley.

Atkinson, A. C. (1972). Planning experiments to detect inadequate regression models. *Biometrika, 59*, 275–293.

Atkinson, A. C., Donev, A. N., & Tobias, R. D. (2007). *Optimum experimental designs, with SAS.* New York, NY: Oxford.

Dobson, A. J., & Barnett, A. G. (2008). *An introduction to generalized linear models* (3rd ed.). Boca Raton, FL: CRC Press.

Fan, S. K., & Chaloner, K. (2001). Optimal design for a continuation-ratio model. In A. C. Atkinson, P. Hackl, & W. G. Müller (Eds.), *MODA6 – Advances in model-oriented design and analysis* (pp. 77–85). Heidelberg: Physica-Verlag.

Finney, D. J. (1978). *Statistical method in biological assay* (3rd ed.). London: Griffin.

Govaerts, B. (1996). Discussion of the papers by Atkinson, and Bates et al. *Journal of the Royal Statistical Society: Series B, 58*, 95–111.

Hyun, S. W., & Wong, W. K. (2015). Multiple-objective optimal designs for studying the dose response function and interesting dose levels. *International Journal of Biostatistics, 11*, 253–271.

Kiefer, J., & Wolfowitz, J. (1960). The equivalence of two extremum problems. *Canadian Journal of Mathematics, 12*, 363–366.

McCullagh, P., & Nelder, J. A. (1989). *Generalized linear models* (2nd ed.). Boca Raton, FL: Chapman & Hall/CRC.

Minkin, S. (1987). Optimal designs for binary data. *Journal of the American Statistical Association, 82*, 1098–1103.

O'Brien, T. E. (2005). Designing for parameter subsets in Gaussian nonlinear regression models. *Journal of Data Science, 3*, 179–197.

O'Brien, T. E., Chooprateep, S., & Homkham, N. (2009). Efficient geometric and uniform design strategies for sigmoidal regression models. *South African Statistical Journal, 43*, 49–83.

O'Brien, T. E., & Funk, G. M. (2003). A gentle introduction to optimal design for regression models. *The American Statistician, 57*, 265–267.

Pawitan, Y. (2013). *All likelihood: Statistical modelling and inference using likelihood.* Oxford: Oxford University Press.

Perevozskaya, I., Rosenberger, W. F., & Haines, L. M. (2003). Optimal design for the proportional odds model. *The Canadian Journal of Statistics, 31*, 225–235.

Price, C. J., Kimmel, C. A., George, J. D., & Marr, M. C. (1987). The developmental toxicity of diethylene glycol dimethyl ether in mice. *Fundamental and Applied Toxicology, 8*, 115–126.

Seber, G. A. F., & Wild, C. J. (1989). *Nonlinear regression.* New York, NY: Wiley.

Silvey, S. D. (1980). *Optimal design.* London: Chapman & Hall.

Zocchi, S. S., & Atkinson, A. C. (1999). optimum experimental designs for multinomial logistic models. *Biometrics, 55*, 437–444.

Testing of Multivariate Spline Growth Model

Tapio Nummi, Jyrki Möttönen, and Martti T. Tuomisto

1 Introduction

Modeling of growth have been of special interest for statisticians over many decades. Many approaches have been proposed for the purpose depending on the research design as well as the assumptions imposed on the data. In our study we focus on methods likely to be especially useful in an experimental situation where more than one variable is measured at each measuring point which is the same for each individual. It is also common in these situations that some experimental groups are tested against each other. One of the most important statistical models for such data is the Growth Curve Model (GCM) of Potthoff and Roy (1964). The early development of this model was mainly based on an unstructured covariance matrix for random vectors (e.g. Khatri 1966 and Grizzle and Allen 1969) with multivariate analysis methods applied after some data transformation. Later developments also introduced some parsimonious models for the covariance matrix (see e.g. Azzalini 1987, Lee 1991 and Nummi 1997). The books by Kshirsagar and Smith (1955) and Pan and Fang (2002) provide comprehensive summaries of the main lines of development under GCM.

The methods introduced in the past have mainly been confined on one-response models. However, our focus is on the situation where more than one response

T. Nummi (✉)
Faculty of Natural Sciences, University of Tampere, FI-33014 Tampere, Finland
e-mail: tapio.nummi@uta.fi; tan@uta.fi

J. Möttönen
Department of Mathematics and Statistics, University of Helsinki, FI-00014 Helsinki, Finland
e-mail: jyrki.mottonen@helsinki.fi

M.T. Tuomisto
Faculty of Social Sciences (Psychology), University of Tampere, FI-33014 Tampere, Finland
e-mail: martti.tuomisto@uta.fi

© Springer International Publishing AG 2017
D.-G. Chen et al. (eds.), *New Advances in Statistics and Data Science*,
ICSA Book Series in Statistics, https://doi.org/10.1007/978-3-319-69416-0_5

variable are involved. Naturally, this also creates a special challenge for modeling the covariance within and between the variables studied. Another challenge is the actual modeling of growth or development that have often been based on the application of parametric linear models. Modeling of growth in this study is based on the use of cubic smoothing splines. For statistical inference with smoothing splines we can refer to Eubank and Spiegelman (1990), Schimek (2000), Cantoni and Hastie (2002), Liu and Wang (2004) and Nummi et al. (2011). The main focus of these studies has been on testing the order of the polynomial model against a spline alternative. However, in a growth modeling context the more important goal is to test whether the mean growth differs in some respect across treatment groups. This topic has been studied in the one-variable situation in Nummi and Koskela (2008) and Nummi and Mesue (2013). The aim of this study is to extend the approach presented in Nummi and Mesue (2013) to the multivariate situation with an application to cardiology testing data.

In Sect. 2 we introduce the basic spline growth model. In Sect. 3 a spline approximation is introduced and a test for mean curves developed. In Sect. 4 the model is extended to the multiple response situation. In Sect. 5 a computational example of multivariate modeling in behavioral cardiology is presented.

2 Modeling Growth with Smooth Functions

We begin by presenting the growth curve model of Potthoff and Roy (1964). This model can be written as

$$\mathbf{Y} = \mathbf{TBA}' + \mathbf{E}, \tag{1}$$

where $\mathbf{Y} = (\mathbf{y}_1, \mathbf{y}_2, \ldots, \mathbf{y}_n)$ is the $q \times n$ matrix of independent $q \times 1$ response vectors, $\mathbf{T}$ is a $q \times p$ within-individual design matrix, $\mathbf{A}$ is an $n \times m$ between-individual design matrix, $\mathbf{B}$ is an unknown $p \times m$ parameter matrix to be estimated and $\mathbf{E}$ is a $q \times n$ matrix of random errors. It is assumed that the columns $\mathbf{e}_1, \ldots, \mathbf{e}_n$ of $\mathbf{E}$ are independently normally distributed as $\mathbf{e}_i \sim N(\mathbf{0}, \boldsymbol{\Sigma})$, $i = 1, \ldots, n$.

In many practical situations, it may be difficult to find a parametric growth model that can be theoretically justified. Often low degree polynomial models are used to summarize the mean growth profiles. Our approach is to use cubic smoothing splines, which are very flexible curves with interesting mathematical properties (see e.g. Green and Silverman 1994). The Spline Growth Model (SGM) (see Nummi and Koskela 2008 and Nummi and Mesue 2013) can be written as

$$\mathbf{Y} = \mathbf{GA}' + \mathbf{E}, \tag{2}$$

where $\mathbf{G} = (\mathbf{g}_1, \ldots, \mathbf{g}_m)$ is the matrix of smooth mean growth curves at time points $t_1, t_2, \ldots, t_q$, where it is assumed that $\boldsymbol{\Sigma}$ follows a parsimonious covariance structure $\boldsymbol{\Sigma} = \sigma^2 \mathbf{R}(\boldsymbol{\theta})$ with covariance parameters $\boldsymbol{\theta}$. The growth curve model of (1) is now the special case $\mathbf{G} = \mathbf{TB}$. Note that our analysis is limited to the situation where measurement points are the same for each individual (complete and balanced data). One of the main advantages of this approach is that certain special covariance structures can be nicely incorporated into the analysis with hypothesis testing using F-test. Smoothing in more general context have been considered by Rice and Silverman (1991), Rice and Wu (2001) and Muller et al. (2005), for example.

The fitted curves can be obtained by minimizing the penalized least squares (PLS) criterion

$$Q = \mathrm{tr}[(\mathbf{Y} - \dot{\mathbf{G}})'\mathbf{H}(\mathbf{Y} - \dot{\mathbf{G}}) + \alpha\dot{\mathbf{G}}'\mathbf{K}\dot{\mathbf{G}}], \tag{3}$$

where we denote $\dot{\mathbf{G}} = \mathbf{GA}'$, $\mathbf{H} = \mathbf{R}^{-1}$ and $\mathbf{K}$ is the roughness matrix from roughness penalty $RP = \int g''^2$ and α is a fixed smoothing parameter. The roughness matrix is now

$$\mathbf{K} = \nabla\Delta^{-1}\nabla', \tag{4}$$

where the non-zero elements of banded $q \times (q-2)$ and $(q-2) \times (q-2)$ matrices ∇ and Δ are respectively

$$\nabla_{k,k} = \frac{1}{h_k}, \ \nabla_{k+1,k} = -\left(\frac{1}{h_k} + \frac{1}{h_{k+1}}\right), \ \nabla_{k+2,k} = \frac{1}{h_{k+1}} \tag{5}$$

and

$$\Delta_{k,k+1} = \Delta_{k+1,k} = \frac{h_{k+1}}{6}, \ \Delta_{k,k} = \frac{h_k + h_{k+1}}{3}, \tag{6}$$

where $h_j = t_{j+1} - t_j, j = 1,2,\ldots,(q-1)$ and $k = 1,2,\ldots,(q-2)$. It can be shown that minimizing Q for given α and $\mathbf{H}$ yields the estimator (Nummi and Mesue 2013)

$$\tilde{\mathbf{G}} = (\mathbf{H} + \alpha\mathbf{K})^{-1}\mathbf{HYA}(\mathbf{A}'\mathbf{A})^{-1}, \tag{7}$$

where the fitted growth curves $\tilde{\mathbf{G}}$ are natural cubic smoothing splines. In practical situations the precision matrix $\mathbf{H}$ may unfortunately not be known. However, if

$$\mathbf{KR} = \mathbf{K} \text{ or equivalently } \mathbf{K} = \mathbf{KH} \tag{8}$$

the spline estimator $\tilde{\mathbf{G}}$ simplifies as

$$\hat{\mathbf{G}} = (\mathbf{I}_q + \alpha\mathbf{K})^{-1}\mathbf{YA}(\mathbf{A}'\mathbf{A})^{-1} = \mathbf{SYA}(\mathbf{A}'\mathbf{A})^{-1}, \tag{9}$$

where the smoother matrix is $\mathbf{S} = (\mathbf{I}_q + \alpha\mathbf{K})^{-1}$. Note that for fixed α the fitted splines are simple linear functions of the observations. If we define $\mathbf{X} = (\mathbf{1}_q, \mathbf{x})$, where $\mathbf{x}$ is a vector of q measuring times, and since ∇' and $\mathbf{X}$ are orthogonal, it is easily seen that the well known structures $\mathbf{R} = \mathbf{I}_q + \sigma_d^2 \mathbf{1}_q \mathbf{1}_q'$, $\mathbf{R} = \mathbf{I}_q + \sigma_{d'}^2 \mathbf{X} \mathbf{X}'$ and $\mathbf{R} = \mathbf{I}_q + \mathbf{X} \mathbf{D} \mathbf{X}'$ meet the condition (8). The Generalized Cross-Validation criteria for choosing the smoothing parameter α can be written as

$$GCV(\alpha) = \frac{\frac{1}{nq} \sum_{i=1}^{n} \sum_{j=1}^{q} [y_{ij} - \hat{y}_{ij}]^2}{(1 - \frac{m \times edf}{nq})^2}, \tag{10}$$

where y_{ij} and $\hat{y}_{ij}$ are observed and smoothed values and $edf = \text{tr}(\mathbf{S})$.

3 Testing of Mean Curves

Testing is an essential part of the analysis of growth curves. This have often been based on some transformed version of the model (e.g. MANCOVA), with MANOVA testing statistics. These methods have been nicely summarized in Seber (1984), Timm (2002), Kollo and Rosen (2005), Kshirsagar and Smith (1955) and Pan and Fang (2002). Testing for multivariate growth curves with certain patterned covariance matrix for random errors is considered in Nummi and Mottonen (2000), for example.

Testing hypotheses with smoothing splines may not be as straightforward as it is with more classical linear models or in a multivariate analysis context. One possible alternative would be to use techniques developed for functional data analysis, see e.g. Ramsay and Silverman (2002). The functional data ANOVA method have been compared with some usual MANOVA tests in Cuesta and Febrero (2010). Here the proposed approach is based on spline approximation. Then more traditional testing methods (Azzalini 1987; Nummi and Mottonen 2000; Nummi and Koskela 2008; Nummi and Mesue 2013) are applied to approximated curves. The advantage is that in some important special cases the test statistic derived has an exact distribution.

3.1 Spline Approximation

The smoother matrix $\mathbf{S}$ is not a projection matrix and therefore certain results developed for linear models are not directly applicable here. Our approach is to approximate the spline fit in such a way that the smoother matrix utilized has the properties of a projection matrix. The smoother matrix can be written as e.g. Hastie (1996)

$$\mathbf{S} = \mathbf{M}(\mathbf{I}_q + \alpha \mathbf{\Lambda})^{-1} \mathbf{M}', \tag{11}$$

where $\mathbf{M}$ is the matrix of q orthogonal eigenvectors of $\mathbf{K}$ and $\mathbf{\Lambda}$ is a diagonal matrix of corresponding q eigenvalues. This shows that $\mathbf{K}$ and $\mathbf{S}$ share the same set of eigenvectors $\mathbf{m}_1, \mathbf{m}_2, \ldots, \mathbf{m}_q$ and the eigenvalues are connected such that the eigenvalues of $\mathbf{S}$ are $\gamma = 1/(1 + \alpha\lambda)$. Here we assume that eigenvectors $\mathbf{m}_1, \mathbf{m}_2, \ldots, \mathbf{m}_q$ are ordered according to the eigenvalues of $\mathbf{S}$. Note that the first two eigenvalues are always 1, and we can set $\mathbf{m}_1 = \mathbf{1}_q/\sqrt{q}$ and $\mathbf{m}_2 = \mathbf{t}_*$, where $\mathbf{t}_* = (\mathbf{t} - \bar{t}\mathbf{1}_q)/S_t$, $\bar{t} = \frac{1}{q}\sum_{i=1}^{q} t_i$ and $S_t = \sqrt{\sum_{i=1}^{q}(t_i - \bar{t})^2}$ are calculated from the time points $t_1, \ldots, t_q$. It is seen that the first two eigenvectors $\mathbf{m}_1$ and $\mathbf{m}_2$ span a straight line model and the sequence of eigenvectors appears to increase in complexity like a sequence of orthogonal polynomials (Ruppert et al. 2005). Therefore one reasonable approximation arises directly from the spline basis $\mathbf{m}_1, \mathbf{m}_2, \ldots, \mathbf{m}_q$ using c first eigenvectors. The smoother matrix $\mathbf{S}$ is substituted by $\mathbf{P}_* = \mathbf{M}_*\mathbf{M}'_*$, where $\mathbf{M}_* = (\mathbf{m}_1, \mathbf{m}_2, \ldots, \mathbf{m}_c)$. This approximation has several advantages. Firstly, $\mathbf{P}_*$ has the properties of a projection matrix, it is computationally very simple (can be obtained directly from $\mathbf{K}$) and provides a good approximation of the spline fit (Nummi et al. 2011). More detailed consideration of spline approximations can be found e.g. in Hastie (1996). The Generalized Cross-Validation criteria for choosing c can be written as

$$GCV(\alpha) = \frac{\frac{1}{nq}\sum_{i=1}^{n}\sum_{j=1}^{q}[y_{ij} - \bar{y}_{ij}]^2}{(1 - \frac{m \times c}{nq})^2}, \tag{12}$$

where fitted values $\bar{y}_{ij}$ are obtained from

$$\bar{\mathbf{Y}} = \mathbf{P}_*\mathbf{Y}\mathbf{P}, \tag{13}$$

where $\mathbf{P} = \mathbf{A}(\mathbf{A}'\mathbf{A})^{-1}\mathbf{A}'$.

3.2 Constructing a Test for Mean Spline Curves

As discussed in the previous section the set of fitted approximation curves can be obtained from

$$\bar{\mathbf{Y}} = \mathbf{P}_*\mathbf{Y}\mathbf{P} = \mathbf{M}_*\hat{\mathbf{\Omega}}\mathbf{A}', \tag{14}$$

where we denoted $\hat{\mathbf{\Omega}} = \mathbf{M}'_*\mathbf{Y}\mathbf{A}(\mathbf{A}'\mathbf{A})^{-1}$. These are just the fitted growth curves when spline basis $\mathbf{M}_*$ is taken as the within-individual model in the growth curve model (1). Therefore all the relevant information for testing mean profiles is in $\hat{\mathbf{\Omega}}$, which can now be considered to be an unbiased estimate of the parameters of the ordinary growth curve model $E(\mathbf{Y}) = \mathbf{M}_*\mathbf{\Omega}\mathbf{A}'$. Testing can be based on the linear hypothesis of the form

$$H_0 : \mathbf{C}\mathbf{\Omega}\mathbf{D} = \mathbf{0},$$

where $\mathbf{C}$ and $\mathbf{D}$ are known $v \times c$ and $m \times g$ matrices with ranks v and g respectively. It is shown in Nummi and Mesue (2013) that testing can based on

$$F = \frac{Q_*/vg}{\hat{\sigma}^2} \sim F[vg, n(q-c)], \tag{15}$$

where

$$Q_* = \mathrm{tr}\{[\mathbf{D}'(\mathbf{A}'\mathbf{A})^{-1}\mathbf{D}]^{-1}[\mathbf{C}\hat{\boldsymbol{\Omega}}\mathbf{D}]'[\mathbf{CM}'_*\mathbf{RM}_*\mathbf{C}']^{-1}[\mathbf{C}\hat{\boldsymbol{\Omega}}\mathbf{D}]\} \tag{16}$$

and

$$\hat{\sigma}^2 = \frac{1}{n(q-c)}\mathrm{tr}\{\mathbf{Y}'(\mathbf{I}_q - \mathbf{P}_*)\mathbf{Y}\} \tag{17}$$

In practical situations $\mathbf{R}$ contains unknown parameters that need to be estimated and therefore the distribution of the F-statistic is only approximate. However, if we are only interested in progression in time we can take $\mathbf{C} = [\mathbf{0}_{v \times (c-v)}, \mathbf{I}_v]$ (constant term dropped) and if we assume the uniform covariance model $\mathbf{R} = d^2 \mathbf{1}_q \mathbf{1}'_q + \mathbf{I}_q$, it can be shown that the distribution of the test statistics is exact. This is an important result since the uniform covariance model is quite common and a good approximation in many situations. In Nummi and Mesue (2013) other kinds of situations are discussed that yield an exact version of the F-test introduced here.

4   Multivariate Spline Growth Curve Model

In this section we generalize the spline growth model to a multivariate response case. The multivariate spline growth curve model is then written as

$$\mathbf{Y} = \mathbf{GA}', \tag{18}$$

where

$$\mathbf{Y} = (\mathbf{y}_1, \ldots, \mathbf{y}_n) = \begin{pmatrix} \mathbf{y}_{11} & \mathbf{y}_{21} & \cdots & \mathbf{y}_{n1} \\ \mathbf{y}_{12} & \mathbf{y}_{22} & \cdots & \mathbf{y}_{n2} \\ \vdots & \vdots & \ddots & \vdots \\ \mathbf{y}_{1s} & \mathbf{y}_{2s} & \cdots & \mathbf{y}_{ns} \end{pmatrix}$$

is a $qs \times n$ matrix of the vectors of measurements of s responses and

$$\mathbf{G} = (\mathbf{g}_1, \ldots, \mathbf{g}_m) = \begin{pmatrix} \mathbf{g}_{11} & \mathbf{g}_{21} & \cdots & \mathbf{g}_{m1} \\ \mathbf{g}_{12} & \mathbf{g}_{22} & \cdots & \mathbf{g}_{m2} \\ \vdots & \vdots & \ddots & \vdots \\ \mathbf{g}_{1s} & \mathbf{g}_{2s} & \cdots & \mathbf{g}_{ms} \end{pmatrix}$$

is the corresponding $qs \times m$ matrix of smooth mean curves. For the covariance matrix $\mathbf{R}$ we can take, for example, a multivariate version of the uniform structure

$$\mathbf{R} = (\mathbf{I}_s \otimes \mathbf{1}_q)\mathbf{D}(\mathbf{I}_s \otimes \mathbf{1}_q)' + \mathbf{I}_{qs}$$

$$= \begin{pmatrix} d_1^2 \mathbf{1}_q \mathbf{1}_q' + \mathbf{I}_q & d_{12} \mathbf{1}_q \mathbf{1}_q' & \cdots & d_{1s} \mathbf{1}_q \mathbf{1}_q' \\ d_{21} \mathbf{1}_q \mathbf{1}_q' & d_2^2 \mathbf{1}_q \mathbf{1}_q' + \mathbf{I}_q & \cdots & d_{2s} \mathbf{1}_q \mathbf{1}_q' \\ \vdots & \vdots & \ddots & \vdots \\ d_{s1} \mathbf{1}_q \mathbf{1}_q' & d_{s2} \mathbf{1}_q \mathbf{1}_q' & \cdots & d_s^2 \mathbf{1}_q \mathbf{1}_q' + \mathbf{I}_q \end{pmatrix}. \qquad (19)$$

If we now define the roughness part of the fitting criteria as

$$\mathbf{K}_s = \mathbf{W} \otimes \mathbf{K},$$

where $\mathbf{W} = \mathrm{diag}(\alpha_1, \ldots, \alpha_s)$ is a diagonal matrix of smoothing parameters $\alpha_1, \ldots, \alpha_s$ and $\mathbf{K}$ is the roughness matrix computed using the time points $t_1, \ldots, t_q$. Then the roughness matrix $\mathbf{K}_s$ meets the multivariate version of the condition (8)

$$\mathbf{R}\mathbf{K}_s = \mathbf{K}_s \qquad (20)$$

and the unweighted spline estimator becomes

$$\hat{\mathbf{G}} = (\mathbf{I}_{qs} + \mathbf{W} \otimes \mathbf{K})^{-1}\mathbf{Y}\mathbf{A}(\mathbf{A}'\mathbf{A})^{-1}$$

$$= \begin{pmatrix} \mathbf{S}(\alpha_1) & \mathbf{O} & \mathbf{O} & \ldots & \mathbf{O} \\ \mathbf{O} & \mathbf{S}(\alpha_2) & \mathbf{O} & \ldots & \mathbf{O} \\ \vdots & & \ddots & & \vdots \\ \mathbf{O} & \mathbf{O} & \mathbf{O} & \ldots & \mathbf{S}(\alpha_s) \end{pmatrix} \mathbf{Y}\mathbf{A}(\mathbf{A}'\mathbf{A})^{-1}, \qquad (21)$$

where $\mathbf{S}(\alpha_j) = (\mathbf{I}_q + \alpha_j \mathbf{K})^{-1}$, for $j = 1, \ldots, s$. If we use the approximation technique introduced earlier we get

$$\hat{\mathbf{G}} = \begin{pmatrix} \mathbf{M}_1\mathbf{M}_1' & \mathbf{O} & \mathbf{O} & \ldots & \mathbf{O} \\ \mathbf{O} & \mathbf{M}_2\mathbf{M}_2' & \mathbf{O} & \ldots & \mathbf{O} \\ \vdots & \vdots & \ddots & & \vdots \\ \mathbf{O} & \mathbf{O} & \mathbf{O} & \ldots & \mathbf{M}_s\mathbf{M}_s' \end{pmatrix} \mathbf{Y}\mathbf{A}(\mathbf{A}'\mathbf{A})^{-1}, \qquad (22)$$

where $\mathbf{M}_j\mathbf{M}_j' = \mathbf{P}_j$ is an approximation matrix for the jth variable. Note that the dimensions needed can be estimated using the generalized cross-validation criteria introduced in Sect. 2. A straightforward generalization of the earlier considerations gives us an estimator

$$\hat{\boldsymbol{\Omega}} = \mathbf{M}_\bullet'\mathbf{Y}\mathbf{A}(\mathbf{A}'\mathbf{A})^{-1}, \qquad (23)$$

where $\mathbf{M}_\bullet = \mathrm{diag}(\mathbf{M}_1, \mathbf{M}_2, \ldots, \mathbf{M}_s)$, of the multivariate growth curve model

$$\mathbf{Y} = \mathbf{M}_\bullet \mathbf{\Omega} \mathbf{A}'. \tag{24}$$

Testing can be based on the linear hypothesis

$$H_0 : \mathbf{C} \mathbf{\Omega} \mathbf{D} = \mathbf{0},$$

where $\mathbf{C}$ and $\mathbf{D}$ are known $v \times c$ and $m \times g$ matrices with ranks v and g, respectively, with

$$F = \frac{Q_*/vg}{\hat{\sigma}^2} \sim F[vg, n(sq - c_{tot})], \tag{25}$$

where $c_{tot} = c_1 + \cdots + c_s$ and

$$Q_* = \mathrm{tr}\left\{ [\mathbf{D}'(\mathbf{A}'\mathbf{A})^{-1}\mathbf{D}]^{-1} [\mathbf{C}\hat{\mathbf{\Omega}}\mathbf{D}]' [\mathbf{C}\mathbf{M}'_*\mathbf{R}\mathbf{M}_*\mathbf{C}']^{-1} [\mathbf{C}\hat{\mathbf{\Omega}}\mathbf{D}] \right\} \tag{26}$$

and

$$\hat{\sigma}^2 = \sum_{l=1}^{s} \frac{1}{n(q - c_l)} \mathrm{tr}\left\{ \mathbf{Y}'_l (\mathbf{I}_q - \mathbf{P}_l) \mathbf{Y}_l \right\}. \tag{27}$$

For an exact version of the F-test it remains to be shown that

$$\mathbf{C}\mathbf{M}'_\bullet \mathbf{R}\mathbf{M}_\bullet \mathbf{C}' = \mathbf{I}_v$$

for the proposed multivariate model. When investigating the progression in a multivariate situation we can take $\mathbf{C} = [\mathbf{I}_s \otimes (\mathbf{0}, \mathbf{I})]$. It is then easily verified that for a multivariate uniform covariance model (19) $\mathbf{C}\mathbf{M}'_\bullet \mathbf{R} = \mathbf{C}\mathbf{M}'_\bullet$ and therefore $\mathbf{C}\mathbf{M}'_\bullet \mathbf{R}\mathbf{M}_\bullet \mathbf{C}' = \mathbf{I}$.

5 Computational Example: Modeling in Behavioral Cardiology

The participants ($n = 95$) of the study were selected from a routine health check-up carried out on 14,215 out of 18,993 men invited through the City of Tampere primary health care in Finland. The participants were from three cohorts aged 35, 40, and 45 years. The inclusion criteria were: healthy on conventional health measures (except for elevated blood pressure) and not on medication. No participants with heavy tobacco or alcohol consumption were included in the study. Twenty-one per cent (2950) met the criteria. The volunteers did no heavy or dirty work on the test day and all fulfilled the following criteria: normal result in physical examination, hematological and biochemical screening tests, chest X-ray, and ECG. The data selected for this study are part of the Tampere Ambulatory Hypertension Study Tuomisto (1997). The variables considered here are systolic blood pressure (SBP), diastolic blood pressure (DBP), and heart rate (HR).

The participants were classified into normotensive (NT), borderline hypertensive (BHT), and hypertensive (HT) groups using World Health Organization (WHO) criteria (WHO, 1978), based on repeated casual blood pressure (BP) measurements in the seated position obtained over 2 months before the experiment. A detailed description of the diagnostic classification procedure is available in Tuomisto (1997). None of the participants took anti-hypertensive medication or any other drugs regularly at the time of the study. The groups, in addition to representing the same age, were similar for participant characteristics such as height, weight, BMI, alcohol consumption, and smoking. They were of the same ethnic, linguistic, and cultural background, and about 90% were of the same religion. However, the effects of possible covariates could also have been tested here by including them into the $\mathbf{A}$ matrix with appropriate choices for $\mathbf{C}$ and $\mathbf{D}$. The data were collected during the years 1987 through 1991. They consist of approximately 100,000 SBP, MAP, DBP, PP, and HR values per participant, respectively, and were reduced to 30 s means and from these means the set of measurements was reduced to means per hour. Figure 1 shows the measurements of the three variables SBP, DPB and HR at 20 different time points during 1 day starting from midnight.

To set up the spline growth model the between-individual design matrix $\mathbf{A}$ was defined as follows. For the normotensive participants (Group 1, $n_1 = 33$) the rows of $\mathbf{A}$ are $(1, 0)$ and for the borderline hypertensive and hypertensive participants (Group 2, $n_2 = 62$) the rows of $\mathbf{A}$ are $(0, 1)$. Using the generalized cross-validation criteria we got the smoothing parameters $\alpha_1 = 0.47$ (SBP), $\alpha_2 = 0.57$ (DPB) and $\alpha_3 = 0.18$ (HR). To use the approximation spline fits we need to determine the dimensions $c_1, \ldots, c_5$. The generalized cross-validation criteria gave the values $c_1 = 12$ (SBP), $c_2 = 10$ (DPB) and $c_3 = 12$ (HR). To test if the progression is the same in both groups we used the matrices $\mathbf{C} = \mathrm{diag}([\mathbf{0}, \mathbf{I}_{c_1-1}], [\mathbf{0}, \mathbf{I}_{c_2-1}], [\mathbf{0}, \mathbf{I}_{c_3-1}])$ and $\mathbf{D} = (1, -1)'$. Then the value of the F-test statistic is

$$F = \frac{1811.041/5}{66.26201} = 5.466301,$$

which gives the P-value $P(F_{52,470} \geq 5.466301) \approx 0$. Therefore the null hypothesis of equal progression of the response variables SBP, DPB and HR in two test groups is clearly rejected. It would also be interesting to further analyze how the response variables differ. For example, whether there is a special daytime or variable, which causes the difference. However, a more detailed further analysis remains a topic of future research.

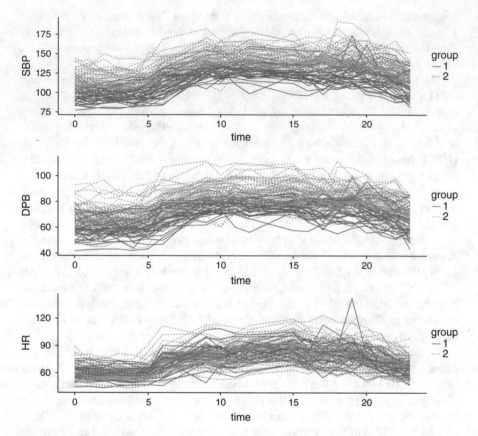

Fig. 1 The measurements of systolic blood pressure (SBP), diastolic blood pressure (DBP) and heart rate (HR) at 20 time points. The group 1 contains the normotensive participants and the group 2 contains the hypertensive participants

Acknowledgements We like to thank the referees for the comments that led to improvements of the manuscript.

References

Azzalini, A. (1987). Growth curves analysis for patterned covariance matrices. In M. L. Puri, J. P. Vilaplana, & W. Wertz (Eds.), *New perspectives in theoretical and applied statistics* (Chap. 3, pp. 63–73). New York, NY: Wiley.

Cantoni, E., & Hastie, T. A. (2002). Degrees-of-freedom tests for smoothing splines. *Biometrika, 89*, 251–263.

Cuesta-Albertos, J. A., & Febrero-Bande, M. (2010). A simple multiway ANOVA for functional data. *Test, 19*, 537–557.

Eubank, R. L., & Spiegelman, C. H. (1990). Testing the goodness of fit of a linear model via nonparametric regression techniques. *Journal of the American Statistical Association, 85,* 387–392.

Green, P. J., & Silverman, B. W. (1994). *Nonparametric regression and generalized linear models.* London: Chapman and Hall.

Grizzle, J. E., & Allen, D. M. (1969). Analysis of growth and dose response curves. *Biometrics, 25,* 357–381.

Hastie, T. (1996). Pseudosplines. *Journal of the Royal Statistical Society, Series B, 58,* 379–396.

Khatri, C. G. (1966) A note on a MANOVA model applied to problems in growth curves. *Annals of the Institute of Statistical Mathematics, 18,* 75–86,

Kollo, T., & von Rosen, D. (2005). *Advanced multivariate statistics with matrices.* Dordrecht: Springer.

Kshirsagar, A. M., & Smith, W. B. (1995). *Growth curves.* New York: Marcel Dekker.

Lee, J. C. (1991). Tests and model solution for general growth curve model. *Biometrics, 47,* 147–159.

Liu, A., & Wang, Y. (2004). Hypothesis testing in smoothing spline models. *Journal of Statistical Computation and Simulation, 74,* 581–597.

Nummi, T. (1997). Estimation in a random effects growth curve model. *Journal of Applied Statistics, 24,* 157–168.

Nummi, T., Jianxin, P., Siren, T., & Liu, K. (2011). Testing for cubic smoothing splines under dependent data. *Biometrics, 67,* 871–875.

Nummi, T., & Koskela, L. (2008). Analysis of growth curve data using cubic smoothing splines. *Journal of Applied Statistics, 35,* 681–691.

Nummi, T., & Mesue, N. (2013). Testing of growth curves with cubic smoothing splines. In R. Dasgupta (Ed.), *Advances in growth curve models. Springer proceedings in mathematics & statistics* (vol. 46, Chap. 3, pp. 49–59). New York, NY: Springer.

Nummi, T., & Möttönen, J. (2000). On the analysis of multivariate growth curves. *Metrika, 52,* 77–89.

Pan, J., & Fang, K. (2002). *Growth curve models.* Springer series in statistics. New York: Springer.

Potthoff, R. F., & Roy, S. N. (1964). A generalized multivariate analysis of variance model useful especially for growth curve problems. *Biometrika, 51,* 313–326.

Ramsay, J. O., & Silverman, B. W. (2002). *Functional data analysis,* 2nd ed. New York: Springer.

Rice, J. A., & Silverman, B. W. (1991). Estimating the mean and covariance structure nonparametrically when the data are curves. *Journal of the Royal Statistical Society, Series B, 53,* 233–243.

Rice, J. A., & Wu, C. O. (2001). Nonparametric mixed effects models for unequally sampled noisy curves. *Biometrics, 57,* 253–259.

Ruppert, D., Wand, M. P., & Carrol, R. J. (2005). *Semiparametric regression.* New York: Cambridge University Press.

Schimek, M. G. (2000). Estimation and inference in partially linear models with smoothing splines. *Journal of Statistical Planning and Inference, 91,* 525–540.

Seber, G. A. F. (1984). *Multivariate observations.* New York: Wiley.

Timm, N. H. (2002). *Applied multivariate analysis.* New York: Springer.

Tuomisto, M. T. (1997). Intra-arterial blood pressure and heart rate reactivity to behavioral stress in normotensive, borderline hypertensive, and mild hypertensive men. *Health Psychology, 16,* 554–565.

Yao, F. Y., Müller, H.-G., & Wang, J.-L. (2005). Functional linear regression analysis for longitudinal data. *The Annals of Statistics, 33,* 2873–2903.

Part II
Complex and Big Data Analysis

Uncertainty Quantification Using the Nearest Neighbor Gaussian Process

Hongxiang Shi, Emily L. Kang, Bledar A. Konomi, Kumar Vemaganti, and Sandeep Madireddy

1 Introduction

Uncertainty quantification plays a vital role in quantitative characterization and reduction of uncertainties in a given system, which has a wide range of applications in various of areas, e.g. engineering and computational experiments. Over the last decades, Gaussian process (GP) based approaches have steadily increased in popularity as prominent tools for data analysis in several fields, including uncertainty quantification. The first attempt of the statistics community to build a computer surrogate with Gaussian process models starts with the seminal papers of Currin et al. (1988) and Sacks et al. (1989) that modeled the computer experiment output as a Gaussian process and developed a comprehensive Bayesian inference for the distributions of the experiment output, based on data comprising observed outputs at a finite number of configurations of the experiment. In addition, Gaussian process models are used to develop surrogate models, called "emulators", to describe the output of experiments as well as computationally expensive simulations in uncertainty quantification (e.g. Craig et al. 2001; Kennedy and O'Hagan 2001; Gramacy and Lee 2008; Liu et al. 2009). These studies have shown that Gaussian process has the advantages to achieve parsimoniousness in the model and to result

H. Shi • E.L. Kang (✉) • B.A. Konomi
Department of Mathematical Sciences, University of Cincinnati, Cincinnati, OH, USA
e-mail: shihn@mail.uc.edu; kangel@ucmail.uc.edu; alex.konomi@uc.edu

K. Vegamanti
Department of Mechanical and Materials Engineering, University of Cincinnati, Cincinnati, OH, USA
e-mail: Kumar.Vemaganti@uc.edu

S. Madireddy
Argonne National Laboratory, Lemont, IL, USA
e-mail: smadireddy@mcs.anl.gov

© Springer International Publishing AG 2017
D.-G. Chen et al. (eds.), *New Advances in Statistics and Data Science*,
ICSA Book Series in Statistics, https://doi.org/10.1007/978-3-319-69416-0_6

in analytically tractable posterior distributions but also possesses the flexibility
to model many stochastic processes in practice. Generally, a Gaussian process
$\{Y(\mathbf{s}) : \mathbf{s} \in \mathscr{D} \subset \mathscr{R}^d\}$ is characterized by its mean function $\mu(\cdot)$ and its covariance
function $c(\cdot, \cdot)$. Usually, a stationary isotropic covariance function with unknown
parameter $\boldsymbol{\theta}$, $c(|| \cdot ||; \boldsymbol{\theta})$, is specified such that the covariance between two locations
$\mathbf{s}_1$ and $\mathbf{s}_2$ only depends on the distance $||\mathbf{s}_1 - \mathbf{s}_2||$, where $\mathbf{s}_1, \mathbf{s}_2 \in \mathscr{D}$. In uncertainty
quantification, the Euclidean distance is often used while other types of distances
can also be applied; for example, it is common to use the great circle distance when
the location coordinates are longitude and latitude.

When the size of data becomes large or massive, modeling with Gaussian process
incurs computational difficulties, which is often referred to as the "big n" problem
for Gaussian problem with n denoting the size of the data set. Classical ways
to make inference for Gaussian process, such as kriging, inevitably involves the
inversion of the $n \times n$ covariance matrix for the data of size n, which requires
$O(n^3)$ operations and $O(n^2)$ storage, thus becoming computationally infeasible for
large n. In recent years, various methods have been proposed to alleviate these
difficulties, including covariance tapering (Furrer et al. 2006), Gaussian predictive
process and its variants (Banerjee et al. 2008; Konomi et al. 2014), and fixed
rank kriging and filtering (Cressie and Johannesson 2008; Cressie et al. 2010).
Recently, Datta et al. (2016) proposed so-called Nearest Neighbor Gaussian Process
(NNGP) and have shown that NNGP possesses some very attractive properties:
NNGP is a valid non-degenerate stochastic process, and the associated computing
complexity is highly scalable for large datasets by introducing sparsity into the
precision matrices. Furthermore, NNGP can be easily adopted in a fully Bayesian
framework to coherently account for uncertainties from various levels including that
from the unknown parameter. Datta et al. (2016) illustrated the computational and
inferential benefits of NNGP when using it to approximate a Gaussian process with
an exponential covariance function and a geostatistical data set.

In this article, we build upon the previous work by Datta et al. (2016) to investigate the potential of NNGP in uncertainty quantification. In particular, we focus
on two important problems common in uncertainty quantification: (1) Smoother
covariance structure: Different from many studies in geostatistics, it is common in
uncertainty quantification to assume a Gaussian process with stronger smoothness,
that is, with the squared-exponential covariance function (Higdon et al. 2008; Qian
et al. 2008; Zhou et al. 2011; Arendt et al. 2012; Santner et al. 2013; Gramacy and
Apley 2015; Crevillen-Garcia et al. 2017). We will show empirically that NNGP
tends to underestimate the range parameter in the squared-exponential covariance
function. As discussed in Kaufman and Shaby (2013), misspecified/estimated range
parameter can be problematic for making predictions. Moreover, we discover that
Bayesian inference needs to be carried out carefully with NNGP. We develop an
algorithm for Bayesian inference that is computationally stable and efficient; (2)
Change-of-support: In physical/computer experiments, sometimes the outputs are
at relatively coarse resolution, due to configurations of the experiment equipment or
the computational cost of the numerical model (e.g. Berrocal et al. 2010; Zaytsev
et al. 2016). However, inference is often preferred at a finer resolution different from

that of data, which is called the "change-of-support" problem. Failure to properly handle this discrepancy of resolutions between data and desirable inference will lead to the so called "ecological fallacy": fallacious conclusions can be reached when inference of individual units is drawn from aggregated data (e.g., Cressie 1996; Nguyen et al. 2012). We will exploit NNGP to demonstrate the importance and benefits of using it when tackling the "change-of-support" problem.

The rest of this article is organized at follows: in Sect. 2, we describe the model of NNGP along with the details on Bayesian inference. Section 3 presents extensive simulation studies to illustrate the performance of NNGP in various scenarios, including different assumptions of the covariance function and assumption of whether or not the observations are aggregated. Section 4 uses the developed techniques to analyze a surface dataset and to make inference for important properties of surface micro-topography. A few concluding remarks are presented in Sect. 5.

2 Methods

In this section, we elaborate the statistical modeling of a latent stochastic process using Gaussian process, briefly describe the Nearest Neighbor Gaussian process (NNGP), and discuss how efficient and stable computational algorithms are developed for fully Bayesian inference.

2.1 Modeling with Gaussian Process

Let $Y(\cdot) \equiv \{Y(\mathbf{s}) : \mathbf{s} \in \mathscr{D}\}$ be the hidden stochastic process of interest over a domain $D \subset \mathscr{R}^d$, where $d \geq 1$ denotes the dimension of space. We assume $Y(\mathbf{s})$ is a Gaussian process with a mean function $\{\mu(\mathbf{s}) : \mathbf{s} \in \mathscr{D}\}$ and a covariance function $C(\mathbf{s}, \mathbf{s}')$. It is equivalent to write the following additive model for $\{Y(\mathbf{s})\}$:

$$Y(\mathbf{s}) = \mu(\mathbf{s}) + w(\mathbf{s}); \quad \mathbf{s} \in \mathscr{D}; \tag{1}$$

where $\{\mu(\cdot)\}$ is called the trend term in geostatistics, and it is modeled as a linear function with p covariates, $\mu(\mathbf{s}) = \mathbf{x}(\mathbf{s})'\boldsymbol{\beta}$ with an unknown p-dimensional vector of coefficients $\boldsymbol{\beta}$. The process $w(\mathbf{s})$ is assumed to be a Gaussian process with mean 0 and the covariance function $C(\mathbf{s}, \mathbf{s}')$ that is known up to a few parameters. To form a valid Gaussian process, the covariance function $C(\cdot, \cdot)$ needs to be symmetric and positive semi-definite (e.g., Cressie 1993). In practice, it is often assumed that the covariance function is isotropic. That is, the covariance function is a function only of the distance, $C(\|\mathbf{s}-\mathbf{s}'\|)$. In geostatistics, the Matérn class of covariance functions are often used: $C(d; \sigma^2, \zeta, \nu) = \frac{\sigma^2}{2^{\nu-1}\Gamma(\nu)} \left(\sqrt{2\nu}\frac{d}{\zeta}\right) K_\nu \left(\sqrt{2\nu}\frac{d}{\zeta}\right)$, where $d = \|\mathbf{s}-\mathbf{s}'\|$;

$\sigma^2 > 0$ is the variance parameter; $\Gamma(\cdot)$ is the gamma function; $K_\nu(\cdot)$ is the modified Bessel function of the second kind and of order ν; the parameter $\zeta > 0$ is called the range parameter, and the parameter $\nu > 0$, is called the smoothness parameter. The Matérn class includes the familiar exponential covariance function with $\nu = \frac{1}{2}$,

$$C(d; \sigma^2, \phi) = \sigma^2 exp\left[-\frac{d}{\phi}\right]. \tag{2}$$

As $\nu \to \infty$, its limit is the squared-exponential covariance function:

$$C(d; \sigma^2, \phi) = \sigma^2 exp\left[-\frac{d^2}{\phi^2}\right]. \tag{3}$$

The Matérn class covariance, especially the exponential covariance function has been widely used in geostatistics (Guttorp and Gneiting 2006). Also Stein (1999) points out that the squared-exponential covariance function ($\nu \to \infty$) is infinitely differentiable and thus is an infinitely smooth process. Although this may be unrealistic for applications in geostatistics, it is often desirable in modeling physical/computer experiment outputs, making the squared-exponential covariance function preferred in uncertainty quantification (e.g. Higdon et al. 2008; Qian et al. 2008; Zhou et al. 2011; Arendt et al. 2012; Santner et al. 2013; Gramacy and Apley 2015).

We assume that potential observations (outputs) have a component of measurement of error term:

$$Z(\mathbf{s}) = Y(\mathbf{s}) + \epsilon(\mathbf{s}); \ \mathbf{s} \in \mathscr{D},$$

where $\{\epsilon(\mathbf{s}) : \mathbf{s} \in \mathscr{D}\}$ is an independent Gaussian white noise that is independent of $Y(\cdot)$ and has mean 0 and $cov(\epsilon(\mathbf{s}), \epsilon(\mathbf{s}')) = \sigma_\epsilon^2 1(\mathbf{s} = \mathbf{s}') > 0$. Data are only observed at a finite set of locations or input configurations of the experiments, $\mathbf{s}_1, \ldots, \mathbf{s}_n$. With these n observations, we define the data vector $\mathbf{Z} = (Z(\mathbf{s}_1), \ldots, Z(\mathbf{s}_n))'$. It is straightforward to observe that

$$\mathbf{Z} \sim MVN(\mathbf{X}\boldsymbol{\beta}, \Sigma_\mathbf{Z}),$$

where $\mathbf{X}$ $MVN(a, \Sigma)$ denotes the multivariate normal distribution with mean $\mathbf{a}$ and covariance matrix Σ; is an $n \times p$ design matrix with its ith row to be $\mathbf{x}(\mathbf{s}_i)'$, and the variance-covariance matrix $\Sigma_\mathbf{Z} \equiv \mathbf{C}(\boldsymbol{\theta}) + \sigma_\epsilon^2 \mathbf{I}_n$ and the $n \times n$ matrix $\mathbf{C}(\boldsymbol{\theta})$ is induced by the latent process $Y(\cdot)$ with entries $C(\mathbf{s}_i, \mathbf{s}_j; \boldsymbol{\theta})$ for $i, j = 1$ to n, and $\boldsymbol{\theta}$ denotes the set of parameters in the covariance function.

To make fully Bayesian inference, we impose priors on the unknown parameters $\boldsymbol{\Omega} = (\boldsymbol{\beta}, \boldsymbol{\theta})$ and then obtain posterior inference usually using Markov chain Monte Carlo (MCMC) methods (Banerjee et al. 2014). However, when n is large, the MCMC algorithm will break down since it requires inverting an $n \times n$ matrix with computational complexity $O(n^3)$ and also requires memory for an $n \times n$ matrix, referred to as the "big n" problem. To alleviate such difficulties, Datta et al.

(2016) propose the Nearest Neighbor Gaussian process (NNGP) to approximate the original Gaussian process by considering the product of low-dimensional conditional densities. Below we briefly describe the NNGP in Datta et al. (2016) and then elaborate on how Bayesian inference can be made and provide guidance when the squared-exponential covariance function is utilized.

We consider a fixed finite collection of locations in $\mathscr{D}$ denoted by $S = \{\mathbf{u}_1, \mathbf{u}_2, \ldots, \mathbf{u}_k\}$, called the reference set. Now given an ordering of the locations, the joint density for $\mathbf{w}_S = (w(\mathbf{u}_1), w(\mathbf{u}_2), \ldots, w(\mathbf{u}_k))'$ can be written as $p(\mathbf{w}_S) = \prod_{i=1}^{k} p(w(\mathbf{u}_i)|\mathbf{w}_{<i})$, where $\mathbf{w}_{<i} = (w(\mathbf{u}_1), w(\mathbf{u}_2), \ldots, w(\mathbf{u}_{i-1}))$ for $2 \leq i \leq k$ and is empty for $i = 1$. To construct NNGP, instead of considering all elements in $\mathbf{w}_{<i}$, we only consider a subset corresponding to $N(\mathbf{u}_i) \subset \{\mathbf{u}_1, \ldots, \mathbf{u}_{i-1}\}$ for every $\mathbf{u}_i \in S$. The locations in $N(\mathbf{u}_i)$ are those close to $\mathbf{u}_i$ and are called neighbors of $\mathbf{u}_i$. Then we replace $\mathbf{w}_{<i}$ with $\mathbf{w}_{N(\mathbf{u}_i)}$ in the conditional densities to obtain the composite likelihood $\tilde{p}(\mathbf{w}_S) = \prod_{i=1}^{k} p(w(\mathbf{u}_i)|\mathbf{w}_{N(\mathbf{u}_i)})$. Datta et al. (2016) prove that $\tilde{p}(\mathbf{w}_S)$ is a valid joint density as long as the directed graph formed with vertices $\mathbf{u}_i$ and directed edges to $\mathbf{u}_i$ from all elements in $N(\mathbf{u}_i)$ is acyclic. The choice of $N(\mathbf{s}_i)$ based upon the "past" locations of $\mathbf{u}_i$, namely $\{\mathbf{u}_1, \mathbf{u}_2, \ldots, \mathbf{u}_{i-1}\}$ guarantees an acyclic specification for the graph. A natural assumption is to define $N(\mathbf{u}_i)$ as the set of m-nearest neighbors of $\mathbf{u}_i$. That is, $N(\mathbf{u}_i)$ is defined as:

$$
N(\mathbf{u}_i) = \begin{cases} \text{empty set,} & \text{for } i = 1 \\ \{\mathbf{u}_1, \mathbf{u}_2, \ldots, \mathbf{u}_{i-1}\}, & \text{for } 2 \leq i \leq m+1 \\ m \text{ nearest neighbors of } \mathbf{u}_i \text{ among } \{\mathbf{u}_1, \mathbf{u}_2, \ldots, \mathbf{u}_{i-1}\}, & \text{for } m+1 < i \leq k. \end{cases}
\tag{4}
$$

Let $\mathbf{C}_{N(\mathbf{u}_i)}$ be the covariance matrix of $\mathbf{w}_{N(\mathbf{u}_i)}$, for $i = 2, \ldots, k$. Thus, $\mathbf{C}_{N(\mathbf{u}_i)}$ is $(i-1) \times (i-1)$ when $2 \leq i \leq m$, and is $m \times m$ when $m+1 \leq i \leq k$. Similarly, denote the cross-covariance vector between $w(\mathbf{u}_i)$ and $\mathbf{w}_{N(\mathbf{u}_i)}$ by $\mathbf{C}_{\mathbf{u}_i, N(\mathbf{u}_i)}$ which is $1 \times (i-1)$ when $2 \leq i \leq m$, and is $1 \times m$ when $m+1 \leq i \leq k$. According to the properties of multivariate normal distribution, it is straightforward to show that $p(w(\mathbf{u}_i)|\mathbf{w}_{N(\mathbf{u}_i)}) = N(w(\mathbf{u}_i)|\mathbf{B}_{\mathbf{u}_i}\mathbf{w}_{N(\mathbf{u}_i)}, F_{\mathbf{u}_i})$, where

$$
\mathbf{B}_{\mathbf{u}_i} = \mathbf{C}_{\mathbf{u}_i, N(\mathbf{u}_i)}\mathbf{C}_{N(\mathbf{u}_i)}^{-1}, \text{ and } F_{\mathbf{u}_i} = C(\mathbf{u}_i, \mathbf{u}_i) - \mathbf{C}_{\mathbf{u}_i, N(\mathbf{u}_i)}\mathbf{C}_{N(\mathbf{u}_i)}^{-1}\mathbf{C}'_{\mathbf{u}_i, N(\mathbf{u}_i)}.
\tag{5}
$$

Then the composite likelihood $\tilde{p}(\mathbf{w}_S)$ is proportional to

$$
\exp\left(-\frac{1}{2} \sum_{i=1}^{k} \left(w(\mathbf{u}_i) - \mathbf{B}_{\mathbf{u}_i}\mathbf{w}_{N(\mathbf{u}_i)}\right)' F_{\mathbf{u}_i}^{-1} \left(w(\mathbf{u}_i) - \mathbf{B}_{\mathbf{u}_i}\mathbf{w}_{N(\mathbf{u}_i)}\right) \right).
\tag{6}
$$

If we write $w(\mathbf{u}_i) - \mathbf{B}_{\mathbf{u}_i}\mathbf{w}_{N(\mathbf{u}_i)} = (\mathbf{B}_{\mathbf{u}_i}^*)'\mathbf{w}_S$, where $\mathbf{B}_{\mathbf{u}_i}^*$ is a k-dimensional vector with $\mathbf{B}_{\mathbf{u}_i}^*[i] = 1$, $\mathbf{B}_{\mathbf{u}_i}^*[\text{index of } N_{(\mathbf{u}_i)} \text{ in } S] = -\mathbf{B}_{\mathbf{u}_i}$, and 0 elsewhere, then (6) is written as:

$$
\sum_{i=1}^{k} \mathbf{w}'_S (\mathbf{B}_{\mathbf{u}_i}^*)' F_{\mathbf{u}_i}^{-1} \mathbf{B}_{\mathbf{u}_i}^* \mathbf{w}_S = \mathbf{w}'_S \mathbf{B}'_S F_S^{-1} \mathbf{B}_S \mathbf{w}_S
\tag{7}
$$

where $\mathbf{F} = \mathrm{diag}(F_{\mathbf{u}_i}, F_{\mathbf{u}_2}, \ldots, F_{\mathbf{u}_k})$ and $\mathbf{B}_S = (\mathbf{B}_{\mathbf{u}_1}^*, \mathbf{B}_{\mathbf{u}_2}^*, \ldots, \mathbf{B}_{\mathbf{u}_k}^*)'$. Therefore, we can derive

$$\mathbf{w}_S \sim MVN(\mathbf{0}, \tilde{\mathbf{C}}_S) \tag{8}$$

where $\tilde{\mathbf{C}}_S = (\mathbf{B}_S' \mathbf{F}_S^{-1} \mathbf{B}_S)^{-1}$. It is easily seen that $\mathbf{B}_S$ has a sparse and low-triangle structure with its diagonal elements equal to 1. Datta et al. (2016) prove that for $m \ll k$, the $k \times k$ precision matrix $\tilde{\mathbf{C}}_S^{-1}$ is sparse with at most $km(m+1)/2$ non-zero entries, thus facilitating efficient computation.

We conclude this section with remarks on NNGP and the methods by Emery (2009) and Gramacy and Apley (2015). The latter two are designed to select an optimal set of locations and to use only the locations in this neighborhood for prediction. It is worth noting that their methods do not guarantee a valid NNGP model and hence prohibit the fully Bayesian inference of the covariance parameters, but they also provide computational advantages as NNGP for making predictions of the underlying process $Y(\cdot)$.

2.2 Bayesian Inference and Computational Considerations

As suggested by Datta et al. (2016), we choose the reference set S to match the set of all observation locations in $\mathscr{D}$. That is, $k = n$, and $S = \{\mathbf{s}_1, \ldots, \mathbf{s}_n\}$. In our study, we order the locations in the reference set according to their distance to the origin in order to reduce possible ties when sorting regular grid points. As illustrated by Datta et al. (2016), various ways of ordering locations in the reference set should have little impact on the performance of NNGP. Different from Datta et al. (2016), we now assume that data are only available at a coarser resolution while the underlying process $Y(\cdot)$ and its inference is at a finer or point-level resolution. This is of practical interest, since the outputs from computer experiments are often at relatively coarse resolution due to configurations of the experiment equipment or the computational cost of the numerical models (e.g. Berrocal et al. 2010; Zaytsev et al. 2016), although inference is preferred at a finer resolution.

We assume that we observe the data process $\{Z(\cdot)\}$ over l blocks:

$$Z(A_i) = \int_{\mathbf{s} \in \mathscr{D} \cap A_i} Z(\mathbf{s}) d\mathbf{s} / |A_i|, \quad i = 1, \ldots, l.$$

where $|A_i|$ denotes the area or volume of the block A_i. As in Cressie (1996) and Nguyen et al. (2012), we impose a lattice over the domain of interest $\mathscr{D}$ and assume that $\mathscr{D} = \cup\{U_i \subset \mathscr{R}^d : i = 1, \ldots, N_D\}$. That is, $\mathscr{D}$ is made up of N_D fine-scale, non-overlapping, basic areal units (BAUs) $\{U_i\}$ with their centroid locations denoted as $\{\mathbf{s}_i : i = 1, \ldots, N_D\}$. For example, the set of BAUs could be a set of tiling squares, and $\{\mathbf{s}_i\}$ is the set of the squares' centers. In practice, the resolution of this lattice $\cup\{U_i\}$ is chosen according to the finest resolution for which inference is desirable.

We model the observation over a block A as the average of the true surface $Y(\cdot)$ over the BAUs within that block plus measurement error:

$$Z(A_i) \equiv \frac{1}{|A_i|} \sum_{s \in A_i} Y(\mathbf{s}) + \epsilon(A_i), \qquad i = 1, \dots, l, \tag{9}$$

where $\epsilon(A_i)$ is also defined as the average of $\epsilon(\cdot)$ over the BAUs within the block A_i, and $|A_i|$ denotes the number of BAUs in A_i. Now define the data vector $\mathbf{Z} = (Z(A_1), Z(A_2), \dots, Z(A_l))'$. Without loss of generality, we assume that these l blocks cover a total of n BAUs, associated with $\{\mathbf{s}_1, \dots, \mathbf{s}_n\}$ with $n \leq N_D$. We then define $\mathbf{Y} = (Y(\mathbf{s}_1), Y(\mathbf{s}_2), \dots, Y(\mathbf{s}_n))'$ and an $l \times n$ aggregation matrix $\mathbf{A}$ such that:

$$\mathbf{Z} = \mathbf{AY} + \mathbf{A}\epsilon = \mathbf{AX}\boldsymbol{\beta} + \mathbf{Aw} + \mathbf{A}\epsilon \tag{10}$$

where the (ij)-th element in $\mathbf{A}$ is $A_{ij} = \frac{1(s_j \in A_i)}{|A_i|}$; $\mathbf{X}$ is the $n \times p$ design matrix for the trend; $\mathbf{w} \equiv (w(\mathbf{s}_1), \dots, w(\mathbf{s}_n))'$, and $\epsilon \sim \mathrm{MVN}(\mathbf{0}, \mathbf{D})$ with $\mathbf{D} = \sigma_\epsilon^2 \mathbf{I}_n$. We then utilize NNGP to specify the distribution of $\mathbf{w}$ and then write the model hierarchically as follows:

$$\mathbf{Z}|\mathbf{w}, \boldsymbol{\beta}, \sigma_\epsilon^2 \sim \mathrm{MVN}(\mathbf{AX}\boldsymbol{\beta} + \mathbf{Aw}, \mathbf{D}_A), \tag{11}$$

$$\mathbf{w}|\boldsymbol{\theta} \sim \mathrm{MVN}(\mathbf{0}, \tilde{\mathbf{C}})), \tag{12}$$

where $\mathbf{D}_A = \mathbf{ADA}'$ and $\tilde{\mathbf{C}}$ is defined in (8) and dependent on $\boldsymbol{\theta}$, the parameters in the covariance function.

In order to make inference, we write out the joint density:

$$p(\boldsymbol{\theta}) \times p(\sigma_\epsilon^2) \times p(\boldsymbol{\beta}) \times p(\mathbf{w}|\boldsymbol{\theta}) \times p(\mathbf{Z}|\mathbf{w}, \boldsymbol{\beta}, \sigma_\epsilon^2) \tag{13}$$

where we assume independence priors for parameters $\{\boldsymbol{\theta}, \sigma_\epsilon^2, \boldsymbol{\beta}\}$; $p(\delta_1)$ denotes the density function of a random variable δ_1 marginally and $p(\delta_1|\delta_2)$ denotes the conditional density function of a random variable δ_1 given δ_2. When implementing our method, we choose priors suggested in previous studies (e.g., Banerjee et al. 2014). For the range parameter ϕ, a uniform prior is assumed. For variance parameters σ^2 and σ_ϵ^2, inverse-Gamma priors are assumed. The full conditional of the unknown parameters as well as the random effects $\mathbf{w}$ can be easily derived analytically and MCMC methods such as the Gibbs sampling can be used to obtain posterior samples of the unknowns. We call this *MCMC Scheme 1*. This is the inference framework suggested in Datta et al. (2016) where interested readers can find more details of MCMC Scheme 1 including all full conditionals.

We now propose an alternative way for Bayesian inference, referred to as *MCMC Scheme* 2. Instead of sampling the random effects $\mathbf{w}$ in MCMC iterations, we integrate them out and obtain the following joint density:

$$p(\boldsymbol{\theta}) \times p(\tau^2) \times p(\boldsymbol{\beta}) \times p(\mathbf{Z}|\boldsymbol{\beta}, \boldsymbol{\theta}, \sigma_\epsilon^2) \tag{14}$$

where it is straightforward that $\mathbf{Z}|\boldsymbol{\beta}, \boldsymbol{\theta}, \sigma_\epsilon^2 \sim \text{MVN}(\mathbf{AX}\boldsymbol{\beta}, \mathbf{A\tilde{C}A'} + \mathbf{D}_A)$. Our motivation is that for a covariance with stronger smoothness such as the squared-exponential covariance function, the matrices $\{\mathbf{C}_{N(\mathbf{s}_i)} : i = 2, \ldots, n\}$ can be close to singular when the locations in $N(\mathbf{s}_i)$ are very close to each other, which makes calculation of $\{\mathbf{C}_{N(\mathbf{s}_i)} : i = 1, \ldots, n\}$ in MCMC iterations computationally unstable. With the random effects $\mathbf{w}$ integrated out, we now combine both $\mathbf{A\tilde{C}A'}$ and the covariance matrix $\mathbf{D}_A$, and the latter is a diagonal matrix and thus can be used as a perturbation term to overcome the potential numerical instability when inverting matrices. This is similar to resolving the numerical instability of kriging predictor by introducing the nugget (Peng and Wu 2004).

In MCMC Scheme 2, the Gibbs sampling proceeds by first updating $\boldsymbol{\beta}$ from its full conditional distribution, $\text{MVN}(\mathbf{V}_\beta^* \boldsymbol{\mu}_\beta^*, \mathbf{V}_\beta^*)$, where

$$\mathbf{V}_\beta^* = (\mathbf{V}_\beta + \mathbf{X}'(\mathbf{A\tilde{C}A'} + \mathbf{D}_A)^{-1}\mathbf{X})^{-1}, \text{ and } \boldsymbol{\mu}_\beta^* = \mathbf{V}_\beta^{-1}\boldsymbol{\mu}_\beta + \mathbf{X}'(\mathbf{A\tilde{C}A'} + \mathbf{D}_A)^{-1}\mathbf{Z}. \tag{15}$$

To invert the $l \times l$ matrix $(\mathbf{A\tilde{C}A} + \mathbf{D}_A)$, we apply the Sherman-Morrison-Woodbury formula:

$$(\mathbf{A\tilde{C}A'} + \mathbf{D}_A)^{-1} = \mathbf{D}_A^{-1} - \mathbf{D}_A^{-1}\mathbf{A}(\tilde{\mathbf{C}}^{-1} + \mathbf{A}'\mathbf{D}_A^{-1}\mathbf{A})^{-1}\mathbf{A}'\mathbf{D}_A^{-1}, \tag{16}$$

which can be calculated efficiently without requiring large memory, since $\tilde{\mathbf{C}}^{-1}$ and $\tilde{\mathbf{C}}^{-1} + \mathbf{A}'\mathbf{D}_A^{-1}\mathbf{A}$ are both sparse matrices and $\mathbf{D}_A$ is a diagonal matrix. Then the covariance parameters σ_ϵ^2 and $\boldsymbol{\theta}$ are updated jointly by using Metropolis-Hastings procedure with the following full conditional as the target density:

$$p(\sigma_\epsilon^2) \times p(\boldsymbol{\theta}) \times |\mathbf{A\tilde{C}A'} + \mathbf{D}_A|^{-1/2} \exp(-\frac{1}{2}(\mathbf{Z} - \mathbf{AX}\boldsymbol{\beta})'(\mathbf{A\tilde{C}A'} + \mathbf{D}_A)^{-1}(\mathbf{Z} - \mathbf{AX}\boldsymbol{\beta})) \tag{17}$$

which involved the determinant $|\mathbf{A\tilde{C}A'} + \mathbf{D}_A|$. Taking advantages of the sparse matrices involved in it, we use a variant of the Sherman-Morrison-Woodbury formula:

$$|\mathbf{A\tilde{C}A'} + \mathbf{D}_A| = \frac{|\tilde{\mathbf{C}}^{-1} + \mathbf{A}'\mathbf{D}_A\mathbf{A}|}{|\tilde{\mathbf{C}}^{-1}|} \times |\mathbf{D}_A|. \tag{18}$$

Notice that our MCMC Scheme 2 can also be used for unaggregated data. In this case, $\mathbf{Z}$ and $\mathbf{Y}$ are at the same resolution, and we have $l = n$. It is easily seen that then the matrix $\mathbf{A}$ will be the $n \times n$ identity matrix. In this case, the matrix $(\mathbf{A}\tilde{\mathbf{C}}\mathbf{A}' + \mathbf{D}_A)^{-1}$ becomes:

$$(\tilde{\mathbf{C}} + \sigma_\epsilon^2 \mathbf{I}_n)^{-1} = \sigma_\epsilon^{-2}\tilde{\mathbf{C}}^{-1}(\tilde{\mathbf{C}}^{-1} + \sigma_\epsilon^{-2}\mathbf{I}_n)^{-1}; \qquad (19)$$

and the determinant $|\tilde{\mathbf{C}}^{-1} + \mathbf{A}'\mathbf{D}_A\mathbf{A}|$ can be calculated as

$$|(\tilde{\mathbf{C}} + \sigma_\epsilon^2 \mathbf{I}_n)^{-1}| = \frac{|\sigma_\epsilon^{-2}\tilde{\mathbf{C}}^{-1}|}{|\tilde{\mathbf{C}}^{-1} + \sigma_\epsilon^{-2}\mathbf{I}_n|}. \qquad (20)$$

Note that although $\mathbf{w}$ is not sampled directly during the sampling procedure in MCMC Scheme 2, it can be easily recovered from $p(\mathbf{w}|\mathbf{Z}) = \int p(\boldsymbol{\theta}|\mathbf{Z})d\boldsymbol{\theta}$ via composition sampling using the posterior realization of $\boldsymbol{\theta}$ (Banerjee et al. 2014). Similarly, posterior samples of $Y(\cdot)$ at any unobserved location $\mathbf{s}$ can also be obtained.

As described above, in iterations from MCMC Scheme 2, we need to obtain the inverse and determinant of $l \times l$ sparse matrices which can be done by calculating the Cholesky factor of sparse matrices, which reduces the computations complexity from $O(l^3)$ to $O(l^{1.5})$ and the storage requirement from $O(l^2)$ to $O(l\log l)$ as noted in Rue and Held (2005). We show in Sect. 3 that the sparsity pattern of $\tilde{\mathbf{C}}_S^{-1}$ grants NNGP substantial computational benefits over the full Gaussian process. Moreover, NNGP only stores the $m \times m$ distance matrices between neighbors for every location rather than the entire $n \times n$ distance matrix.

3   Simulation Experiments

In this section, we demonstrate the performance and computational efficiency of NNGP using MCMC Schemes 1 and 2 under various scenarios in simulation studies. The computation is carried out in Matlab on a 4-core HP system with Intel Xeon x5650 CPU and 12 Gigabytes memory.

We simulate the latent process $Y(\mathbf{s})$ using the model in (1) at $70 \times 70 = 4900$ regularly spaced locations within a unit square $\mathscr{D} = [0, 1] \times [0, 1] \subset \mathscr{R}^2$. We assume a constant trend for $Y(\cdot)$, i.e, $\mu(\mathbf{s}) = \beta$ for any $\mathbf{s} \in \mathscr{D}$. We simulate $w(\mathbf{s})$ from a Gaussian process with mean 0 and the covariance function to be either the exponential covariance function in (2) or the squared-exponential covariance function in (3). The former is often used when analyzing geostatistical data in environmental sciences, while the latter is widely used in uncertainty quantification for physical and computer experiments. The true values of the parameters for the covariance functions are shown in Table 1. To generate the data $Z(\mathbf{s})$, we added a white noise term $\epsilon(\mathbf{s})$ to $Y(\mathbf{s})$ where $\epsilon(\mathbf{s})$ is generated from $N(0, \sigma_\epsilon^2)$ independently. To obtain the aggregated data at a coarse resolution, we use the 70×70 grids as the BAUs and to obtain $Z(A)$ we aggregate $Z(\mathbf{s})$ to a coarser resolution using (9)

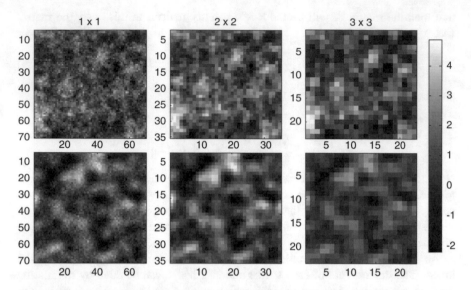

Fig. 1 Simulated data using the exponential covariance function (upper panels) and the squared-exponential covariance function (lower panels) at the BAU resolution of 70×70 (left panels), the coarse resolution of 35×35 (middle panels), and the coarser resolution of 23×23 (right panels)

with A contains four adjacent BAUs in 2×2 blocks. Thus, there are a total of $35 \times 35 = 1225$ blocks in the domain of interest. We also consider a coarser resolution with A contains nine adjacent BAUs in 3×3 blocks. For convenience, we remove the last column and the last row of the data at the original resolution to obtain the aggregated data which has a total of $23 \times 23 = 529$ blocks of size 3×3. We use $\mathbf{Z}_f$, $\mathbf{Z}_{c_1}$ and $\mathbf{Z}_{c_2}$ to denote the data vector at the fine resolution ($n = 4900$), the data vector at the coarse resolution ($l = 1225$), and the data at the coarser resolution ($l = 529$), respectively. Figure 1 presents simulated data at these three resolutions using the exponential covariance function (upper panels) and the squared-exponential covariance function (lower-panels).

We first use the data at the BAU resolution, $\mathbf{Z}_f$ to make Bayesian inference. We consider three methods, the full Gaussian process, NNGP with MCMC Scheme 1, and NNGP with MCMC Scheme 2, called Full GP, NNGP, and mNNGP, respectively. For all of the three methods, we give flat prior distribution for the intercept β_0, inverse-Gamma IG(2, 1) and IG(2, 0.1) prior for σ^2 and σ_ϵ^2, respectively, and a uniform prior $U(1/30, 1/3)$ for the range parameter ϕ, since $(1/30, 1/3)$ corresponds to the effective range between 0.1 to 1 domain distance units roughly. When implementing NNGP, we choose the set of observations as the reference set, and set $m = 10$ as suggested by Datta et al. (2016).

Parameter estimates and 95% credible intervals are shown in Table 1. With the exponential covariance function, all of three methods, Full GP, NNGP, and mNNGP, give very similar posterior inference of the parameters. The posterior median and 95% credible intervals are consistent with the true values. We also

Table 1 Summaries of inference with three methods, NNGP, mNNGP, and Full GP, using simulated data $\mathbf{Z}_f$

Parameter	True	NNGP	mNNGP	Full GP
Exponential				
β	1	1.23 (0.97, 1.53)	1.18 (0.94, 1.43)	1.20 (0.95, 1.45)
σ_ϵ^2	0.1	0.11 (0.09, 0.14)	0.11 (0.09, 0.13)	0.11 (0.08, 0.13)
σ^2	1	1.01 (0.85, 1.28)	0.98(0.83, 1.22)	0.97 (0.82, 1.21)
ϕ	0.06	0.061 (0.049,0.085)	0.058 (0.046, 0.078)	0.057 (0.046, 0.076)
Time	–	183.57	399.12	1843.75
Squared-exponential				
β	1	–	0.94 (0.81, 1.07)	0.88 (0.67, 1.11)
σ_ϵ^2	0.1	–	0.10 (0.10, 0.11)	0.10 (0.10, 0.11)
σ^2	1	–	1.06 (0.89, 1.28)	0.81 (0.65, 1.00)
ϕ	0.08	–	0.066 (0.063, 0.069)	0.078 (0.074, 0.081)

Posterior median of the parameters and a 95% creditable interval using 2.5th and 97.5th percentiles are presented. Computing time (in minutes) for running one chain of 25,000 iterations using data with the exponential covariance function is given

record the computing times (in minutes) of running an MCMC chain of 25,000 iterations for the Full GP, NNGP, and mNNGP. It demonstrates the enormous computational advantage of NNGP and mNNGP over Full GP, verifying that using NNGP facilitates efficient computation. NNGP requires the shortest computing time since it just requires inverting $m \times m$ matrices, while mNNGP requires inverting not only these $m \times m$ matrices to construct $\tilde{\mathbf{C}}$ but also sparse matrices as described in Sect. 2.2. With the squared-exponential covariance function, NNGP (MCMC Scheme 1, without integrating out $\mathbf{w}$) fails to produce any estimates as the covariance matrices of the neighbor set are very close to singular. Note that the squared-exponential covariance function produces smoother response surface compared to those covariance functions in the Matérn family (including the exponential function as a special case). In particular, for the squared-exponential covariance, the responses within small distance are highly correlated, and such correlation goes to zero slowly when the distance increases. Therefore, if the points in the reference set are closely spaced, the covariance matrices can be very close to singular, making the computation of NNGP unstable. Meanwhile, we notice that although mNNGP generates similar estimates for β and σ_ϵ^2 as Full GP does, it tends to underestimate the range parameter ϕ in particular, and the 95% credible interval does not include the true value of ϕ. This discrepancy between mNNGP and Full GP can also be explained by the stronger smoothness of the squared-exponential covariance function.

Although the non-marginalized NNGP requires even less computing time, it cannot guarantee stable computation, and thus we use mNNGP for the rest of our simulation and the real data analysis. We proceed to analyze the data at the coarse resolution $\mathbf{Z}_{c_1}$ and the data at the coarser resolution $\mathbf{Z}_{c_2}$. In order to demonstrate the importance of handling the "change-of-support" problem, we implement the model in (10) that takes into consideration the change-of-support, and denote the methods as $mNNGP_C$ and Full GP_C, corresponding to whether mNNGP or the full Gaussian process is used to model $w(\cdot)$, respectively. Meanwhile, we implement mGGNP and Full GP as in analyzing $\mathbf{Z}_f$, i.e., ignoring the fact that data $\mathbf{Z}_{c_1}$ and $\mathbf{Z}_{c_2}$ are from a coarser resolution. We call them $mNNGP_{NC}$ and Full GP_{NC}, respectively, where NC means not taking into account the change-of-support problem. The priors for unknown parameters are kept the same for all the methods. The results for $\mathbf{Z}_{c_1}$ and $\mathbf{Z}_{c_2}$ are summarized in Tables 2 and 3, correspondingly. With the

Table 2 Summaries of inference with four methods, $mNNGP_C$, Full GP_C, $mNNGP_{NC}$, Full GP_{NC}, using $\mathbf{Z}_{c_1}$ at the coarse resolution (2×2) with the exponential covariance function and the squared-exponential covariance function

		Handling "change-of-support"		Not handling "change-of-support"	
	True	$mNNGP_C$	Full GP_C	$mNNGP_{NC}$	Full GP_{NC}
Exponential					
β	1	1.16 (0.92, 1.40)	1.17 (0.94, 1.40)	1.12 (0.82, 1.66)	1.19 (0.85, 1.55)
τ^2	0.1	0.05 (0.02, 0.13)	0.06 (0.02, 0.14)	01 (0.01, 0.03)	0.02 (0.01, 0.03)
σ^2	1	1.00 (0.86, 1.28)	0.96 (0.82, 1.18)	0.94 (0.70, 1.46)	0.81 (0.62, 1.10)
ϕ	0.06	0.055 (0.044, 0.076)	0.052 (0.042, 0.069)	0.108 (0.079, 0.175)	0.090 (0.066, 0.128)
Squared-exponential					
β	1	0.98 (0.85, 1.12)	0.89 (0.67, 1.11)	0.89 (0.67, 1.11)	0.89 (0.67, 1.12)
τ^2	0.1	0.09 (0.08, 0.11)	0.10 (0.09, 0.11)	0.02 (0.02, 0.03)	0.03 (0.02, 0.03)
σ^2	1	1.04 (0.87, 1.24)	0.80 (0.64, 1.01)	0.93 (0.74, 1.18)	0.79 (0.64, 1.02)
ϕ	0.08	0.064 (0.061, 0.067)	0.078 (0.074, 0.082)	0.076 (0.072, 0.080)	0.080 (0.076, 0.084)

Posterior median of the parameters and a 95% creditable interval using 2.5th and 97.5th percentiles are presented

Table 3 Summaries of inference with four methods, $mNNGP_C$, Full GP_C, $mNNGP_{NC}$, Full GP_{NC}, using $\mathbf{Z}_{c_2}$ at the coarse resolution (3×3) with the exponential covariance function and the squared-exponential covariance function

		Handling "change-of-support"		Not handling "change-of-support"	
	True	$mNNGP_C$	Full GP_C	$mNNGP_{NC}$	Full GP_{NC}
Exponential					
β	1	1.16 (0.95, 1.37)	1.15 (0.93, 1.37)	1.17 (0.77, 1.60)	1.18 (0.81, 1.58)
τ^2	0.1	0.06 (0.02, 0.27)	0.06 (0.02, 0.30)	0.02 (0.01, 0.05)	0.02 (0.01, 0.05)
σ^2	1	0.95 (0.81, 1.17)	0.92 (0.77, 1.13)	0.70 (0.52, 1.15)	0.68 (0.50, 1.10)
ϕ	0.06	0.050 (0.039, 0.071)	0.049 (0.038, 0.067)	0.108 (0.075, 0.192)	0.103 (0.072, 0.180)
Squared-exponential					
β	1	0.90 (0.76, 1.04)	0.87 (0.64, 1.11)	0.97 (0.73, 1.21)	0.88 (0.64, 1.12)
τ^2	0.1	0.07 (0.04, 0.11)	0.09 (0.06, 0.13)	0.01 (0.01, 0.02)	0.01 (0.01, 0.02)
σ^2	1	1.35 (1.10, 1.68)	0.86 (0.68, 1.12)	0.78 (0.61, 1.07)	0.81 (0.64, 1.06)
ϕ	0.08	0.064 (0.060, 0.068)	0.079 (0.074, 0.084)	0.078 (0.074, 0.084)	0.083 (0.079, 0.088)

Posterior median of the parameters and a 95% creditable interval using 2.5th and 97.5th percentiles are presented

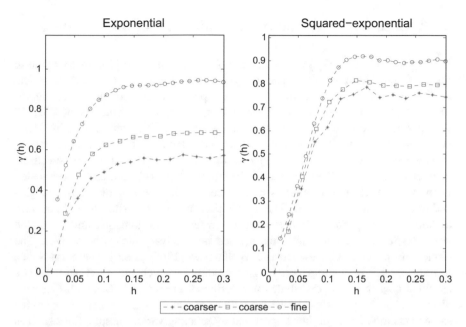

Fig. 2 Empirical semivariograms obtained using fine-resolution data $\mathbf{Z}_f$ (circle), coarse-resolution data $\mathbf{Z}_{c_1}$ (square), and coarser-resolution data $\mathbf{Z}_{c_2}$ (asterisk) from the exponential (left panel) and squared-exponential covariance function (right panel), respectively

exponential covariance function, failing to handle the change-of-support problem results in severe overestimation of the range parameter ϕ and underestimation of the measurement error variance σ_ϵ^2, no matter which model between Full and mNNGP is used. However, with the squared-exponential covariance function, the estimate for the range parameter ϕ from Full GP does not change much no matter whether or not the change-of-support problem is handled. To investigate the reason behind this situation, we plot the empirical semivariograms from $\mathbf{Z}_f$, $\mathbf{Z}_{c_1}$ and $\mathbf{Z}_{c_2}$ for both the exponential covariance function and the squared-exponential covariance function as shown in Fig. 2. It can be easily seen that the difference of the empirical semivariograms from the fine and the coarse resolutions is more substantial and obvious for the exponential covariance function compared to that for the squared-exponential covariance function. In fact, the empirical semivariograms from $\mathbf{Z}_f$, $\mathbf{Z}_{c_1}$ and $\mathbf{Z}_{c_2}$ with squared-exponential covariance are very close especially when the lag distance is small. As for the parameter σ_ϵ^2, Tables 2 and 3 show that even with the squared-exponential covariance function, it is still important to deal with the change-of-support; failing to do so will result in severely underestimated parameter. As expected, we have less confidence in the estimation of σ_ϵ^2 at a coarser resolution as the confidence interval becomes wider as the resolution becomes coarser.

4   Application: Uncertainty Quantification for Surface Data

In this section, we briefly present an example of applying the proposed method in
Sect. 2 to an Aluminum 6061 surface which is measured by non-contact optical
profilometry at a sampling interval of 6.67 μm. The measured surface micro-
topography of Al 6061 surface is shown in Fig. 3, which consists of 251,856
data points. Due to random nature of the contact surface, micro-asperity based
statistical models are extensively used to understand the role of surface microstructure on the contact phenomena such as friction, wear, thermal and electrical
contact conductance. The parameters for these statistical models are calculated
from two fundamental properties of surface: the distribution of surface heights
and their covariance functions. The distribution function describes how the surface
heights vary perpendicular to the surface whereas the autocorrelation function
describes the manner in which the surface heights vary along the surface. The
pioneering paper of Greenwood and Williamson (1966) is an important advance
in development of micro-asperity based models in which the rough surfaces are
assumed as a randomly distributed population of elastic asperities with Gaussian
distributed asperity heights., while the radii of curvature of all the asperities are the
same. This model was further improvised by relaxing various assumptions such as
constant mean curvature and elastic deformation (Bush et al. 1975; Tworzydlo et al.

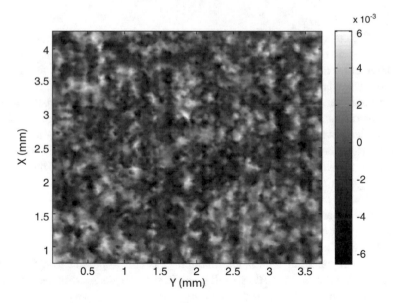

Fig. 3 Micro-topography of the Al 6061 surface

1988). Uncertainty quantification for contact surfaces involves understanding the properties of rough surfaces that are commonly reported including RMS roughness, mean slope and mean curvature. These quantities are generally calculated from the spectral moments of surfaces. Sista and Vemaganti (2014) recently propose the squared-exponential covariance function motivated by its insensitivity to smaller asperities that are registered at higher resolutions, and they have derived explicitly the formulas of the power spectral moments for the squared-exponential covariance function:

$$m_0 = \frac{\sigma^2 \phi}{2\sqrt{\pi}} \int_{-\infty}^{\infty} \exp(-\frac{k^2\phi^2}{4})dk = \sigma^2, \tag{21}$$

$$m_2 = \frac{\sigma^2 \phi}{2\sqrt{\pi}} \int_{-\infty}^{\infty} \exp(-\frac{k^2\phi^2}{4})(k^2)dk = \frac{2\sigma^2}{\phi^2}, \tag{22}$$

$$m_4 = \frac{\sigma^2 \phi}{2\sqrt{\pi}} \int_{-\infty}^{\infty} \exp(-\frac{k^2\phi^2}{4})(k^2)dk = \frac{2\sigma^2}{\phi^4} = \frac{12\sigma^2}{\phi^4}. \tag{23}$$

From above equations, we can see that the power spectral moments, m_0, m_2, and m_4 are functions of only the covariance parameters σ^2 and ϕ. This means that to obtain these important features of surfaces, we simply obtain inference of functions of parameters σ^2 and ϕ. Given the surface data, we thus model $\mathbf{Z}$ as described in Sect. 2.1 where the covariance function takes the form of the squared-exponential function as suggested by Sista and Vemaganti (2014). In addition, we assume a constant trend term and assign a flat prior. For covariance parameters, we impose inverse-Gamma prior IG(2,0.02) for σ^2 and the uniform prior for ϕ. Given the large size of data, the full Gaussian process cannot be implemented due to the "big n" problem. We first carry out a pilot study on a subset of data and find that both $m = 10$ and $m = 20$ give similar inference results (not presented). For more efficient computation, we thus decide to use the NNGP with $m = 10$ when analyzing the complete surface data. We integrate out the random effects $\mathbf{w}$ in MCMC to obtain fully Bayesian inference, and we obtain the posterior samples of the unknown parameters σ^2 and ϕ, based on which we generate posterior samples of these spectral moments m_0, m_2, and m_4, presented in Table 4 and Fig. 4.

Table 4 Posterior median and 5th and 95th percentiles for the spectral moments of the Aluminum 6061 surface described in Sect. 4

Parameter	Median	5th percentile	95th percentile
σ^2	2.1093(−6)	2.0139(−6)	2.2152(−6)
ϕ	0.4325(−1)	0.4269(−1)	0.4217(−1)
m_0	2.1093(−6)	2.0139(−6)	2.2152(−6)
m_2	2.3110(−3)	2.2136(−3)	2.4249(−3)
m_4	7.6077(0)	7.2446(0)	8.0252(0)

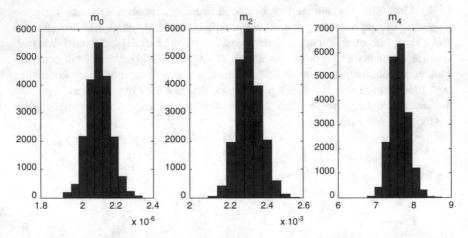

Fig. 4 Histograms of the posterior samples of the spectral moments, m_0 (left), m_2 (middle), and m_4 (right) for the Aluminum 6061 surface

5 Conclusions and Discussion

In this study, we investigate the performance of NNGP related to the squared-exponential covariance function, a commonly used function in uncertainty quantification and the capability of NNGP to handle the "change-of-support" problem with the exponential covariance function and the squared-exponential covariance function. Through the simulation studies, we find that with the exponential covariance function, NNGP performs consistently well; it can produce accurate parameter estimates and it can successfully handle the "change-of-support" problem. With the squared-exponential covariance function, we suggest an alternative MCMC framework that can overcome computational instability by integrating out the random effects. Meanwhile, we discover that NNGP tends to slightly underestimate the range parameter in the squared-exponential covariance function. Moreover, for the squared-exponential covariance function, we find through our simulation experiments that the change-of-support problem is not as severe as that with the exponential covariance function. That is, the parameter estimates obtained via handling the change-of-support problem do not differ much from those obtained without handling the problem, which may be due to the very strong smoothness of the squared-exponential covariance function. Although we focus on only the exponential and squared-exponential covariance functions, since the latter is the limit of the Maérn family with the smoothness parameter going to infinity, we expect our findings to be applicable for a Matérn covariance function with a very large smoothness parameter.

Our findings show that NNGP can be potentially used in uncertainty quantification when the physical/computer experiment outputs are of large or massive size, as illustrated by the real data example in Sect. 4. Meanwhile, there are still a few problems requiring further investigation. For example, in experiments with p input and q output variables, the outputs will be assumed to be a Gaussian process over $\mathscr{D} \subset \mathscr{R}^{p+q}$. When separability is assumed, NNGP can be implemented to each dimension, and tensor products of matrices can be utilized to achieve efficient computation. However, without separability, how to sort locations in such a ultra high-dimensional space and/or to define the so-called nearest neighbors is not obvious. For example, it is not desirable to choose the m nearest neighbors in each dimension, since it can result a total of m^{p+q} neighbors and inverting an $m^{p+q} \times m^{p+q}$ matrix can be computationally infeasible even when m, p and q are moderate.

Furthermore, NNGP can also be applied to analyze outputs from multiple experiment outputs and/or multiple field datasets. The model in Sect. 2.2 can be used as a building block to describe data resources at different resolutions, and thus provide a way to model outputs from different scales directly instead of treating the coarse ones (sometimes, also called the low-fidelity ones) as a regression covariate (e.g. Kennedy and O'Hagon 2000; Perditaris et al. 2015) Another direction is to extent the NNGP model to the context of multivariate analysis. Specifically, a valid cross-covariance function can be used to specify the dependence structure, not only within each output variable, but across these variables as well. A common way to guarantee the validity of a cross-covariance function is through linear models of coregionalization (LMC) where each component is represented as a linear combination of latent, independent univariate spatial processes (Goulard and Marc 1992; Wackernagel 2013). The multivariate Matérn covariance function proposed by Gneiting et al. (2010) can also be used alternatively to construct a valid cross-covariance function. These topics are currently under investigation.

Acknowledgements This work was supported in part by an allocation of computing time from the Ohio Supercomputer Center (OSC 1987). Shi's research was supported by the Taft Research Center at the University of Cincinnati. Kang's research was partially supported by the Simons Foundation's Collaboration Award (#317298) and the Taft Research Center at the University of Cincinnati. Vemaganti's work was partially supported by the University of Cincinnati Simulation Center.

References

Arendt, P. D., Apley, D. W., & Chen, W. (2012). Quantification of model uncertainty: Calibration, model discrepancy, and identifiability. *Journal of Mechanical Design, 134*, 100908-100908-12.

Banerjee, S., Carlin, B. P., & Gelfand, A. E. (2014). *Hierarchical modeling and analysis for spatial data*. Boca Raton: CRC Press.

Banerjee, S., Gelfand, A. E., Finley, A. O., & Sang, H. (2008). Gaussian predictive process models for large spatial data sets. *Journal of the Royal Statistical Society B, 70*, 825–848.

Berrocal, V. J., Gelfand, A. E., & Holland, D. M. (2010). A spatio-temporal downscaler for output from numerical models. *Journal of Agricultural, Biological, and Environmental Statistics, 15*, 176–197.

Bush, A., Gibson, R., & Thomas, T. (1975). The elastic contact of a rough surface. *Wear, 35*, 87–111.

Craig, P. S., Goldstein, M., Rougier, J. C., & Seheult, A. H. (2001). Bayesian forecasting for complex systems using computer simulators. *Journal of the American Statistical Association, 96*, 717–729.

Cressie, N. (1993). *Statistics for spatial data*, revised ed. New York: Wiley.

Cressie, N. (1996). Change of support and the modifiable areal unit problem. *Geographical Systems, 3*, 159–180.

Cressie, N., & Johannesson, G. (2008). Fixed rank kriging for very large spatial data sets. *Journal of the Royal Statistical Society: Series B (Statistical Methodology), 70*, 209–226.

Cressie, N., Shi, T., & Kang, E. K. (2010). Fixed rank filtering for spatio-temporal data. *Journal of Computational and Graphical Statistics, 19*, 724–745.

Crevillen-Garcia, D., Wilkinson, R. D., Shah, A. A., & Power, H. (2017). Gaussian process modelling for uncertainty quantification in convectively-enhanced dissolution processes in porous media. *Advances in Water Resources, 99*, 1–14.

Currin, C., Mitchell, T, Morris, M., & Ylvisaker, D. (1988). *A Bayesian approach to the design and analysis of computer experiments*. Technical Report, ORNL498, Oak Ridge Laboratory.

Datta, A., Banerjee, S., Finley, A. O., & Gelfand, A. E. (2016). Hierarchical nearest-neighbor Gaussian process models for large geostatistical datasets. *Journal of the American Statistical Association, 111*, 800–812.

Emery, X. (2009). The kriging update equations and their application to the selection of neighboring data. *Computational Geosciences, 13*, 269–280.

Furrer, R., Genton, M. G., & Nychka, D. (2006). Covariance tapering for interpolation of large spatial datasets. *Journal of Computational and Graphical Statistics, 15*, 502–523.

Gneiting, T., Kleiber, W., & Schlather, M. (2010). Matérn cross-covariance functions for multivariate random fields. *Journal of the American Statistical Association, 105*, 1167–1177.

Goulard, M., & Voltz, M. (1992). Linear coregionalization model: Tools for estimation and choice of cross-variogram matrix. *Mathematical Geology, 24*, 269–286.

Gramacy, R. B., & Apley, D. W. (2015). Local Gaussian process approximation for large computer experiments. *Journal of Computational and Graphical Statistics, 24*, 561–578.

Gramacy, R. B., & Lee, H. K. H. (2008). Bayesian treed Gaussian process models with an application to computer modeling. *Journal of the American Statistical Association, 103*, 1119–1130.

Greenwood, J. A., & Williamson, J. B. P. (1966). Contact of nominally flat surfaces. In *Proceedings of the Royal Society of London A: Mathematical, Physical and Engineering Sciences. The Royal Society* (Vol. 295, pp. 300–319).

Guttorp, P., & Gneiting, T. (2006). Studies in the history of probability and statistics XLIX: On the Matérn correlation family. *Biometrika, 93*, 989–995.

Higdon, D., Nakhleh, C., Gattiker, J., & Williams, B. (2008). A Bayesian calibration approach to the thermal problem. *Computer Methods in Applied Mechanics and Engineering, 1976*, 2431–2441.

Kaufman, C. G., & Shaby, B. A. (2013). The role of the range parameter for estimation and prediction in geostatistics. *Biometrika, 100*, 473–484.

Kennedy, M. C., & O'Hagan, A. (2000). Predicting the output from a complex computer code when fast approximations are available. *Biometrika, 87*, 1–13.

Kennedy, M. C., & O'Hagan, A. (2001). Bayesian calibration of computer models. *Journal of the Royal Statistical Society: Series B (Statistical Methodology), 63*, 425–464.

Konomi, B., Sang, H., & Mallick, B. (2014). Adaptive Bayesian nonstationary modeling for large spatial datasets using covariance approximations. *Journal of Computational and Graphical Statistics, 23*, 802–829.

Liu, F., Bayarri, M. J., & Berger, J. O. (2009). Modularization in Bayesian analysis, with emphasis on analysis of computer models. *Bayesian Analysis, 4*, 119–150.

Nguyen, H., Cressie, N., & Braverman, A. (2012). Spatial statistical data fusion for remote sensing applications. *Journal of the American Statistical Association, 107*, 1004–1018.

Ohio Supercomputer Center (OSC). (1987). Columbus OH: Ohio Supercomputer Center. http://osc.edu/ark:/19495/f5s1ph73

Peng, C. Y., & Wu, J. (2004). On the choice of nugget in kriging modeling for deterministic computer experiments. *Journal of Computational and Graphical Statistics, 23,* 151–168.

Perdikaris, P., Venturi, D., Royset, J. O., & Karniadakis, G. E. (2015). Multi-fidelity modelling via recursive co-kriging and Gaussian Markov random fields. *Proceedings of the Royal Society of London A, 471,* 20150018.

Qian, P. Z. G., Wu, H., & Wu, C. F. J. (2008). Gaussian process Models for computer experiments with qualitative and quantitative factors. *Technometrics, 50,* 383–396.

Rue, H., & Held, L. (2005). *Gaussian Markov random fields: Theory and applications.* Boca Raton: Chapman and Hall.

Sacks, J., Welch, W. J., Mitchell, T. J., & Wynn, H. P. (1989). Design and analysis of computer experiments. *Statistical Science, 4,* 409–423.

Santner, T. J., Williams, B. J., & Notz, W. I. (2013). *The design and analysis of computer experiments.* New York: Springer Science & Business Media.

Sista, B., & Vemaganti, K. (2014). Estimation of statistical parameters of rough surfaces suitable for developing micro-asperity friction models. *Wear, 316,* 6–18.

Stein, M. L. (1999). *Interpolation of spatial data: Some theory for kriging.* New York: Springer.

Tworzydlo, W. W., Cecot, W., Oden, J. T., & Yew, C. H. (1988). Computational micro-and macroscopic models of contact and friction: Formulation, approach and applications. *Wear, 220,* 113–140.

Wackernagel, H. (2003). *Multivariate geostatistics: An introduction with applications,* 3rd ed. Berlin: Springer.

Zaytsev, V., Biver, P., Wachernagel, H., & Allard, D. (2016). Change-of-support models on irregular grids for geostatistical simulation. *Mathematical Geosciences, 48,* 353–369.

Zhou, Q., Qian, P. Z. G., & Zhou, S. (2011). A simple approach to emulation for computer models with qualitative and quantitative factors. *Technometrics, 53,* 266–273.

Tuning Parameter Selection in the LASSO with Unspecified Propensity

Jiwei Zhao and Yang Yang

1 Introduction

Nowadays advances in technologies have led to an emerging demand for statistical strategies to analyze data with complex structure. For instance, in a biomedical study the number of explanatory variables could be relatively large, or even larger than the sample size. In these settings, it is usually believed that only a small number of variables are truly informative while others are irrelevant. An underfitted model excluding some of the truly informative variables may lead to severe estimation bias in model fitting, whereas an overfitted model including some of the irrelevant variables may enlarge the estimation variance and hinder the model interpretation. Therefore, it is the primary goal to identify the truly informative variables.

Regularization is a popular and powerful method to achieve this goal. Although there exist various regularization methods through different penalty functions, the least absolute shrinkage and selection operator (LASSO; Tibshirani 1996) is still one of the most useful and representative approaches in regularization. The key idea of the original LASSO is to put an L_1 penalty on the least square objective function to attain a sparse estimator for the unknown parameter. Compared with traditional estimation methods, LASSO's major advantage is its simultaneous execution of both parameter estimation and variable selection. Furthermore, the LASSO has very nice computational properties. Using the technique of coordinate descent, Friedman et al. (2010) implemented a very fast and efficient algorithm to solving LASSO-type problems. In recent years, there has been an enormous amount of research activity devoted to the extension of the LASSO and the related regularization methods.

J. Zhao (✉) • Y. Yang
Department of Biostatistics, State University of New York at Buffalo, Buffalo, NY 14214, USA
e-mail: zhaoj@buffalo.edu

© Springer International Publishing AG 2017
D.-G. Chen et al. (eds.), *New Advances in Statistics and Data Science*,
ICSA Book Series in Statistics, https://doi.org/10.1007/978-3-319-69416-0_7

In biomedical studies with human being's behaviors involved, missing-data is the rule rather than the exception. Lots of settings can be named, for example, nonresponse in a health survey (Zhao and Shao 2015), missing covariate values (Fang et al. 2017), or dropout in a follow-up study (Shao and Zhao 2013). Statistical methods handling missing data relies on the assumption imposed on the probability of having a missing value conditioned on all the data, termed as propensity. It is called ignorable when the propensity doesn't depend on any unobserved data; otherwise it is called nonignorable. In general different statistical methods have to be created based on different assumptions on the propensity. In reality, however, the assumption imposed on the propensity is often unverifiable. Therefore, a more flexible propensity is ideal. In this paper we study the variable selection through the LASSO when the data have missing values and the propensity is not fully specified.

With a flexible and generally applicable propensity that is not fully specified, the main idea is to create a pseudo likelihood function for the parameter (of main interest) in the regression model treating the propensity model as a nuisance. In this paper we consider the conditional likelihood applying the idea of Kalbfleisch (1978) to a regression setting. We also approximate this conditional likelihood to a computational feasible version (Liang and Qin 2000). Through this technique, the propensity model, as a nuisance, is canceled out and disappears in the likelihood. Hence, this method is propensity free. To some extend, this method can be regarded as a universal solution under a large family of different assumptions on the propensity. Furthermore, after some data manipulation, we transform the pseudo likelihood function to the likelihood function of a classic logistic regression without the intercept term. This is a paramount breakthrough since instead of using Newton-type algorithm for maximizing the likelihood function, we can adopt the common software designed for the logistic regression to optimize our pseudo likelihood function. To perform variable selection, we extend the idea of the LASSO to the penalized likelihood and put the L_1 penalty function in our pseudo likelihood, and in computation it can be treated as a logistic regression with the LASSO. We will detail this part in Sect. 2.

In penalized likelihood method with the LASSO, the performance of its corresponding estimator depends on the choice of the tuning parameter, which is employed to control the trade-off between model fitting and model sparsity. Theoretically the optimal property of the penalized likelihood method requires certain specification of the optimal tuning parameter. For example, Zhao and Yu (2006) showed that, under the irrepresentable condition, the linear regression with the LASSO is selection consistent when the tuning parameter converges to zero at a rate slower than $O(n^{-1/2})$, where n is the sample size. These results guarantee the existence of the λ needed, but offer little guidance on how to find the desired λ in practice. Indeed, data-driven regularization parameter selection with guaranteed theoretical performance turns out to be a particularly difficult problem. Therefore, in practical implementations, penalized likelihood methods are usually applied with a sequence of tuning parameters resulting in a corresponding collection of models. Therefore, it is of crucial importance to select the appropriate tuning parameter so that the performance of the penalized regression model can be optimized.

The multifold cross validation (CV; Stone 1974; Arlot and Celisse 2010) is a popular model-free criterion for tuning parameter selection. It relies on data resampling technique to minimize the prediction error of a collection of candidate solutions. However, it's known that in many situations, the CV fails to identify all of the truly informative variables consistently (Shao 1993, 1997). On the other hand, Wang et al. (2007) showed that the tuning parameter that is selected by the Bayesian information criterion (BIC; Schwarz et al. 1978) can identify all of the truly informative variables consistently for the smoothly clipped absolute deviation (SCAD) approach in Fan and Li (2001). For non-fixed dimensionality, Wang et al. (2009) showed that a modified BIC continues to work for tuning parameter selection consistency with diverging dimensionality and Fan and Tang (2013) studied the generalized information criterion for tuning parameter selection consistency when allowing the number of parameters to grow exponentially fast with the sample size.

Statisticians also propose tuning parameter selection methods based on stability. Sun et al. (2013) proposed a tuning parameter selection criterion based on variable selection stability (VSS). The key idea is that if multiple samples are available from the same distribution, a good variable selection method should yield similar sets of informative variables that do not vary much from one sample to another. The similarity between two informative variable sets is measured by Cohen's kappa coefficient (Kohen 1960), which adjusts the actual variable selection agreement relative to the possible agreement by chance. Using the similar idea and focusing on the estimation instead of variable selection, Lim and Yu (2016) proposed a tuning parameter selection method based on estimation stability and CV (ESCV). Clearly, variable selection stability and estimation stability are model-free and can be used to tune any penalized regression model.

In this paper, we focus on the tuning parameter selection in the LASSO when the data have missing values and the propensity is unspecified. We introduce the four aforementioned tuning parameter selection methods into our penalized pseudo likelihood function with the LASSO. We detail this part in Sect. 3. In Sects. 4 and 5 respectively, we conduct comprehensive simulation studies including both low and high dimensional settings, and a melanoma data study to examine the performance of different tuning parameter selection methods in real applications. We provide some final remarks in Sect. 6 to conclude our paper.

2   Model and Method

To fix our idea, we let Y denote the scalar response variable, and X be a p-dimensional covariate variable. For simplicity, we assume that, with a canonical link, the conditional distribution of Y given X belongs to a generalized linear model (GLM) with the following density:

$$p(Y|X; \theta) = \exp[\phi^{-1}\{Y\eta - b(\eta)\} + c(y; \phi)], \tag{1}$$

where b and c are known functions, $\eta = \alpha + \boldsymbol{\beta}^T \boldsymbol{X}$, $\boldsymbol{\theta} = (\alpha, \boldsymbol{\beta}^T, \phi)^T$, ϕ represents the positive dispersion parameter. Assume that we have independent and identically distributed observations $\{y_i, \boldsymbol{x}_i\}$, $i = 1, \ldots, N$. When variables from (Y, X) have missing values, we use the indicator $R = 1$ to represent that, the data from that subject are completely observed, and $R = 0$ otherwise. Without loss of generality, we assume the first n subjects are fully observed with $r_i = 1$, $i = 1, \ldots, n$, and the remaining $N - n$ subjects may contain missing components with $r_i = 0, i = n+1, \ldots, N$.

For the propensity $\Pr(R = 1|Y, X)$, since its underlying truth is unknown and its assumption is unverifiable, it is ideal to impose an assumption, that is more robust than a single parametric model, and is as flexible and generally applicable as possible. In this paper, we impose a general assumption as follows

$$\Pr(R = 1|Y, X) = s(Y)t(X), \tag{2}$$

where s and t are some functions, not necessarily to be known or specified. The assumption (2) is very flexible and generally applicable. The situations we concern include: only Y has missing values (missing response); only X has missing values (missing covariate); both Y and X have missing values. It also includes both ignorable and nonignorable cases. For example, for the case of missing response, if s=constant, (2) is covariate-dependent and hence ignorable; if t=constant, (2) is outcome-dependent and hence nonignorable; for the case of missing covariate, if s=constant, (2) is nonignorable while if t=constant, (2) is ignorable. Furthermore, (2) only assumes that $\Pr(R = 1|Y, X)$ can be written as the multiplier of an X-only function and a Y-only function. We do not impose any concrete form on s or t, therefore, it is robust to misspecification of s or t function.

Due to the complexity of the missing data structure and the presence of unknown functions s and t, we propose the following pseudo likelihood function. Notice that

$$p(Y|X, R = 1) = \frac{\Pr(R = 1|Y, X)}{\Pr(R = 1|X)} p(Y|X), \tag{3}$$

which reveals that, the direct maximum likelihood estimate from a biased sample (the fully observed subjects) will result in biased estimates and incorrect conclusions unless $\Pr(R = 1|Y, X) = \Pr(R = 1|X)$. Under the separable propensity assumption (2), $\Pr(R = 1|Y, X)/\Pr(R = 1|X)$ in (3) preserves to be the multiplier of an X-only function and a Y-only function. Therefore, following Kalbfleisch (1978) and Liang and Qin (2000), restricting attention to completely observed subjects with subscripts ranging from $\{1, \ldots, n\}$, decomposing $\{y_1, \ldots, y_n\}$ as rank statistics and order statistics, and conditioning on the order statistics $\{y_{(1)}, \ldots, y_{(n)}\}$, we have the following for $\boldsymbol{\theta}$:

$$p(y_1, \ldots, y_n | r_1 = \ldots = r_n = 1, \boldsymbol{x}_1, \ldots, \boldsymbol{x}_n, y_{(1)}, \ldots, y_{(n)}) = \frac{\prod_{i=1}^n p(y_i | \boldsymbol{x}_i; \boldsymbol{\theta})}{\sum_c \prod_{i=1}^n p(y_{(i)} | \boldsymbol{x}_i; \boldsymbol{\theta})}, \tag{4}$$

where the summation in the denominator corresponds to all possible permutations of $\{1, \ldots, n\}$. An appealing feature of this method is that, it is now nuisance free: all s, t functions are all canceled out through conditioning. Furthermore, to reduce the computational burden, Liang and Qin (2000) advocated the following pairwise pseudo likelihood

$$\prod_{1 \leq i < j \leq n} \frac{p(y_i|x_i; \theta)p(y_j|x_j; \theta)}{p(y_i|x_i; \theta)p(y_j|x_j; \theta) + p(y_i|x_j; \theta)p(y_j|x_i; \theta)}. \tag{5}$$

Under the GLM assumption, the negative part of the log-version of (5), after adding a normalizing constant, can be written as

$$\mathscr{L}(\gamma) = \frac{1}{n(n-1)/2} \sum_{1 \leq i < j \leq n} \log\{1 + \exp(-y_{i\backslash j}x_{i\backslash j}^T \gamma)\}, \tag{6}$$

where $y_{i\backslash j} = y_i - y_j$, $x_{i\backslash j} = x_i - x_j$ and $\gamma = \beta/\phi$. To perform variable selection with the LASSO, we propose to minimize the penalized pseudo likelihood

$$\mathscr{L}(\gamma) + \lambda \sum_{j=1}^{p} |\gamma_j| = \frac{1}{n(n-1)/2} \sum_{1 \leq i < j \leq n} \log\{1 + \exp(-y_{i\backslash j}x_{i\backslash j}^T \gamma)\} + \lambda \sum_{j=1}^{p} |\gamma_j|, \tag{7}$$

and we denote the minimizer as $\widehat{\gamma}$.

It can be seen that, the unpenalized component $\mathscr{L}(\gamma)$ is a U-statistic, in which even the original b function in the definition of GLM disappears. Since our method is under a very flexible and generally applicable assumption (2), to compensate for missing data, not surprisingly, we may not be able to estimate the whole unknown parameter θ itself. Instead, we can only estimate a scaled parameter $\gamma = \beta/\phi$. Denote the true value of β and γ as β^* and γ^* respectively. It's clear that each coordinate $\beta_j^* = 0$ if and only if $\gamma_j^* = 0$. Therefore, we can carry out variable selection through the scaled parameter γ.

For computation, note that

$$\mathscr{L}(\gamma) = \frac{1}{n(n-1)/2} \sum_{1 \leq i < j \leq n} \log\{1 + \exp(-y_{i\backslash j}x_{i\backslash j}^T \gamma)\}$$

$$= \frac{1}{n(n-1)/2} \sum_{1 \leq i < j \leq n} \log\{1 + \exp(-\text{sign}(y_{i\backslash j})|y_{i\backslash j}|x_{i\backslash j}^T \gamma)\}$$

$$= \frac{1}{T} \sum_{k=1}^{T} \log\{1 + \exp(z_k v_k^T \gamma)\},$$

where we let $\text{sign}(\cdot)$ denote the sign function, $z_k = -\text{sign}(y_{i\backslash j})$ and $v_k = x_{i\backslash j}|y_{i\backslash j}|$, $T = n(n-1)/2$. If we define

$$u_k = \begin{cases} 1 & \text{if } y_{i\setminus j} > 0 \\ 0 & \text{if } y_{i\setminus j} < 0, \end{cases}$$

it can be seen that, $\mathscr{L}(\gamma)$ can be regarded as the negative log-likelihood function of a regular logistic regression with response u_k, covariate v_k, without the intercept term. Hence, the minimization of (7) can be achieved in any available software for solving penalized logistic regression by forcing the intercept term to zero.

3 Tuning Parameter Selection in the LASSO

How to select the regularization parameter λ is of paramount importance in penalized likelihood estimation since λ governs the complexity of the selected model. A large value of λ tends to choose a simple model, whereas a small value of λ inclines to a complex model. Theoretically quantified optimal tuning parameters are not practically feasible, because they are valid only asymptotically and usually depend on unknown nuisance parameters in the true model. Therefore, in practical implementations, penalized likelihood methods are usually applied with a sequence of tuning parameters resulting in a corresponding collection of models. The trade-off between the model complexity and the prediction accuracy yields an optimal choice of λ. In this Section, we introduce four different tuning parameter selection methods in our proposed penalized pseudo likelihood function with the LASSO.

3.1 Multifold Cross Validation (CV)

The multifold cross validation (CV; Stone 1974) is one of the most frequently used tuning parameter selection methods in regularization. It optimizes the prediction error of a collection of candidate models based on some data resampling techniques. Specifically, we denote the data set indexed by $\{1, \ldots, n\}$ as T, and randomly partition this set into K equally sized subsets $T^{(v)}$, $v = 1, \ldots, K$. We denote the cross validation training and test sets by $T \setminus T^{(v)}$ and $T^{(v)}$, for $v = 1, \ldots, K$, where the usual choice of K is 5 or 10. Each time, for fixed λ and v, we find the minimizer $\widehat{\gamma}_\lambda^{(-v)}$ of $\mathscr{L}(\gamma) + \lambda \|\gamma\|_1$ using the training set $T \setminus T^{(v)}$. Finally, we choose λ_{CV} to be the minimizer of the following cross validation function

$$\text{CV}(\lambda) = \frac{1}{K} \sum_{v=1}^{K} \mathscr{L}^{(v)}(\widehat{\gamma}_\lambda^{(-v)}),$$

where $\mathscr{L}^{(v)}(\cdot)$ represents the evaluation of $\mathscr{L}(\cdot)$ using the test set $T^{(v)}$.

Although computationally convenient, the literature showed that, in many situation the CV failed to identify all of the truly informative variables consistently and often overfitted the model (Shao 1993, 1997). On the other hand, under some regularity conditions the Bayesian information criterion (BIC; Schwarz et al. 1978) was shown to be selection consistent.

3.2 Bayesian Information Criterion (BIC)

Information criterion is a traditional method for variable selection, especially the Bayesian information criterion (BIC). To be more specific, for each fixed tuning parameter λ, we find the minimizer $\widehat{\boldsymbol{\gamma}}_\lambda$ of the objective function $\mathscr{L}(\boldsymbol{\gamma}) + \lambda \|\boldsymbol{\gamma}\|_1$. Then we choose λ to be the minimizer of the following BIC function

$$\mathrm{BIC}(\lambda) = 2\mathscr{L}(\widehat{\boldsymbol{\gamma}}_\lambda) + p_\lambda \frac{\log(n)}{n},$$

where p_λ is the number of nonzero coordinates in $\widehat{\boldsymbol{\gamma}}_\lambda$. Wang et al. (2007) showed that the tuning parameter that is selected by the BIC can identify all of the truly informative variables consistently for the smoothly clipped absolute deviation (SCAD) approach in Fan and Li (2001). The BIC method was well accepted to result a more parsimonious model than the CV.

In high dimensional settings, for regression models without missing data, to preserve to be selection consistent, it was shown that some modifications are needed for the definition of the BIC. Wang et al. (2009) considered the situation with diverging dimensionality $p \propto n^\alpha$ and showed that the second component in the classic BIC function should be changed to $p_\lambda \log(n) \log\{\log(p)\}/n$ to continue to be selection consistent; while Fan and Tang (2013) considered the so-called ultrahigh dimensionality $\log p \propto n^\alpha, 0 < \alpha < 1$ and showed that the second component in the classic BIC function should be changed to $p_\lambda \log\{\log(n)\} \log(p)/n$ to continue to be selection consistent. In our proposal, we modify the BIC as the following two functions and we term them as BIC1 and BIC2 respectively:

$$\mathrm{BIC1}(\lambda) = 2\mathscr{L}(\widehat{\boldsymbol{\gamma}}_\lambda) + p_\lambda \frac{\log(n) \log\{\log(p)\}}{n},$$

and

$$\mathrm{BIC2}(\lambda) = 2\mathscr{L}(\widehat{\boldsymbol{\gamma}}_\lambda) + p_\lambda \frac{\log\{\log(n)\} \log(p)}{n}.$$

In the current literature, CV and BIC are the most two dominating tuning parameter selection methods. Statisticians also propose tuning parameter selection methods based on stability. We review one for estimation stability and the other for variable selection stability.

3.3 Variable Selection Stability (VSS)

Sun et al. (2013) proposed a tuning parameter selection criterion based on variable selection stability (VSS). The key idea is that if we repeatedly draw samples from the population and apply the candidate variable selection methods, a desirable method should produce the informative variable set that does not vary much from one sample to another. The similarity between two informative variable sets can be measured by Cohen's kappa coefficient (Kohen 1960), which adjusts the actual variable selection agreement relative to the possible agreement by chance.

To be more detailed, we denote the data set indexed by $\{1, \ldots, n\}$ as T. Each time, we randomly partition T into two subsets T_1^b and T_2^b. For a fixed λ and one subset T_1^b (or T_2^b), we optimize the proposed penalized pseudo likelihood function and obtain $\widehat{\gamma}_\lambda^{1b}$ (or $\widehat{\gamma}_\lambda^{2b}$), each yielding a set of selected informative variables $\mathscr{A}_\lambda^{1b}$ (or $\mathscr{A}_\lambda^{2b}$). We measure the agreement between $\mathscr{A}_\lambda^{1b}$ and $\mathscr{A}_\lambda^{2b}$ by the Cohen's kappa coefficient:

$$\kappa(\mathscr{A}_\lambda^{1b}, \mathscr{A}_\lambda^{2b}) = \frac{\Pr(a) - \Pr(e)}{1 - \Pr(e)},$$

where $\Pr(a) = (n_{11} + n_{22})/p$ and $\Pr(e) = (n_{11} + n_{12})(n_{11} + n_{21})/p^2 + (n_{12} + n_{22})(n_{21} + n_{22})/p^2$, with $n_{11} = |\mathscr{A}_\lambda^{1b} \cap \mathscr{A}_\lambda^{2b}|$, $n_{12} = |\mathscr{A}_\lambda^{1b} \cap \overline{\mathscr{A}_\lambda^{2b}}|$, $n_{21} = |\overline{\mathscr{A}_\lambda^{1b}} \cap \mathscr{A}_\lambda^{2b}|$, $n_{22} = |\overline{\mathscr{A}_\lambda^{1b}} \cap \overline{\mathscr{A}_\lambda^{2b}}|$, and $|\cdot|$ being the set cardinality. We repeat this procedure B times and we define the variable selection stability at this fixed λ as

$$\Psi(\lambda) = \frac{1}{B} \sum_{b=1}^{B} \kappa(\mathscr{A}_\lambda^{1b}, \mathscr{A}_\lambda^{2b}).$$

Finally we select

$$\lambda_{\mathrm{VSS}} = \min \left\{ \lambda : \frac{\Psi(\lambda)}{\max_{\lambda'} \Psi(\lambda')} \geq 1 - \alpha \right\}.$$

Note that, the adoption of α in the last step is necessary since some informative variables may have relatively weak effect compared with others. Following Sun et al. (2013), we take $\alpha = 0.1$ and $B = 20$ in our numerical studies.

3.4 Estimation Stability (ESCV)

The last tuning parameter selection method we are introducing is motivated from estimation stability and the cross validation (Lim and Yu 2016). The intuition is the same as VSS but the focus changes to estimation. Note that since the model we concern is semiparametric, and it may have arbitrary missing values in the samples $i = n + 1, \ldots, N$, the procedure proposed by Lim and Yu (2016) cannot be applied directly. Instead, what we do is the following.

Similar to the CV, we denote the data set indexed by $\{1, \ldots, n\}$ as T, and randomly partition this set into K equally sized subsets $T^{(v)}$, $v = 1, \ldots, K$. We denote the cross validation training and test sets by $T \backslash T^{(v)}$ and $T^{(v)}$ for $v = 1, \ldots, K$. Each time, for fixed λ and v, we find the minimizer $\widehat{\boldsymbol{\gamma}}_\lambda^{(-v)}$ of $\mathscr{L}(\boldsymbol{\gamma}) + \lambda \|\boldsymbol{\gamma}\|_1$ using the training set $T \backslash T^{(v)}$. Then we compute the estimates $\boldsymbol{x}_{i \backslash j}^T \widehat{\boldsymbol{\gamma}}_\lambda^{(-v)}$ for $i, j = 1, \ldots, n$ and form it to an S-dimensional vector $z_\lambda^{(-v)}$, where $S = n(n-1)/2$. We define

$$\bar{z}_\lambda = \frac{1}{K} \sum_{v=1}^{K} z_\lambda^{(-v)},$$

and

$$\text{ESCV}(\lambda) = \frac{\frac{1}{K} \sum_{v=1}^{K} \|z_\lambda^{(-v)} - \bar{z}_\lambda\|_2^2}{\|\bar{z}_\lambda\|_2^2}.$$

We denote $\lambda_{\text{escv}} = \arg \min_\lambda \text{ESCV}(\lambda)$ and due to the same reason as in Lim and Yu (2016), our final choice of the tuning parameter is $\lambda_{\text{ESCV}} = \lambda_{\text{escv}} \vee \lambda_{\text{CV}}$.

One advantage of the stability motivated tuning parameter selection methods is that, they are model-free and can be used to tune any penalized regression model.

4 Simulation Studies

In this Section, we conduct simulation studies to examine the finite sample performance of our proposed method. We mainly compare the performance in terms of estimation and variable selection under different tuning parameter selection methods: CV, the multi-fold cross validation; BIC, the Bayesian information criterion; VSS, the variable selection stability; and ESCV, the estimation stability based on cross validation. We consider the classic BIC for low-dimensional case and BIC1 and BIC2, the two modified criteria for high-dimensional case. We examine two commonly used models: linear regression and logistic regression.

For linear regression, we generate the response Y following GLM with $\eta = \alpha + \boldsymbol{\beta}^T \boldsymbol{X}$, $\alpha = 0$, $\boldsymbol{\beta} = (2, 1.5, 0.5, 0, \ldots, 0)^T$, the dispersion parameter $\phi = 1$. We generate the covariate $\boldsymbol{X}$ from $N(\boldsymbol{0}, \boldsymbol{\Sigma})$, where $\boldsymbol{\Sigma}_{ij} = 0.5^{|i-j|}$. We consider the total sample size $N = 200$ and $p = 8$ for low dimension and $p = 200$ for high dimension, and in both cases the number of truly informative variables is 3. For the propensity, we consider the following assumption

$$\Pr(R = 1 | Y, \boldsymbol{X}) = I_{\{Y > \gamma_1\}} I_{\{X_1 > \gamma_2\}},$$

which means the propensity depends on both response Y and the covariate variable X_1. The choices of γ_1 and γ_2 are as follows: for either low or high dimensional case, $\gamma_1 = 0.7$, $\gamma_2 = -0.3$ to achieve around 40% completely observed samples; $\gamma_1 = -1.1$, $\gamma_2 = -0.8$ to achieve around 60%; and $\gamma_1 = -3.2$, $\gamma_2 = -1.3$ to achieve around 80%.

For logistic regression, we set $\alpha = 0$, $\boldsymbol{\beta} = (3, 2, 1, 0, \ldots, 0)^T$. Same as above, we generate the covariate $\boldsymbol{X}$ from $N(\boldsymbol{0}, \boldsymbol{\Sigma})$, where $\boldsymbol{\Sigma}_{ij} = 0.5^{|i-j|}$. We consider the total sample size $N = 500$ and $p = 8$ for low dimension and $p = 500$ for high dimension, and in both cases the number of truly informative variables is 3. For the propensity, we consider

$$\Pr(R = 1 | Y, X) = I_{\{X_1 > \gamma\}} s(Y).$$

The specific choices of γ and $s(Y)$ are as follows: for either low or high dimensional case, $\gamma = 0.2$ and $s(Y) = (2Y + 3)/5$ for 40% observed proportion, $\gamma = -0.5$ and $s(Y) = (2Y + 3)/5$ for 60% observed proportion, and $\gamma = -1$ and $s(Y) = (Y + 9)/10$ for 80% observed proportion.

For the performance of estimation, we consider three measures: L_1, L_2 and L_∞ norms of the estimation bias. To be more specific, if we have the estimator $\widehat{\boldsymbol{\beta}}$ and the true value $\boldsymbol{\beta}^*$, the L_1 norm is defined as $\|\widehat{\boldsymbol{\beta}} - \boldsymbol{\beta}^*\|_1 = \sum_{i=1}^p |\widehat{\beta}_i - \beta_i^*|$, the L_2 norm is defined as $\|\widehat{\boldsymbol{\beta}} - \boldsymbol{\beta}^*\|_2 = \left(\sum_{i=1}^p |\widehat{\beta}_i - \beta_i^*|^2\right)^{1/2}$, and the L_∞ norm is defined as $\|\widehat{\boldsymbol{\beta}} - \boldsymbol{\beta}^*\|_\infty = \max_i |\widehat{\beta}_i - \beta_i^*|$. In this paper, following Sun et al. (2013), we report the results on the estimation based on the estimators by maximizing the pairwise pseudo likelihood function, or equivalently, minimizing (6), only with the selected informative variables, after the standard minimization of (7) has been executed. In terms of variable selection, we consider the following measures: #FP, the number of false positives (the ones with true zero value but falsely estimated as nonzero); #FN, the number of false negatives (the ones with true nonzero value but falsely estimated as zero); F-measure, the harmonic mean of precision and sensitivity, which is defined as

$$F = \frac{2\#\text{TP}}{2\#\text{TP} + \#\text{FP} + \#\text{FN}},$$

in which TP stands for true positive (the one with true nonzero value and also correctly estimated as nonzero). We also consider the proportion of under-fit, correct-fit and over-fit, where under-fit represents the situation of excluding any nonzero coefficients, correct-fit means the situation of selecting the exact subset model, and over-fit stands for the situation of including all three significant variables and some noise variables.

For linear regression, we report a boxplot of the three norms for estimation in Fig. 1 and summarize the other measures for variable selection in Table 1. Similarly, Fig. 2 and Table 2 are for logistic regression respectively. We report the results based on 100 replications in each setting.

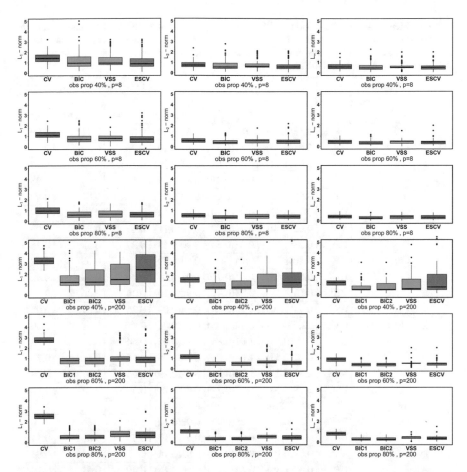

Fig. 1 The L_1 (1st column), L_2 (2nd column) and L_∞ (3rd column) norms of the estimation bias through different tuning parameter selection methods (CV, BIC (or BIC1, BIC2), VSS, ESCV) for linear regression with dimensionality $p = 8$ (1st, 2nd and 3rd rows), $p = 200$ (4th, 5th and 6th rows), and observed proportion 40% (1st and 4th rows), 60% (2nd and 5th rows) and 80% (3rd and 6th rows)

Our conclusions from the simulation studies are as follows. For estimation, when the number of the observed samples gets increase, the L_1, L_2 and L_∞ norms become smaller and the contrast among different tuning parameter selection methods becomes clearer. At 80% observed proportion level, the CV performs worse than all other methods BIC, VSS and ESCV. The difference among BIC, VSS and ESCV are quite indistinguishable. For variable selection, the CV performs much worse than all the other methods. It always overfits the model. Under low dimensionality, the performance of BIC, ESCV and VSS are comparable, while under high dimensionality, BIC is slightly better than the other two. The behaviors of BIC1 and BIC2 under high dimensionality are almost always exactly the same.

Table 1 Mean and standard deviation (SD; in parentheses) of #FP, #FN and F-measure and the proportion of under-fit, correct-fit and over-fit through different tuning parameter selection methods (CV, BIC (or BIC1, BIC2), VSS, ESCV) for linear regression with dimensionality $p = 8$ or $p = 200$, and observed proportion 40%, 60% or 80%

| | Observed proportion (%) | | #FP | #FN | F-measure | Proportion of | | |
						under-fit	correct-fit	over-fit
$p = 8$	40	CV	3.13(1.25)	0(0)	0.67(0.10)	0	0.01	0.99
		BIC	0.81(0.86)	0.11(0.31)	0.87(0.12)	0.06	0.39	0.55
		VSS	0.09(0.32)	0.67(0.62)	0.85(0.14)	0.59	0.33	0.08
		ESCV	0.50(0.72)	0.24(0.49)	0.88(0.12)	0.18	0.44	0.38
	60	CV	3.50(1.22)	0.00(0.00)	0.64(0.09)	0	0.01	0.99
		BIC	0.73(0.92)	0.02(0.14)	0.90(0.11)	0	0.52	0.48
		VSS	0.02(0.14)	0.48(0.52)	0.90(0.11)	0.47	0.51	0.02
		ESCV	0.23(0.60)	0.31(0.54)	0.90(0.13)	0.27	0.57	0.16
	80	CV	3.40(1.23)	0(0)	0.65(0.09)	0	0.02	0.98
		BIC	0.51(0.66)	0.01(0.10)	0.93(0.09)	0	0.58	0.42
		VSS	0(0)	0.34(0.48)	0.93(0.10)	0.34	0.66	0
		ESCV	0.11(0.40)	0.25(0.44)	0.94(0.09)	0.25	0.67	0.08
$p = 200$	40	CV	22.78(6.81)	0.14(0.35)	0.21(0.06)	0	0	1.00
		BIC1	0.29(0.54)	1.01(0.81)	0.72(0.25)	0.64	0.11	0.25
		BIC2	0.27(0.53)	1.06(0.84)	0.71(0.26)	0.66	0.11	0.23
		VSS	1.47(4.22)	1.04(0.70)	0.67(0.19)	0.64	0.07	0.29
		ESCV	3.99(6.30)	0.67(0.74)	0.60(0.21)	0.34	0.04	0.62
	60	CV	27.62(8.93)	0.01(0.10)	0.19(0.06)	0	0	1.00
		BIC1	0.19(0.46)	0.26(0.44)	0.92(0.10)	0.24	0.60	0.16
		BIC2	0.17(0.45)	0.27(0.45)	0.92(0.10)	0.25	0.61	0.14
		VSS	0.01(0.10)	0.85(0.58)	0.82(0.14)	0.75	0.24	0.01
		ESCV	0.42(1.36)	0.46(0.58)	0.86(0.15)	0.40	0.41	0.19
	80	CV	29.14(9.02)	0.01(0.10)	0.18(0.06)	0	0	1.00
		BIC1	0.14(0.38)	0.08(0.27)	0.96(0.07)	0.07	0.80	0.13
		BIC2	0.13(0.37)	0.09(0.29)	0.96(0.08)	0.08	0.80	0.12
		VSS	0(0)	0.60(0.49)	0.88(0.10)	0.60	0.40	0
		ESCV	0.06(0.24)	0.38(0.53)	0.91(0.11)	0.36	0.58	0.06

5 Melanoma Study

Melanoma is the most dangerous type of skin cancer. Melanoma incidence is increasing at a rate that exceeds all solid tumors. High-risk melanoma patients, although education efforts have resulted in earlier detection of melanoma, continue to have high relapse and mortality rate of 50% or higher. Several post-operative (adjuvant) chemotherapies have been proposed for this class of melanoma patients, and the one which seems to provide the most significant impact on relapse-free

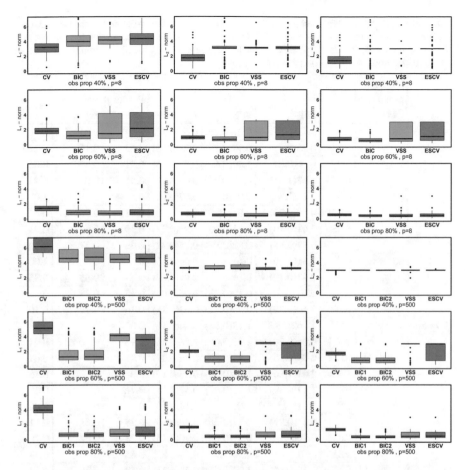

Fig. 2 The L_1 (1st column), L_2 (2nd column) and L_∞ (3rd column) norms of the estimation bias through different tuning parameter selection methods (CV, BIC (or BIC1, BIC2), VSS, ESCV) for logistic regression with dimensionality $p = 8$ (1st, 2nd and 3rd rows), $p = 500$ (4th, 5th and 6th rows), and observed proportion 40% (1st and 4th rows), 60% (2nd and 5th rows) and 80% (3rd and 6th rows)

survival is Interferon Alpha-2b (IFN). This immunotherapy was evaluated in E1690, an observation-controlled Eastern Cooperative Oncology Group (ECOG) phase III clinical trial (Kirkwood et al. 2000).

In this trial as we consider, there are in total $N = 427$ patients and all the patients were randomized to one of two treatment trials: high dose interferon or observation. In this analysis, the outcome variable Y, was taken to be binary, and was assigned a 1 if the patient had an overall survival greater than or equal to 0.55 years, and 0 otherwise. There are several prognostic factors that were identified as potentially important predictors: X_1, treatment (two levels); X_2, age (in years); X_3, nodes1 (four levels); X_4, sex (two levels); X_5, perform (two levels); and X_6, logarithm of Breslow

Table 2 Mean and standard deviation (SD; in parentheses) of #FP, #FN and F-measure and the proportion of under-fit, correct-fit and over-fit through different tuning parameter selection methods (CV, BIC (or BIC1, BIC2), VSS, ESCV) for logistic regression with dimensionality $p = 8$ or $p = 500$, and observed proportion 40%, 60% or 80%

	Observed proportion (%)		#FP	#FN	F-measure	Proportion of under-fit	correct-fit	over-fit
$p = 8$	40	CV	3.12(1.36)	0.07(0.29)	0.66(0.12)	0	0.04	0.96
		BIC	0.23(0.45)	0.94(0.75)	0.75(0.18)	0.62	0.16	0.22
		VSS	0.06(0.24)	1.40(0.60)	0.67(0.16)	0.91	0.03	0.06
		ESCV	1.07(1.51)	0.97(0.81)	0.66(0.14)	0.55	0.01	0.44
	60	CV	3.15(1.31)	0.01(0.10)	0.67(0.10)	0	0	1.00
		BIC	0.59(0.79)	0.01(0.10)	0.92(0.10)	0.01	0.55	0.44
		VSS	0.01(0.10)	0.71(0.92)	0.82(0.23)	0.39	0.60	0.01
		ESCV	0.37(0.85)	0.82(0.97)	0.75(0.22)	0.43	0.37	0.20
	80	CV	3.31(1.29)	0(0)	0.66(0.10)	0	0	1.00
		BIC	0.47(0.73)	0(0)	0.94(0.09)	0	0.65	0.35
		VSS	0(0)	0.17(0.43)	0.96(0.09)	0.15	0.85	0
		ESCV	0.10(0.30)	0.25(0.61)	0.93(0.15)	0.16	0.74	0.10
$p = 500$	40	CV	17.62(13.37)	1.13(0.58)	0.24(0.16)	0.02	0	0.98
		BIC1	0.04(0.20)	1.92(0.66)	0.48(0.26)	0.96	0	0.04
		BIC2	0.04(0.20)	1.97(0.67)	0.46(0.27)	0.96	0	0.04
		VSS	2.81(10.64)	1.55(0.58)	0.56(0.19)	0.84	0	0.16
		ESCV	1.12(4.39)	1.56(0.52)	0.57(0.15)	0.72	0	0.28
	60	CV	35.19(15.83)	0(0)	0.18(0.10)	0	0	1.00
		BIC1	0.11(0.31)	0.37(0.63)	0.90(0.15)	0.28	0.61	0.11
		BIC2	0.10(0.30)	0.37(0.63)	0.90(0.15)	0.28	0.62	0.10
		VSS	0(0)	1.50(0.75)	0.64(0.19)	0.85	0.15	0
		ESCV	0.19(0.60)	1.09(0.91)	0.71(0.21)	0.62	0.26	0.12
	80	CV	33.38(19.52)	0(0)	0.19(0.10)	0	0	1.00
		BIC1	0.09(0.29)	0.02(0.14)	0.98(0.05)	0.02	0.89	0.09
		BIC2	0.07(0.26)	0.02(0.14)	0.99(0.05)	0.02	0.91	0.07
		VSS	0(0)	0.30(0.54)	0.94(0.12)	0.26	0.74	0
		ESCV	0.10(0.33)	0.47(0.78)	0.87(0.19)	0.29	0.62	0.09

thickness (in mm). Among all six covariates, only X_6 has missing values and the total number of completely observed samples is $n = 417$. The data set is available from Ibrahim et al. (2001).

We adopt the logistic regression and we minimize the following penalized likelihood function

$$\frac{1}{n(n-1)/2} \sum_{1 \le i < j \le n} \log\{1 + \exp(-y_{i\backslash j} \boldsymbol{x}_{i\backslash j}^T \boldsymbol{\beta})\} + \lambda \sum_{j=1}^{p} |\beta_j|.$$

Table 3 The parameter estimation and the number of selected informative variables in the Melanoma study based on different tuning parameter selection methods: CV, BIC, VSS and ESCV

	TRT	AGE	NODES1	SEX	PERFORM	log(BRESLOW)	p_λ
CV	−0.080	0.018	0.499	−0.052	0.000	0.267	5
BIC	0.000	0.018	0.464	0.000	0.000	0.226	3
VSS	0.000	0.017	0.212	0.000	0.000	0.000	2
ESCV	0.000	0.018	0.396	0.000	0.000	0.137	3

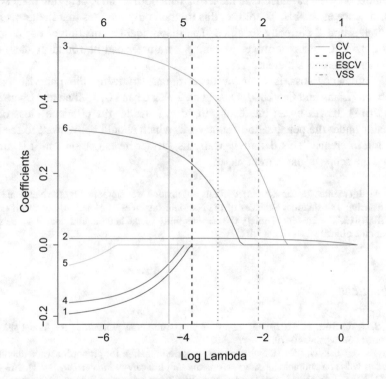

Fig. 3 The solution path for the proposed penalized pseudo likelihood in the Melanoma study and the determination of the tuning parameter based on different methods: CV, BIC, VSS and ESCV, where 1=TRT, 2=AGE, 3=NODES1, 4=SEX, 5=PERFORM, 6=log(BRESLOW)

We examine the four methods to select the tuning parameter λ: CV, BIC, VSS and ESCV. We report the estimation result in Table 3 and visualize the solution path in Fig. 3. It can be seen that, out of six variables, the CV chooses five as informative ones, while BIC, ESCV and VSS choose three, three and two variables respectively. This is consistent with the simulation studies in the sense that CV tends to overfit the model. The performance of BIC, ESCV and VSS are similar. The variables age and nodes1 are always significant, and the variable logarithm of Breslow is significant when using BIC or ESCV.

6 Discussion

In this paper, we mainly evaluate the numerical performance among various tuning parameter selection methods under an arbitrary and unspecified propensity assumption. The key idea is to use a conditional argument and then obtain a pseudo likelihood function in a pairwise fashion. During this conditional argument procedure, only the parameters in the terms with both Y and X in (1) are preserved in (6), and hence estimable. Therefore, this method only requires that the terms in (1) with both Y and X correctly specified. The theoretical justification of our proposed method using CV to determine the tuning parameter can be found in Zhao et al. (2017) and references therein.

The efficiency loss is a major disadvantage of using the pairwise pseudo likelihood (Liang and Qin 2000; Diao et al. 2012; Chan 2013; Zhao and Shao 2017; Zhao 2017). It will be an interesting topic to consider the efficiency loss of this estimator under the penalization framework, which should be relevant to the post-selection inference. This definitely warrants further investigation and it is already beyond the scope of the current paper.

Acknowledgements Research reported in this publication was supported by the National Center for Advancing Translational Sciences of the National Institutes of Health under award number UL1TR001412. The content is solely the responsibility of the authors and does not necessarily represent the official views of the NIH.

References

Arlot, S., & Celisse, A. (2010). A survey of cross-validation procedures for model selection. *Statistics Surveys, 4*, 40–79.

Chuen, K., & Chan, G. (2013). Nuisance parameter elimination for proportional likelihood ratio models with nonignorable missingness and random truncation. *Biometrika, 100*(1), 269–276.

Diao, G., Ning, J., & Qin, J. (2012). Maximum likelihood estimation for semiparametric density ratio model. *The International Journal of Biostatistics, 8*(1). https://doi.org/10.1515/1557-4679.1372

Fan, J., & Li, R. (2001). Variable selection via nonconcave penalized likelihood and its oracle properties. *Journal of the American Statistical Association, 96*(456), 1348–1360.

Fan, Y., & Tang, C. Y. (2013). Tuning parameter selection in high dimensional penalized likelihood. *Journal of the Royal Statistical Society: Series B (Statistical Methodology), 75*(3), 531–552.

Fang, F., Zhao, J., & Shao, J. (2017). Imputation-based adjusted score equations in generalized linear models with nonignorable missing covariate values. *Statistica Sinica, 27*. https://doi.org/doi:10.5705/ss.202015.0437

Friedman, J., Hastie, T., & Tibshirani, R. (2010). Regularization paths for generalized linear models via coordinate descent. *Journal of Statistical Software, 33*(1), 1.

Ibrahim, J. G., Chen, M.-H., & Sinha, D. (2001). *Bayesian survival analysis*. Berlin: Springer.

Kalbfleisch, J. D. (1978). Likelihood methods and nonparametric tests. *Journal of the American Statistical Association, 73*(361), 167–170.

Kirkwood, J.M., Ibrahim, J.G., Sondak, V.K., Richards, J., Flaherty, L.E. & Ernstoff, M.S., et al. (2000). High-and low-dose interferon alfa-2b in high-risk melanoma: first analysis of intergroup trial E1690/S9111/C9190. *Journal of Clinical Oncology: Official Journal of the American Society of Clinical Oncology, 18*(12), 2444.

Kohen, J. (1960). A coefficient of agreement for nominal scales. *Educational and Psychological Measurement, 20,* 37–46.

Liang, K.-Y., & Qin, J. (2000). Regression analysis under non-standard situations: A pairwise pseudolikelihood approach. *Journal of the Royal Statistical Society: Series B (Statistical Methodology), 62*(4), 773–786.

Lim, C., & Yu, B. (2016). Estimation stability with cross-validation (ESCV). *Journal of Computational and Graphical Statistics, 25*(2), 464–492.

Schwarz, G. (1978). Estimating the dimension of a model. *The Annals of Statistics, 6*(2), 461–464.

Shao, J. (1993). Linear model selection by cross-validation. *Journal of the American statistical Association, 88*(422), 486–494.

Shao, J. (1997). An asymptotic theory for linear model selection. *Statistica Sinica, 7,* 221–264.

Shao, J., & Zhao, J. (2013). Estimation in longitudinal studies with nonignorable dropout. *Statistics and Its Interface, 6,* 303–313.

Stone, M. (1974). Cross-validatory choice and assessment of statistical predictions. *Journal of the Royal Statistical Society. Series B (Methodological), 36,* 111–147.

Sun, W., Wang, J., & Fang, Y. (2013). Consistent selection of tuning parameters via variable selection stability. *Journal of Machine Learning Research, 14*(1), 3419–3440.

Tibshirani, R. (1996). Regression shrinkage and selection via the lasso. *Journal of the Royal Statistical Society. Series B (Methodological), 58,* 267–288.

Wang, H., Li, B., & Leng, C. (2009). Shrinkage tuning parameter selection with a diverging number of parameters. *Journal of the Royal Statistical Society: Series B (Statistical Methodology), 71*(3), 671–683.

Wang, H., Li, R., & Tsai, C.-L. (2007). Tuning parameter selectors for the smoothly clipped absolute deviation method. *Biometrika, 94*(3), 553–568.

Zhao, J. (2017). Reducing bias for maximum approximate conditional likelihood estimator with general missing data mechanism. *Journal of Nonparametric Statistics, 29,* 577–593.

Zhao, J., & Shao, J. (2015). Semiparametric pseudo-likelihoods in generalized linear models with nonignorable missing data. *Journal of the American Statistical Association, 110*(512), 1577–1590.

Zhao, J., & Shao, J. (2017). Approximate conditional likelihood for generalized linear models with general missing data mechanism. *Journal of Systems Science and Complexity, 30*(1), 139–153.

Zhao, J., Yang, Y., & Ning, Y. (2017). Penalized pairwise pseudo likelihood for variable selection with nonignorable missing data. arXiv preprint arXiv:1703.06379.

Zhao, P., & Yu, B. (2006). On model selection consistency of Lasso. *The Journal of Machine Learning Research, 7,* 2541–2563.

Adaptive Filtering Increases Power to Detect Differentially Expressed Genes

Zixin Nie and Kun Liang

1 Introduction

Detecting differentially expressed genes between conditions is a fundamental task in biomedical research. With the advent of the high-throughput technology such as microarray, the task becomes more challenging due to the large number of tests performed simultaneously. Typical microarray datasets contain measurements on thousands of genes, with a comparatively small number of samples.

One method to determine whether a gene is differentially expressed (DE) versus equivalently expressed (EE) is to perform variable-by-variable hypothesis testing (Dudoit et al. 2003; Kerr et al. 2000; Bourgon et al. 2010). The null hypothesis is no differential expression, for example, there is no difference in the mean measurements of a gene between a treatment group and a control group. Assuming the expression data are distributed normally, which is a reasonable assumption after a log transformation, t-tests can be performed and p-values can be computed accordingly.

When performing a large number of hypothesis tests simultaneously we need to adjust for multiplicity. Suppose we have m null hypotheses under consideration, of which m_0 are true nulls and m_1 are false nulls. Let $\pi_0 = m_0/m$ denote the true null proportion. Suppose the p-values associated with the m null hypotheses are $p_1, \ldots, p_m$, respectively. Furthermore, let $p_{(1)} \leq \ldots \leq p_{(m)}$ denote these p-values in ascending order. We can reject some null hypotheses, i.e., declare them significant, and the resulting classification is shown in Table 1. Two global error rates can be considered, the family-wise error rate (FWER), and the false discovery rate (FDR) due to Benjamini and Hochberg (1995). The FWER is defined to be $P(V \geq 1)$, or

Z. Nie • K. Liang (✉)
University of Waterloo, 200 University Ave W, Waterloo, ON, Canada
e-mail: zixinnie@gmail.com; kun.liang@uwaterloo.ca

© Springer International Publishing AG 2017   127
D.-G. Chen et al. (eds.), *New Advances in Statistics and Data Science*,
ICSA Book Series in Statistics, https://doi.org/10.1007/978-3-319-69416-0_8

Table 1 Classification of m		True null	False null	Total
null hypotheses	Declared significant	V	S	R
	Declared non-significant	U	T	$m - R$
	Total	m_0	$m - m_0$	m

the probability of having at least 1 false discovery. Controlling the FWER at level α means the probability of making even one false discovery is controlled at α. The FDR is defined to be the expected proportion of false discoveries, or $E[\frac{V}{R \vee 1}]$.

Controlling the FDR instead of the FWER will result in more detections (Benjamini and Hochberg 1995). The Benjamini-Hochberg (BH) procedure is the most commonly used method for controlling the FDR, which operates as follows:

1. For a given FDR target level α, let $k = \max\{i : p_{(i)} \leq i\alpha/m\}$.
2. Reject all hypotheses whose p-values $\leq p_{(k)}$.

The BH procedure controls the FDR at level $\pi_0 \alpha$ under independence and a special positive dependence condition (Benjamini and Yekutieli 2001). This motivates the more powerful *adaptive* procedures that apply the BH procedure at level $\alpha/\hat{\pi}_0$, where $\hat{\pi}_0$ is an estimator of π_0. A widely used π_0-estimator (Storey 2002) is

$$\hat{\pi}_0(\lambda) = \frac{\#\{p_i > \lambda\}}{(1 - \lambda)m},$$

where λ is a tuning parameter in $[0, 1)$ to be specified. Liang and Nettleton (2012) proposed the right-boundary (RB) procedure that selects λ from a candidate set according the observed p-values and guarantees that the resulting $\hat{\pi}_0(\lambda)$ is a conservative estimator of π_0. Briefly, for a λ candidate set $\Lambda = \{\lambda_1, \ldots, \lambda_J\}$ such that $0 \equiv \lambda_0 < \lambda_1 < \ldots < \lambda_J < 1$, the λ chosen is the first λ_j such that $\hat{\pi}_0(\lambda_j) \geq \hat{\pi}_0(\lambda_{j-1})$.

An alternative method for increasing the number of discoveries is to reduce the number of tests to perform. This is achieved by filtering hypotheses whose filtering statistics are below a certain threshold. In this paper, we will investigate the filtering approach in detail.

In Sect. 2, we briefly review the existing literature of filtering. We propose a novel adaptive filtering method in Sect. 3 and evaluate its performance in Sect. 4. Summaries and discussions are presented in Sect. 5.

2 Existing Filtering Methods

In the context of detecting differentially expressed genes, the filtering method can at least be traced back to Scholtens and Von Heydebreck (2005). Hackstadt and Hess (2009) performed simulation studies to compare different filtering methods.

When comparing two or more groups, Bourgon et al. (2010) first pointed out that, according to Basu's theorem, the overall mean and variance are independent of the test statistic when the null hypothesis is true. Thus, the overall mean and variance can serve as independent filter statistics without affecting the distribution of the test statistic under the null. Farcomeni and Finos (2013) further show that such independent filter statistics exist under a general linear model where nuisance parameters can be incorporated. On the other hand, the independent filter statistics can be correlated with the test statistic under the alternative and be useful to improve power, see Section 3 of Farcomeni and Finos (2013) for details. In the rest of the paper, we will work with the independent filter statistics.

When using the BH procedure to control the FDR, Hackstadt and Hess (2009) show that the realized FDR level can decrease as more tests are filtered out. If the EE genes are more likely to be filtered, then the true null proportion among the remaining hypotheses is likely to decrease and so is the FDR level if the BH procedure is used. This phenomenon calls for an adjustment of the true null proportion after filtering.

More importantly, it is unclear from the literature what fraction of genes should be filtered out. Ideally, we want to maximize the power or the number of the true positives. In practice, we do not know the true status of hypotheses, and a natural substitute is to maximize the number of rejections. However, Ignatiadis et al. (2016) show that a greedy filtering procedure that maximize the number of rejections over all possible filtering fractions leads to inflated FDR levels.

In the next section, we propose a novel method to address the true null proportion correction and filtering fraction selection simultaneously.

3 Proposed Method

Suppose in addition to the p-values, the filtering statistics associated with the m null hypotheses are $s_1, \ldots, s_m$, respectively. We consider selecting filter threshold θ from a candidate set $\Theta = \{\theta_i, i = 1, \ldots, I\}$. After filtering at threshold $\theta_i, i \in \{1, \ldots, I\}$, suppose there are m_i hypotheses left, among which m_{0i} are true nulls and m_{1i} are false nulls.

Definition 1 (Adaptive Filtering Procedure) For each $\theta_i, i \in \{1, \ldots, I\}$,

1. Filter hypotheses with filtering statistics $\leq \theta_i$.
2. Apply RB on the remaining p-values with a candidate λ set $\Lambda = \{\lambda_1, \ldots, \lambda_J\}$ to obtain $\hat{\pi}_{0i}^{RB}$.
3. Apply BH on the remaining p-values with target level of $\alpha / \hat{\pi}_{0i}^{RB}$.

Among all possible filter thresholds, choose the one with the largest # of rejections. We denote the index of the selected filter threshold as i^* and the corresponding λ chosen by RB as $\lambda_{i^*}^{RB}$.

After filtering at θ_i, $i \in \{1, \ldots, I\}$, for $t \in [0, 1]$, define the following empirical processes:

$$V_i(t) = \#\{\text{null} p_k : p_k \leq t \text{ and } s_k > \theta_i\},$$

$$S_i(t) = \#\{\text{alternative} p_k : p_k \leq t \text{ and } s_k > \theta_i\},$$

$$R_i(t) = V_i(t) + S_i(t).$$

Then the FDR at a fixed p-value cut-off $t \in (0, 1]$, denoted by $\text{FDR}(t)$, can be defined from the above processes as

$$\text{FDR}_i(t) = E\left[\frac{V_i(t)}{R_i(t) \vee 1}\right].$$

We also define the π_0-estimator after filtering as

$$\hat{\pi}_{0i}(\lambda) = \frac{\#\{p_k > \lambda \text{ and } s_k > \theta_i\}}{(1 - \lambda)m_i} = \frac{m_i - R_i(\lambda)}{(1 - \lambda)m_i}.$$

Assuming null p-values are independent and uniformly distributed on $(0, 1)$, a natural estimator of $\text{FDR}_i(t)$ is

$$\widehat{\text{FDR}}_{i,\lambda}(t) = \frac{m_i \hat{\pi}_{0i}(\lambda)t}{R_i(t) \vee 1}.$$

And the FDR estimator for the selected filter threshold according to our adaptive filtering procedure is

$$\widehat{\text{FDR}}_{i*,\lambda_{i*}^{RB}}(t) = \frac{m_{i*} \hat{\pi}_{0i*}(\lambda_{i*}^{RB})t}{R_{i*}(t) \vee 1}.$$

Consider the following conditions: for each $i \in \{1, \ldots, I\}$,

$$\lim_{m \to \infty} \frac{V_i(t)}{m_{0i}} = t \text{ almost surely for each } t \in (0, 1], \tag{1}$$

$$\lim_{m \to \infty} \frac{S_i(t)}{m_{1i}} = G_i(t) \text{ almost surely for each } t \in (0, 1]. \tag{2}$$

where G_i is a continuous function.

$$\lim_{m \to \infty} m_{0i}/m_i \equiv \pi_{0i} \text{ exists.} \tag{3}$$

We require these conditions to hold for each filter threshold, and they are parallel to the conditions (1)–(3) in Liang and Nettleton (2012). Condition 1 can be easily satisfied by the independence between null p-values and the filtering statistics and the uniform distribution of null p-values. Define the pointwise limit of $\widehat{FDR}_{i,\lambda}(t)$ under the conditions of (1)–(3) as

$$\widehat{FDR}_{i,\lambda}^{\infty}(t) \equiv \frac{\left\{\pi_{0i} + \frac{1-G_i(\lambda)}{1-\lambda}\pi_{1i}\right\} t}{\pi_{0i}t + \pi_{1i}G_i(t)},$$

where $\pi_{1i} = 1 - \pi_{0i}$. Furthermore, for any function $0 \leq F \leq 1$, define the step-up threshold function

$$t_\alpha(F) = \sup\{0 \leq t \leq 1 : F(t) \leq \alpha\}.$$

Then the adaptive filtering procedure controls the FDR asymptotically.

Theorem 1 *Suppose that conditions (1)–(3) hold. Also suppose there is a θ candidate set $\Theta = \{\theta_i, i = 1, \ldots, I\}$ and a λ candidate set $\Lambda = \{\lambda_j, j = 1, \ldots, J\} \in [0, 1)^J$, and the set size I and J are fixed finite integers. If for each $\theta_i \in \Theta$ and $\lambda_j \in \Lambda$ there exists a $t_{i,j} \in (0, 1]$ such that $\widehat{FDR}_{i,\lambda_j}^{\infty}(t_{i,j}) < \alpha$, then,*

$$\limsup_{m\to\infty} FDR\left\{t_\alpha(\widehat{FDR}_{i^*,\lambda_{i^*}^{RB}})\right\} \leq \alpha.$$

Proof Abbreviate $t_\alpha(\widehat{FDR}_{i,\lambda})$ by $t_\alpha^{i,\lambda}$. According to the conditions of the theorem, for each θ_i and λ_j there exist a $t_{i,j} > 0$ such that $\alpha - \widehat{FDR}_{i,\lambda_j}^{\infty}(t_{i,j}) = \varepsilon_{i,j} > 0$. We can let m be sufficiently large so that $|\widehat{FDR}_{i,\lambda_j}^{\infty}(t_{i,j}) - \widehat{FDR}_{i,\lambda_j}(t_{i,j})| < \varepsilon_{i,j}$, which implies that $\widehat{FDR}_{i,\lambda_j}(t_{i,j}) < \alpha$ and $t_\alpha^{i,\lambda_j} \geq t_{i,j}$. Therefore, $\liminf_{m\to\infty} t_\alpha^{i,\lambda_j} \geq t_{i,j}$ with probability 1. Similar to the proof of Theorem 5 of Liang and Nettleton (2012), it is straightforward to show

$$\liminf_{m\to\infty}\left[\widehat{FDR}_{i,\lambda_j}(t_\alpha^{i,\lambda_j}) - \frac{V_i(t_\alpha^{i,\lambda_j})}{R_i(t_\alpha^{i,\lambda_j}) \vee 1}\right] \geq \lim_{m\to\infty}\inf_{t \geq \delta_{i,j}}\left[\widehat{FDR}_{i,\lambda_j}(t) - \frac{V_i(t)}{R_i(t) \vee 1}\right] \geq 0$$

with probability 1 for $\delta_{i,j} = t_{i,j}/2$. By definition, $\widehat{FDR}_{i,\lambda_j}(t_\alpha^{i,\lambda_j}) \leq \alpha$, and it follows that

$$\limsup_{m\to\infty}\left[\frac{V_i(t_\alpha^{i,\lambda_j})}{R_i(t_\alpha^{i,\lambda_j}) \vee 1}\right] \leq \alpha,$$

with probability 1. Then,

$$\limsup_{m\to\infty}\left[\frac{V_{i^*}(t_\alpha^{i^*,\lambda_{i^*}^{RB}})}{R_{i^*}(t_\alpha^{i^*,\lambda_{i^*}^{RB}}) \vee 1}\right] \leq \limsup_{m\to\infty}\left[\max_{1\leq i\leq I, 1\leq j\leq J}\left\{\frac{V_i(t_\alpha^{i,\lambda_j})}{R_i(t_\alpha^{i,\lambda_j}) \vee 1}\right\}\right]$$

$$\leq \alpha,$$

with probability 1. Then by Fatou's lemma,

$$\limsup_{m \to \infty} \left(E\left[\frac{V_{i*}(t_\alpha^{i*,\lambda_{i*}^{RB}})}{R_{i*}(t_\alpha^{i*,\lambda_{i*}^{RB}}) \vee 1} \right] \right) \leq E\left[\limsup_{m \to \infty} \left[\frac{V_{i*}(t_\alpha^{i*,\lambda_{i*}^{RB}})}{R_{i*}(t_\alpha^{i*,\lambda_{i*}^{RB}}) \vee 1} \right] \right] \leq \alpha.$$

$\square$

On the surface, the adaptive filtering procedure is similar to the greedy filtering procedure proposed in Ignatiadis et al. (2016) that they both maximize the number of rejections across candidate filter thresholds. However, the two procedures are different in the number of candidates they consider. Ignatiadis et al. (2016) consider all possible filtering fractions, i.e., the θ candidate set size is the same as m. On the other hand, Theorem 1 requires that the θ candidate set size I be fixed and let m tend to infinity, which means in practice I should be small relative to m. For gene expression data where the number of genes are in the thousands, we propose to set $I = 20$.

4 A Data-Based Simulation Study

To mimic the characteristic of real gene expression data, we generate gene expression levels based on existing microarray data similar to the simulation schemes in Nettleton et al. (2008), Liang and Nettleton (2010), and Benidt and Nettleton (2015). Suppose we have an existing microarray dataset with a treatment group and a control group. To simulate G gene expression levels with G_0 EE genes and G_1 DE genes in a two-group setting with sample size of n in each group, we perform the following steps:

1. For each gene, calculate a p-value for differential expression using a regular two-sample t-test.
2. Calculate for each gene the probability of being DE using the fdrtool package (Strimmer 2008).
3. Compute the sampling weight vector w by subtracting the probability of DE from 1, and then normalize the weights so that they sum to unity.
4. Randomly select G_1 genes without replacement to be DE based on the sampling weights in w.
5. Randomly select G_0 genes without replacement to be EE. Thus, in total, we have $G = G_1 + G_0$ genes selected.
6. Randomly select n samples without replacement from the treatment group, subsetting to the set of G_1 DE genes. This will be our swap set.
7. Randomly select $2n$ samples without replacement from the control group, subsetting to the set of G selected genes. We will treat the first n samples as the simulated control group and the second n samples as the simulated treatment group.

8. Swap the G_1 genes in the swap set with the G_1 genes in the simulated treatment group.
9. Keep only the gene expressions in the simulated treatment and control groups.

The gene expression levels of G_0 genes are sampled from the same population (the original control group) and are EE by construction. On the other hand, the gene expression levels of G_1 genes are sampled from different populations and are DE. This simulation scheme is nonparametric and maintains the correlation structure among genes.

We could also simulate data parametrically with the parameters estimated from the original dataset. More specifically, we conduct the following steps:

1. For each gene, estimate its mean and variance in the original treatment and control groups, respectively.
2. Follow the steps 1–5 of the nonparametric simulation procedure to generate G_1 DE genes and G_0 EE genes.
3. For each EE gene, generate expression levels for $2n$ samples across both the simulated treatment and control groups by sampling from a normal distribution using the mean and variance of the same gene in the original control group.
4. For each DE gene, simulate expression levels from different normal distributions in the simulated treatment and control groups. First calculate the pooled variance across the original treatment and control groups to use as the variance, then generate expression levels for the n samples in the simulated control group using the mean of the original control group, and generate expression levels for the n samples in the simulated treatment group using the mean of the original treatment group.

In the parametric simulation setting, the gene expressions are independent between genes, which is the biggest difference comparing to the nonparametric simulation setting.

We use both the parametric and nonparametric settings to create simulated datasets, and compare the performances of the following four procedures:

(a) `Variance Filter`: the adaptive filtering procedure with overall variance as the filter statistic
(b) `Mean Filter`: the adaptive filtering procedure with overall mean as the filter statistic
(c) `limma`: with more than 5000 citations as of December, 2016, `limma` (Smyth 2004) is the most widely used method for detecting DE genes.
(d) `limma_RB`: `limma` using the right-boundary correction from Liang and Nettleton (2012).

Note that `limma` by default use the BH procedure to control FDR.

We used the B- and T-cell Acute Lymphocytic Leukemia dataset (Chiaretti et al. 2004) as our basis for simulation. Similar to Bourgon et al. (2010), we used the 37 samples with the BCR/ABL mutation as our treatment group and the 42 samples with no observed cytogenetic abnormalities as our control group.

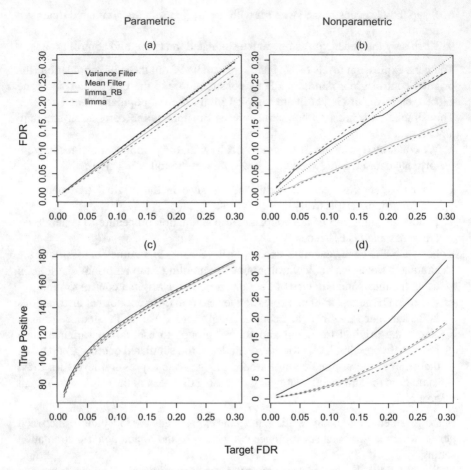

Fig. 1 Simulation results. Top row: realized FDR; dotted lines indicate diagonal lines. Bottom row: the number of true positives

Simulation settings are as follows: 5000 genes are simulated from the two datasets, with 500 set as DE. The sample size $n = 10$. Results were averaged over 1000 repeats. We search over the filtering fraction of 0%, 5%, ..., 95%. For the RB, we set $\Lambda = \{0.05, 0.1, \ldots, 0.95\}$ for parametric simulation and $\Lambda = \{0.05\}$ for nonparametric simulation, where the latter was suggested by Blanchard and Roquain (2009) for adaptive false discovery rate control under dependence. Figure 1 shows the realized FDR and the number of true positives as functions of the target FDR levels.

Under the parametric simulation setting, the realized FDR levels of Variance Filter and Mean Filter match precisely to the target FDR levels. Under the nonparametric simulation setting, the realized FDR levels of Variance Filter and Mean Filter only loosely follow the target FDR levelswith much more variations, likely due to the correlation among genes. In both settings, `Variance Filter` is the most powerful procedure, followed by `Mean Filter`, `limma_RB`, and `limma`.

The overall results show that filtering can lead to more powerful tests than `limma`. Although the best method for analyzing microarray data may depend on the dataset, filtering can be a simple yet effective approach to increase the power of detecting DE genes.

5 Conclusion

To increase the power of finding DE genes, we investigate the method of adaptive filtering to reduce the number of statistical tests and adapt to the true null proportion after filtering. We show that our proposed adaptive filtering procedure controls the FDR asymptotically. Using a data-based simulation method to mimic the characteristic of the real data, we conduct simulations to investigate whether filtering can detect more DE genes compared to other methods while maintaining proper FDR control. Simulation results show that filtering methods can maintain their FDR levels closely to the target FDR levels, while increasing the power of the test beyond that of `limma`.

Although we focus on the detection of DE genes, the proposed adaptive filter procedure can potentially be used in other settings, such as in chromatin immuno-precipitation with sequencing (Liang and Keleş 2012) and hypothesis testing with discrete data (Gilbert 2005), provided a good filtering statistic exists.

Acknowledgements Kun Liang is supported by Canada NSERC grant 435666-2013.

References

Benidt, S., & Nettleton, D. (2015). Simseq: A nonparametric approach to simulation of rna-sequence datasets. *Bioinformatics, 31*(13), 2131–2140.

Benjamini, Y., & Hochberg, Y. (1995). Controlling the false discovery rate: A practical and powerful approach to multiple testing. *Journal of the Royal Statistical Society: Series B, 57*, 289–300.

Benjamini, Y., & Yekutieli, D. (2001). The control of the false discovery rate in multiple testing under dependency. *Annals of Statistics, 29*, 1165–1188.

Blanchard, G., & Roquain, E. (2009). Adaptive false discovery rate control under independence and dependence. *Journal of Machine Learning Research, 10*, 2837–2871.

Bourgon, R., Gentleman, R., & Huber, W. (2010). Independent filtering increases detection power for high-throughput experiments. *Proceedings of the National Academy of Sciences, 107*(21), 9546–9551.

Chiaretti, S., Li, X., Gentleman, R., Vitale, A., Vignetti, M., Mandelli, F., et al. (2004). Gene expression profile of adult T-cell acute lymphocytic leukemia identifies distinct subsets of patients with different response to therapy and survival. *Blood, 103*(7), 2771–2778.

Dudoit, S., Shaffer, J. P., & Boldrick, J. C. (2003). Multiple hypothesis testing in microarray experiments. *Statistical Science, 18*, 71–103.

Farcomeni, A., & Finos, L. (2013). FDR control with pseudo-gatekeeping based on a possibly data driven order of the hypotheses. *Biometrics, 69*(3), 606–613.

Gilbert, P. B. (2005). A modified false discovery rate multiple-comparisons procedure for discrete data, applied to human immunodeficiency virus genetics. *Journal of the Royal Statistical Society: Series C, 54*(1), 143–158.

Hackstadt, A. J., & Hess, A. M. (2009). Filtering for increased power for microarray data analysis. *BMC Bioinformatics, 10*(1), 11.

Ignatiadis, N., Klaus, B., Zaugg, J. B., & Huber, W. (2016). Data-driven hypothesis weighting increases detection power in genome-scale multiple testing. *Nature Methods, 13*(7), 577–580.

Kerr, M. K., Martin, M., & Churchill, G. A. (2000). Analysis of variance for gene expression microarray data. *Journal of Computational Biology, 7*(6), 819–837.

Liang, K., & Keleş, S. (2012). Detecting differential binding of transcription factors with ChIP-seq. *Bioinformatics, 28*(1), 121–122.

Liang, K., & Nettleton, D. (2010). A hidden Markov model approach to testing multiple hypotheses on a tree-transformed gene ontology graph. *Journal of the American Statistical Association, 105*(492), 1444–1454.

Liang, K., & Nettleton, D. (2012). Adaptive and dynamic adaptive procedures for false discovery rate control and estimation. *Journal of the Royal Statistical Society: Series B, 74*(1), 163–182.

Nettleton, D., Recknor, J., & Reecy, J. M. (2008). Identification of differentially expressed gene categories in microarray studies using nonparametric multivariate analysis. *Bioinformatics, 24*(2), 192–201.

Scholtens, D., & Von Heydebreck, A. (2005). Analysis of differential gene expression studies. In *Bioinformatics and computational biology solutions using R and Bioconductor* (pp. 229–248). New York: Springer.

Smyth, G. (2004). Linear models and empirical Bayes methods for assessing differential expression in microarray experiments linear models and empirical Bayes methods for assessing differential expression in microarray experiments. *Statistical Applications in Genetics and Molecular Biology, 3*(1), 1–26.

Storey, J. (2002). A direct approach to false discovery rates. *Journal of the Royal Statistical Society: Series B, 64*(3), 479–498.

Strimmer, K. (2008). Fdrtool: A versatile R package for estimating local and tail area-based false discovery rates. *Bioinformatics, 24*(12), 1461–1462.

Estimating Parameters in Complex Systems with Functional Outputs: A Wavelet-Based Approximate Bayesian Computation Approach

Hongxiao Zhu, Ruijin Lu, Chen Ming, Anupam K. Gupta, and Rolf Müller

1 Introduction

Functional data, such as signals, surfaces, and images, are frequently encountered in many scientific disciplines. The increased prevalence of such data promotes the development of *functional data analysis* (Ferraty and Vieu 2006; Horváth and Kokoszka 2012; Ramsay and Silverman 1997; Wang et al. 2016). While considerable efforts have been made to the preprocessing (Ramsay and Li 1998; Tang and Müller 2008), estimation (Rice and Silverman 1991; Yang et al. 2016; Yao et al. 2005), and regression analysis (Cardot 2005; Chiou et al. 2003; Morris 2015; Scheipl et al. 2014; Zhu et al. 2011) of functional data, existing approaches primarily rely on linking functional observations with the unknown parameters via a likelihood or an objective function. Many applications, however, involve inferring parameters when such linkage is implicit or difficult to specify. In this paper, we consider a family of parameter estimation problems under such situations.

Hongxiao Zhu and Ruijin Lu contributed equally to this work.

H. Zhu (✉) • R. Lu
Department of Statistics, Virginia Tech, 250 Drillfield Drive, MC0439, Blacksburg, VA 24061, USA
e-mail: hongxiao@vt.edu; lruijin@vt.edu

C. Ming • A.K. Gupta • R. Müller
Department of Mechanical Engineering, Virginia Tech, 1075 Life Science Cir, MC0917, Blacksburg, VA 24061, USA
e-mail: cming@vt.edu; anupamkg@vt.edu; rolf.mueller@vt.edu

© Springer International Publishing AG 2017
D.-G. Chen et al. (eds.), *New Advances in Statistics and Data Science*,
ICSA Book Series in Statistics, https://doi.org/10.1007/978-3-319-69416-0_9

137

Fig. 1 A conceptual
demonstration of the
parameter estimation
problems we consider

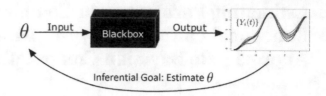

Figure 1 provides a conceptual demonstration of the estimation problems we consider. The black box represents an unknown complex system that takes the parameter θ as input and produces functional observations $\{Y_i(t)\}$ as outputs. Our goal is to estimate the underlying parameter θ based on the observed functional outputs. If the relationship between $\{Y_i(t)\}$ and θ is known, for example, if $\{Y_i(t)\}$ are independent and identically distributed Gaussian processes with mean zero and a covariance kernel that depends on θ, we can estimate θ through maximum likelihood or Bayesian method. There are, however, many other situations in which the true linkage between $\{Y_i(t)\}$ and θ is more complicated, and scientists use physical rules and/or mathematical equations to model such linkage. To illustrate these situations, we provide two examples—the light detection and ranging (LIDAR) data and the foliage-echo data.

1. *The LIDAR data.* LIDAR is an optical remote-sensing technique that uses laser light to measure targets and produces high-resolution functional data. For example, authors in Xun et al. (2013) considered LIDAR data measured on an aerosol cloud. During the measurement, a point source laser was transmitted into an aerosol cloud at multiple wavelengths and over multiple time points. The laser light was then scattered by the aerosol cloud and reflected back to a receiver. The resulting data can be modeled by $Y(t, z) = g(t, z) + \varepsilon(t, z)$, where t is time, z is the range value, $Y(t, z)$ is the random surface that can be observed, $g(t, z)$ is the underlying true signal, and $\varepsilon(t, z)$ is the random measurement error. The linkage between $g(t, z)$ and the parameters of interest is implicit, described by a partial differential equation (PDE):

$$\frac{\partial g(t, z)}{\partial t} - \theta_D \frac{\partial^2 g(t, z)}{\partial z^2} - \theta_S \frac{\partial g(t, z)}{\partial z} - \theta_A g(t, z) = 0,$$

   subject to boundary conditions. Here, the parameters θ_D, θ_S, and θ_A denote the diffusion rate, the drift shift, and the reaction rate respectively, which reflect the physical properties of the laser light reflection. Consequently, the relationship between the functional observation $Y(t, z)$ and the parameters is implicit, and one cannot write the likelihood of $Y(t, z)$ in terms of the parameters explicitly.

2. *The foliage-echo data.* The foliage-echo data represents a more general situation when functional data is produced by a complicated system which cannot be described using a single formula (e.g., a PDE). During the measurement, an active sonar system transmits acoustic waves into tree foliages, and the waves reflected back from the foliages (i.e. the echoes) are received. While the

mechanism of sound propagation and reflection is complicated, we are able to simulate echoes using a simulator by applying acoustic laws under simplified assumptions. Details of the simulation are described in Sect. 2 and the Appendix. Our goal is to estimate properties of the foliages, such as the density of the leaves (i.e., how many leaves per cubic meter), based on the echoes.

The above two examples demonstrate functional data produced by complex systems. These systems have the following characteristics: (1) Due to the complexity of the underlying physical rules, the parameter estimation is a difficult inverse problem which may be ill-posed, meaning that the solution to the parameter estimation may not be unique. For example, both LIDAR and foliage-echo examples are remote sensing problems in which the data are aggregations of reflected waveforms from numerous reflectors; therefore, it is possible that different combinations of the model parameters result in the same/similar data outputs. Furthermore, analytical or numerical solution to these inverse problems is often hard to find. (2) One can numerically simulate data from a physical/mathematical model (e.g., a PDE or a more complicated simulator), but the simulation may be computationally intensive. (3) The data-generation procedure of the complex system involves random variables, hence, it produces random functional outputs for a given set of parameters. For example, in both LIDAR and foliage-echo examples, randomness may be caused by measurement error and/or numerous reflecting facets whose size, location, and orientation follow certain probability distributions. (4) It is often difficult to explicitly link the functional outputs with the underlying parameters via a likelihood or an objective function. (5) The functional outputs are often measured on a dense, high-dimensional grid.

For systems that can be described using ordinary differential equations (ODEs) or PDEs, such as the LIDAR data case, estimation approaches based on regularized optimization, also called *parameter cascading*, have been proposed (Ramsay et al. 2007; Lu et al. 2011; Xun et al. 2013; Zhang et al. 2017). These methods, however, are not suitable for systems that cannot be described by ODEs or PDEs. In this paper, we propose a wavelet-based approximate Bayesian computation (wABC) approach that is applicable to general complex systems—systems that include ODE and PDE as special cases. For this reason, we will use the more general foliage-echo data as our primary example.

The proposed wABC approach inherits the "likelihood-free" property of the traditional approximate Bayesian computation (ABC) (Marin et al. 2012; Turner and Van Zandt 2012) through bypassing analytical evaluations of the likelihood function. The bypassing is achieved through approximating the likelihood function evaluation by simulation. The basic idea is illustrated in Fig. 2. Specifically, instead of evaluating the likelihood, the ABC approach first samples a candidate parameter θ^* from the prior distribution $\pi(\theta)$, then simulates data $\{X_i\}$ from a "simulator" of the system by treating θ^* as the input. If the simulated data is "close to" the observed data, the candidate parameter θ^* is accepted, otherwise it is rejected. A more detailed review of ABC can be found in Sect. 3.1.

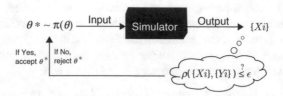

Fig. 2 The basic idea of the ABC method. Here, $\{X_i\}$ represent the simulated data, $\{Y_i\}$ represent the observed data, and $\rho(\cdot, \cdot)$ measures how "close" the simulated data are to the observed data

Despite their flexibility in handling complex systems, as a simulation-based approach, the ABC method suffers from low efficiency when the dimension of the observed data increases and when the "simulator" becomes computationally expensive. As the dimension of the data increases, the criterion $\rho(\{X_i(t)\}, \{Y_i(t)\}) \leq \varepsilon$ is harder to be satisfied, resulting in lower acceptance rate. When the "simulator" becomes moderately expensive, even on the scale of a few seconds per simulation, accepting 1000 samples of θ would require hours of calculation, and the computation quickly becomes intractable when the acceptance rate drops. Our proposed wABC approach extends beyond existing ABC by allowing functional outputs measured on high-dimensional grid, yet still remains computationally tractable. It relies on the near-lossless wavelet decomposition and compression to reduce the high-correlation between measurement points and the high-dimensionality, and adopts a Markov chain Monte Carlo algorithm with a Metropolis-Hastings sampler to obtain posterior samples of the parameters. To avoid expensive simulations, a Gaussian process surrogate for the simulator is introduced, and the uncertainty of the resulting sampler is controlled by calculating the expected error rate of the acceptance probability.

To our knowledge, the proposed wABC approach is the first that estimates parameters in complex systems based on functional outputs measured on a dense, high-dimensional grid. It is generally applicable to various physical, chemical, and biological systems that facilitate numerical simulations. Compared with existing functional data analytical tools, our approach has the following advantages: (1) It is likelihood-free. It takes full advantages of the physical/mathematical rules that connect data with the parameter. (2) It can characterize various linear or nonlinear data-parameter relationships. (3) It produces the joint posterior distribution of the parameters with various multi-modality and shape structures. (4) It is scalable to functional outputs measured on high-dimensional grids as well as expensive simulations. Our results for the simulated foliage-echo data demonstrate the effectiveness of the proposed method in estimating parameters.

2 A Motivating Example: The Foliage-Echo Simulation System

While the method we propose is generally applicable to various complex systems, it is initially motivated by the foliage-echo study. The goal of the study is to estimate the statistical properties of tree foliages, i.e., the density of the leaves, the average size of the leaves, and the average orientation of the leaves, based on the echo signals captured by a sonar device.

Figure 3 shows the working mechanism of an active sonar, which consists of an emitter that ensonifies the environment and a receiver that records the returning echoes. The transmitter emits acoustic waves and the receiver collects echoes reflected from objects in the environment. The echo signals carry information about the targets, hence have been used for various identification and navigation tasks (Vanderelst et al. 2016). In natural environments, an echo signal is the superposition of reflected waveforms from numerous scatterers, e.g., foliage leaves, rocks in uneven natural terrains, thus is highly stochastic.

To study the foliage echoes, we establish a computational model to simulate a natural sonar scene in a three-dimensional (3-d) space. The scene is demonstrated in Fig. 4a, which consists of an active sonar sensor and a cluster of tree leaves. The sensor is located at the origin. It emits ultrasonic waves towards the positive x-axis direction. The tree foliages are uniformly located in a $[1, 10] \times [-2, 2] \times [-2, 2]$ region in 3-d. The total number of leaves is determined by the leaf density—the number of leaves per cubic meter, denoted by θ_1. The leaf shapes are approximated by planar circular disks with radius (denoted by a) randomly sampled from a normal distribution $N(\theta_2, 0.1\theta_2)$, where θ_2 denotes the mean radius. The orientation of each leaf relative to the sonar is determined by two angles: (1) the angle between the leaf normal vector and pulse direction (the positive x-axis direction), which follows a truncated normal distribution $N(x|\theta_3, 5)1_{\{0<x<90\}}$ with θ_3 the mean angle and 5 the variance; and (2) the angle that describes the rotation of the leaf normal vector around the pulse direction clockwisely, which follows a uniform distribution in the range of $[0, 2\pi)$. Based on these two angles, we further calculate the incident angle—the angle between the leaf's normal direction and the sonar-leaf center line. We denote the incident angle by β. With these setups and the specification of

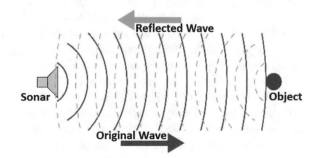

Fig. 3 The principle of an active sonar. This figure was created based on an online figure available at the Wikipedia website on Sonar (Wikipedia 2017) (https://en. wikipedia.org/wiki/Sonar)

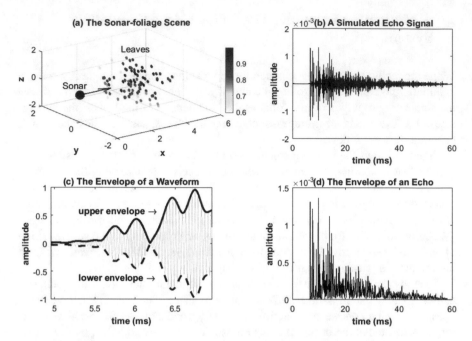

Fig. 4 The Foliage-echo Simulation. (**a**) The sonar scene in 3-d. The color indicates the sound intensity leaves receive/reflect (scaled to $[0, 1]$). (**b**) A simulated echo signal with leaf density of 30 (in number of leaves per cubic meter), leaf radius of 0.0171 (in meter), and leaf orientation of 45 (in degree). (**c**) A demonstration of the upper and lower envelopes of the waveform. (**d**) The echo envelope extracted from the echo signal in (**b**)

acoustic properties of the sonar, echoes are simulated following acoustic laws of sound emission, propagation, and reflection (Bowman et al. 1987). More technical details of the simulator are described in the Appendix.

The above simulation model constitutes a physical system with three inputs: the leaf density (θ_1), the mean leaf radius (θ_2), and the mean leaf orientation (θ_3). The output is an echo signal as demonstrated in Fig. 4b. The output echo signal is a temporal waveform measured from 0 to 60 ms with a sampling rate of 400 kHz. The total number of measurement points is 24,000 for each echo. The parameters ($\theta_1, \theta_2, \theta_3$) summarize statistical properties of the foliage targets. Therefore, estimating these parameters based on the echo signals provides us knowledge of the targets. While the current study only involves echoes simulated from a physical model, our ultimate hope is to use the proposed estimation approach to infer target properties based on echoes collected in a real scene.

Directly modeling the echo signals is difficult because the echoes contain information about both emitted signals and the target properties. Since sound reflection from stationary targets does not change the carrier frequency of the emitted signal, information about targets is contained in the amplitude modulation, which is captured by the *envelopes* of the echo signals. We therefore perform a preprocessing step to extract the echo envelopes, and use this data for our analysis. The envelope of a signal is the boundary curve within which all amplitude values of the signal are contained. A conceptual demonstration is shown in Fig. 4c. The envelope of an echo retains the target-specific information by capturing the low frequency amplitude variations, which makes it an ideal representation of echo signals. In the sonar echo data, since the upper and the lower envelopes are always symmetric, we only consider the upper envelopes in our data analysis. The envelope signal extracted from the echo in Fig. 4b is shown in Fig. 4d.

3 Wavelet-Based Approximate Bayesian Computation

The foliage-echo data example demonstrated in Sect. 2 represents a family of parameter estimation problems involving functional data. In these problems, functional data is related to the parameters of interest through a complex system guided by physical or mathematical rules. As a result, one cannot explicitly write the likelihood of the functional outputs as a function of the parameters. To facilitate parameter estimation under these scenarios, we propose a wavelet-based Approximate Bayesian Computation (wABC) approach. The logic behind the main concepts introduced in Sects. 3.1–3.4 and their connections with wABC are illustrated in Fig. 5. Section 3.1 reviews the general ABC approach, which is the foundation for the proposed wABC approach. In order to facilitate functional outputs measured on a dense, high-dimensional grid, we represent functional data through wavelet basis expansion and perform a wavelet compression to reduce dimension; details are in Sect. 3.2. For simulators that are computationally expensive, we further introduce the Gaussian process surrogate for the simulator to enable fast simulation; this is discussed in Sect. 3.3. Sections 3.1–3.3 constitute the general framework of wABC. Finally, in Sect. 3.4, we introduce a method to control the uncertainty of the decision-making in wABC.

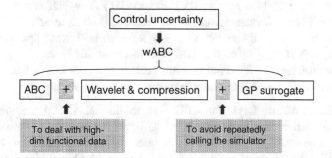

Fig. 5 The logic behind the concepts introduced in Sects. 3.1–3.4 and their connections with wABC

3.1 Review of Approximate Bayesian Computation

Let Y denote a random element whose realizations are the observed data and let θ denote a parameter that determines the distribution of Y. In a typical Bayesian setup, one computes the posterior distribution $\pi(\theta|Y) \propto \pi(Y|\theta)\pi(\theta)$, where $\pi(Y|\theta)$ is the likelihood that relates Y to the parameter θ and $\pi(\theta)$ is the prior distribution for θ. Approximate Bayesian Computation (ABC), initially proposed by Pritchard et al. (1999), aims to approximate the posterior distribution $\pi(\theta|Y)$ without explicitly specifying the likelihood $\pi(Y|\theta)$. In particular, we assume that $\pi(Y|\theta)$ is unknown, but there is a simulation model, often denoted by $\pi(X|\theta)$, that produces simulated data X given θ^*. We sometimes call X the pseudo-data. Here, θ^* is an arbitrary sample from the prior distribution $\pi(\theta)$. If X is "close to" Y, we retain θ^* as a sample of $\pi(\theta|Y)$, otherwise we reject θ^* and repeat the procedure with a new θ^*. This procedure, as illustrated in Fig. 2, will be repeated until the desired amount of "good samples" is collected. In ABC, we often use a distance measure $\rho(\cdot, \cdot)$ to determine how close X is to Y. For example, in the univariate case, by letting $\rho(X, Y) = |X - Y|$, we will retain θ^* when $|X - Y| \le \varepsilon$ for a small ε.

The above procedure indeed produces samples for the distribution $\pi(\theta|\{\rho(X, Y) \le \varepsilon\})$, a distribution that is identical to $\pi(\theta|Y)$ when $\varepsilon = 0$ (i.e., $X = Y$). However, since $\{X=Y\}$ happens with probability 0 for continuous random variables, in practice, we can only require $\rho(X, Y) \le \varepsilon$ for a small discrepancy ε, which results in $\pi(\theta|\{\rho(X, Y) \le \varepsilon\})$. The distribution $\pi(\theta|\{\rho(X, Y) \le \varepsilon\})$ serves as an approximation of $\pi(\theta|Y)$ when ε is small, i.e.,

$$\pi(\theta|Y) \approx \pi(\theta|\rho(X, Y) \le \varepsilon), \text{ for a small } \varepsilon.$$

When multiple samples are observed, we index the data by Y_i, $i = 1, \ldots, n$ and denote $\mathbf{Y} = \{Y_1, \ldots, Y_n\}$. In this case, ABC can be performed by sampling $\mathbf{X} = \{X_1, \ldots, X_m\}$ based on each θ^*, and define $\rho(\cdot, \cdot)$ based on a summary statistic $S(\cdot)$ of the samples. If $S(\mathbf{Y})$ is a sufficient statistic for θ, then $S(\mathbf{Y})$ contains all information about θ, therefore $\pi(\theta|\mathbf{Y}) = \pi(\theta|S(\mathbf{Y}))$, which can be shown by applying the Fisher-Neyman factorization theorem (Lehmann and Casella 1998). The right-hand side of the equation $\pi(\theta|S(\mathbf{Y}))$ can be further approximated by $\pi(\theta|\rho(S(\mathbf{X}), S(\mathbf{Y})) \le \varepsilon)$ using the ABC. For example, if $\{Y_1, \ldots, Y_n\}$ is a random sample from a Bernoulli distribution with mean θ, then one can define $\rho(\mathbf{X}, \mathbf{Y}) = |\bar{Y} - \bar{X}|$, where $S(\mathbf{Y}) = \bar{Y}$ is the sample mean, a sufficient statistic for θ.

Markov Chain Monte Carlo for ABC The traditional ABC procedure relies on accepting θ^* when $\rho(S(\mathbf{X}), S(\mathbf{Y})) \le \varepsilon$. This procedure can be embarrassingly inefficient because of two reasons: (1) A good sufficient statistic can be hard to find. Sometimes one has to use the original data set as the sufficient statistic. (2) The acceptance rate can be extremely low especially when the statistic $S(\cdot)$ or the parameter θ is of high dimension. Various alternative algorithms have been proposed to improve the computational efficiency of ABC. Here, we review an Markov chain Monte Carlo (MCMC) algorithm using the Metropolis-Hastings (MH) sampler.

More discussions of the MCMC algorithm for ABC can be found in Wegmann et al. (2009), Didelot et al. (2011), Meeds and Welling (2014), and Sadegh and Vrugt (2014), among others. First, we transfer the acceptance criterion $\rho(S(\mathbf{X}), S(\mathbf{Y})) \leq \varepsilon$ to a probability density function $\pi_\varepsilon(S(\mathbf{Y}) \mid S(\mathbf{X}))$ controlled by the discrepancy parameter ε. For example, with an independent Gaussian assumption, we may write

$$\pi_\varepsilon(S(\mathbf{Y}) \mid S(\mathbf{X})) = (2\pi\varepsilon)^{-J/2} \exp\{-\frac{1}{2\varepsilon^2}(S(\mathbf{X}) - S(\mathbf{Y}))^T (S(\mathbf{X}) - S(\mathbf{Y}))\}, \quad (1)$$

where J is the dimension of the sufficient statistic $S(\cdot)$. With this representation, we can approximate the likelihood $\pi(S(\mathbf{Y}) \mid \theta)$ by $\pi_\varepsilon(S(\mathbf{Y}) \mid \theta)$, and the latter can be approximated using the Monte Carlo integration

$$\pi_\varepsilon(S(\mathbf{Y}) \mid \theta) = \int \pi_\varepsilon(S(\mathbf{Y}) \mid S(\mathbf{X}))\pi(S(\mathbf{X}) \mid \theta) \, dS(\mathbf{X})$$

$$\approx \frac{1}{H} \sum_{g=1}^{H} \pi_\varepsilon(S(\mathbf{Y}) \mid S(\mathbf{X}^{(g)})). \quad (2)$$

Here, $\{\mathbf{X}^{(g)}, g = 1, \ldots, H\}$ denote H samples of the pseudo-data generated from the simulator, $\pi(\mathbf{X} \mid \theta)$. Note that we do not need to evaluate $\pi(S(\mathbf{X}) \mid \theta)$ in Eq. (2). We just need to sample from it. Based on the approximated likelihood, we can design a MCMC algorithm by assuming an proposal distribution $q(\theta^*|\theta)$. We accept the proposed θ^* with probability

$$\alpha(\theta^*|\theta) = \min\left\{1, \frac{\pi(\theta^*)\pi_\varepsilon(S(\mathbf{Y}) \mid \theta^*)q(\theta|\theta^*)}{\pi(\theta)\pi_\varepsilon(S(\mathbf{Y}) \mid \theta)q(\theta^*|\theta)}\right\}.$$

The above MCMC algorithm provides improved mixing for the posterior samples than the traditional rejection-based ABC algorithm. However, it requires H repeated calls to the simulator in order to compute the approximation in Eq. (2), and this has to be performed during each MCMC iteration. Here, H needs to be large enough to guarantee a good approximation, e.g., $H = 1000$ is reasonable if $\pi(S(\mathbf{X}) \mid \theta)$ is a Gamma distribution. Repeated sampling can be a computational burden when the simulator runs slow. In Sect. 3.3, we adopt a Gaussian process surrogate (GPS) for the simulator following the idea of Meeds and Welling (2014), which substantially reduces the number of simulation calls.

3.2 Wavelet Representation and Compression of Functional Data

While the idea of ABC is straightforward to follow, it can be inefficient due to a number of assumptions and approximations that may not be easily satisfied. One assumption is the existence of a sufficient statistic for the parameters of interest.

Given a random sample $\mathbf{Y} = \{Y_1, \ldots, Y_n\}$, the determination of a sufficient statistic $S(\mathbf{Y})$ for θ is often difficult without knowing the distribution of Y_i. Although one can always choose the data itself as the sufficient statistic, doing so only makes the specification of the distance measure $\rho(\cdot, \cdot)$ extremely difficult (because the dimension of $\mathbf{Y}$ is high). This issue is particularly severe for high dimensional vectors and functional data. In our foliage-echo example, an echo envelope is of dimension 24,000, therefore, the data $\mathbf{Y}$ can be written as a n-by-24,000 matrix. Given that the relationship between the data and the parameters is implicit, determining a sufficient statistics for $(\theta_1, \theta_2, \theta_3)$ given $\mathbf{Y}$ is practically intractable.

To facilitate the efficient performance of ABC for functional data measured on a dense, high-dimensional grid, we adopt a strategy that achieves de-correlation and compression so that functional observations can be parsimoniously represented in a much lower dimensional setting. In particular, we represent the functional data by a multi-scale wavelet basis. Given a set of multi-scale wavelet basis functions $\{\psi_{jk}; j = 1, \ldots, J, \ k = 1, \ldots, K_j\}$ and a scale function (the father wavelet) $\{\psi_{0k}; k = 1, \ldots, K_0\}$, we can expand a functional observation $Y(t)$ by $Y(t) = \sum_{j=0}^{J} \sum_{k=1}^{K_j} d_{jk} \psi_{jk}(t)$. Here, d_{jk} is the wavelet coefficient at scale j and location k. For functional data measured on an equally spaced grid, this representation is *lossless*, i.e., providing an exact representation of the original data. Therefore, $\{d_{jk}\}$ contain the same amount of information as $Y(t)$ thus can be treated as a sufficient statistic for θ. We can denote the sufficient statistics of $\mathbf{Y}$ as $S(\mathbf{Y}) = \mathbf{D}$, where $\mathbf{D} = (d_{ijk})$ is a n-by-K matrix and $K = \sum_{j=0}^{J} K_j$. In general, the wavelet transformation is not the only option. It is possible to construct lossless transforms with other basis functions (e.g. Spline or Fourier bases), or construct an approximately lossless transformation with a basis $\{B_k(t), k = 1, \ldots, K\}$ that satisfies $|Y(t) - \sum_{k=1}^{K} d_k B_k(t)| < \delta$ for all t and a small δ.

The wavelet representation has two advantages: the coefficients $\{d_{jk}\}$ are sparse, meaning that most coefficients are zero or close-to-zero, and they are approximately uncorrelated. These properties bring two types of convenience to the specification of the distance measure in ABC. First, since components in $\{d_{jk}\}$ are approximately uncorrelated, the conditional distribution $\pi_\varepsilon(S(\mathbf{Y}) \mid S(\mathbf{X}))$ can be specified following Eq. (1), i.e., assuming that components of $S(\mathbf{Y})$ (or $S(\mathbf{X})$) are mutually independent of each other. Second, the sparsity of the wavelet coefficients makes the wavelet compression feasible.

Wavelet Compression For many high-dimensional problems, representing the data in a much lower dimensional space brings tremendous convenience to data storage and processing. This is also true in the ABC context. Let $\mathbf{D} = (d_{ijk})$ denote the n by K matrix of wavelet coefficients, and the ith row corresponds to the wavelet coefficients of the ith functional observation. Since $\mathbf{D}$ is sparse, many components of $\mathbf{D}$ are zero or close-to-zero, therefore do not contain essential information about the parameter. Wavelet compression removes zero or close-to-zero components while retaining large components. The compressed matrix, denoted by $\widetilde{\mathbf{D}}$, is nearly lossless, thus can be used as an approximately sufficient statistic for θ. To compress $\mathbf{D}$, we retain K_1 columns of $\mathbf{D}$ so that the proportion of energy retained is greater than (or equal to) a threshold δ_1 (e.g., $\delta_1 = 0.999$) for each function. Here, the proportion of energy retained for a function $Y_i(t)$ is defined by $\sum_{(j,k) \in C_1} d_{ijk}^2 / \sum_{(j,k)} d_{ijk}^2$, where C_1 is the set of scale and location indices that correspond to columns retained in $\widetilde{\mathbf{D}}$.

The wavelet representation and compression introduced above provide an effective way to transform the functional observation $\mathbf{Y}$ to wavelet coefficient matrix $\mathbf{D}$ in the wavelet domain, and to reduce the dimension of $\mathbf{D}$ from n-by-K to n-by-K_1. The compression also has the effect of removing high frequency noise in functional data. The reduced data $\widetilde{\mathbf{D}}$ will be treated as a sufficient statistics of $\mathbf{Y}$ to be used in the MCMC sampling scheme for wABC.

3.3 A Gaussian Process Surrogate for the Simulator

As discussed in Sect. 3.1, although the MCMC method can provide better mixing than the traditional rejection-based ABC method, it requires sampling from the simulator H times during each MCMC iteration. Even if each simulation only requires a moderate amount of time, running a large amount of MCMC iterations can be computationally intractable. For example, our foliage-echo simulator takes 2.3 s to simulate one echo envelope. If the MCMC algorithm has an acceptance rate of 30%, $H = 100$, and the number of independent samples in $\mathbf{X}$ is $m = 3$, the expected time needed to obtain 1000 posterior samples of θ is around 639 h (26.6 days). It is possible to use parallel computing at the stage of computing $\pi_\varepsilon(S(\mathbf{Y}) \mid \theta)$, i.e., during each MCMC, the H samples of $\mathbf{X}$ (which contain Hm echoes) can be performed in parallel using a multi-core computing server. However, it may still take days to obtain 1000 posterior samples of θ because the number of computing cores one has access to is often limited. The modern graphics processing units (GPU) based computing system provides far more computing cores (Sanders and Kandrot 2010), but each core can only deal with relatively simple calculation, therefore may not be suitable for the large-scale matrix calculations required by our simulator. When the speed of the simulator cannot be improved any further, a good solution is to adopt a strategy that requires less calls of the simulator. We now introduce a GPS for the simulator following the idea of Meeds and Welling (2014). GPS can substantially reduce the number of simulation calls in the MCMC.

We explain the GPS in the context of the foliage-echo example. Suppose that J columns of $\mathbf{D}$ are retained after wavelet compression. Let $\widetilde{\mathbf{D}}_y = (\mathbf{d}_y^1, \ldots, \mathbf{d}_y^J)$ denote the n-by-J matrix of wavelet coefficients after compression, where each $\mathbf{d}_y^j$ is an n-by-1 vector. The randomness in the leaf location, orientation, and radius causes random fluctuations in the n samples. These fluctuations reflect the leaf-specific information, i.e., exact locations, orientations, and radii of leaves in a scene, which is not relevant to the population parameters $(\theta_1, \theta_2, \theta_3)$. Therefore, we remove the random fluctuation by averaging each $\mathbf{d}_y^j$ across its n entries, resulting in a scalar $\bar{d}_y^j$. Denote the averaged wavelet coefficients by $\bar{\mathbf{D}}_y = (\bar{d}_y^1, \ldots, \bar{d}_y^J)^T$. We will use $S(\mathbf{Y}) = \bar{\mathbf{D}}_y$ in the analysis of foliage-sonar data. Since the wavelet coefficients in

$\mathbf{D}_y$ are approximately independent of each other, we will calculate the likelihood $\pi_\varepsilon(\overline{d}_y^j \mid \theta)$ for each j independently. We assume that

$$\overline{d}_y^j = \overline{d}_x^j + e^j, \quad e^j \sim N(0, \varepsilon^2). \tag{3}$$

Here, $\overline{d}_x^j$ is the jth averaged wavelet coefficients based on the simulated samples $\mathbf{X} = \{X_1, \ldots, X_m\}$. Model (3) is equivalent to assuming that $\pi_\varepsilon(\overline{d}_y^j \mid \overline{d}_x^j)$ corresponds to a $N(\overline{d}_x^j, \varepsilon^2)$ distribution. We further approximate the simulator distribution $\pi(\overline{d}_x^j \mid \theta)$ by assuming that $\overline{d}_x^j$ follows a Gaussian process (GP) regression model:

$$\overline{d}_x^j = f_j(\theta) + r_j, \quad f_j(\theta) \sim GP(0, k_j(\theta, \theta^*)), \quad r_j \sim N(0, \sigma_j^2), \tag{4}$$

where $f_j(\theta)$ is an unknown GP with mean zero and a pre-specified covariance kernel $k_j(\theta, \theta^*)$. For example, a commonly used covariance kernel is the squared exponential kernel $k_j(\theta, \theta^*) = \phi_j^2 \exp\{-||\theta - \theta^*||^2/(2\tau_j^2)\}$. Since both (3) and (4) induce Gaussian distributions, we can analytically calculate $\pi_\varepsilon(\overline{d}_y^j \mid \theta)$ by integrating out $\overline{d}_x^j$. This analytical integration avoids the need to perform approximation using Monte Carlo integration as described in Eq. (2). We call the GP regression model (4) a GPS. The main idea is to train a GP model on a grid of θ and use it to replace the simulation distribution $\pi_\varepsilon(\overline{d}_y^j \mid \theta)$. This strategy avoids the need of frequently calling the simulator during the MCMC iteration.

Specifically, we calculate $\pi_\varepsilon(\overline{d}_y^j \mid \theta)$ following a three-step procedure.

1. Produce a grid of values $\Theta = (\theta_1, \ldots, \theta_A)^T$ on the domain of θ, generate $\mathbf{X} = \{X_1, \ldots, X_m\}$ at each grid point, perform wavelet decomposition and compression of $\mathbf{X}$, and average the wavelets coefficients across the m samples. This results in a list of "input-output" pairs $\{(\theta_i, \overline{d}_{x,i}^j), i = 1, \ldots, A\}$, which will be treated as the training data for estimating the function $f_j(\theta)$.
2. Given a pair of values (θ^*, θ), we will calculate the GP predictive distribution on (θ^*, θ) using the conditional distribution, which gives $N(\mu_{(\theta^*,\theta)|\Theta}^j, \Sigma_{(\theta^*,\theta)|\Theta}^j)$, where

$$\mu_{(\theta^*,\theta)|\Theta}^j = \begin{pmatrix} \mathbf{k}_{\theta^*,\Theta} \\ \mathbf{k}_{\theta,\Theta} \end{pmatrix} \left(\mathbf{K}_{\Theta,\Theta} + \sigma_j^2 \mathbf{I}\right)^{-1} \overline{\mathbf{d}}_x^j, \tag{5}$$

$$\Sigma_{(\theta^*,\theta)|\Theta}^j = \begin{pmatrix} k_{\theta^*,\theta^*} & k_{\theta^*,\theta} \\ k_{\theta,\theta^*} & k_{\theta,\theta} \end{pmatrix} - \begin{pmatrix} \mathbf{k}_{\theta^*,\Theta} \\ \mathbf{k}_{\theta,\Theta} \end{pmatrix} \left(\mathbf{K}_{\Theta,\Theta} + \sigma_j^2 \mathbf{I}\right)^{-1} \begin{pmatrix} \mathbf{k}_{\theta^*,\Theta} \\ \mathbf{k}_{\theta,\Theta} \end{pmatrix}^T. \tag{6}$$

Here, $\overline{\mathbf{d}}_x^j = (\overline{d}_{x,1}^j, \ldots, \overline{d}_{x,A}^j)^T$ is an A-by-1 vector of training points, $\mathbf{k}_{\theta^*,\Theta}$ is a 1-by-A vector consisting of kernel evaluations at θ^* and components in Θ, $\mathbf{K}_{\Theta,\Theta}$ is an A-by-A matrix consisting of kernel evaluations at two components in Θ, and $k_{\theta^*,\theta} = k(\theta^*, \theta)$. We treat the above GP conditional distribution as a *surrogate* of the simulator. In Fig. 6, we compared the prediction performance of the GPS at a test value of θ_1 with the sample estimate obtained from data directly sampled

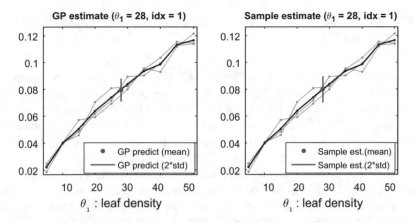

Fig. 6 A one-dimensional demonstration of the GP prediction using the sonar-foliage simulator. Here, we have fixed $\theta_2 = 0.017$ and $\theta_3 = 45$, and treated θ_1 as the unknown parameter. Left panel: the gray lines are the first wavelet coefficient of $m = 3$ simulated echo envelopes at $A = 10$ grid points on the domain $[5, 50]$; the black lines are the average of the three gray lines; the magenta dot and line are the predictive mean and the confidence interval (*mean* $\pm$ 2 *std*) calculated using the GPS. Right panel: the gray lines and the black lines are the same as the left panel. The magenta dot is the sample estimate of the mean, and the magenta bar is the confidence interval based on 100 echoes sampled directly from the simulator

from the simulator. Here, we have fixed θ_2 and θ_3, treating θ_1 as the parameter to be estimated. Figure 6 demonstrates that the GPS gives as accurate prediction as the sample estimates (which are based on 100 samples) using only 10 training locations on the support of θ_1.

3. Based on the GPS, the likelihoods $\pi_\varepsilon(\bar{d}_y^j \mid \theta^*)$ and $\pi_\varepsilon(\bar{d}_y^j \mid \theta)$ can be approximated by $N(\bar{d}_y^j|\mu_{\theta*}^{j,\dagger}, \sigma_j^2 + \varepsilon^2)$ and $N(\bar{d}_y^j|\mu_\theta^{j,\dagger}, \sigma_j^2 + \varepsilon^2)$ respectively, where $(\mu_{\theta*}^{j,\dagger}, \mu_\theta^{j,\dagger})$ is a sample from $N(\mu_{(\theta*,\theta)|\Theta}^j, \Sigma_{(\theta*,\theta)|\Theta}^j)$. The acceptance probability of the MCMC can be calculated by

$$\alpha(\theta^*|\theta) = \min\left\{1, \frac{\pi(\theta^*)\prod_{j=1}^{J}N(\bar{d}_y^j|\mu_{\theta*}^{j,\dagger}, \sigma_j^2 + \varepsilon^2)q(\theta|\theta^*)}{\pi(\theta)\prod_{j=1}^{J}N(\bar{d}_y^j|\mu_\theta^{j,\dagger}, \sigma_j^2 + \varepsilon^2)\ q(\theta^*|\theta)}\right\}. \qquad (7)$$

Note that if the function $f_j(\cdot)$ is known, we can replace $\mu_{\theta*}^{j,\dagger}$ and $\mu_\theta^{j,\dagger}$ by the true values of $f_j(\theta^*)$ and $f_j(\theta)$ respectively, in which case $\alpha(\theta^*|\theta)$ is a deterministic value. However, since we have used GPS, the randomness of $\mu_{\theta*}^{j,\dagger}$ and $\mu_\theta^{j,\dagger}$ introduces uncertainty to $\alpha(\theta^*|\theta)$. This uncertainty may cause an error for decision-making in the MCMC algorithm. Therefore, we need to control the uncertainty so that the probability of making a wrong decision based on $\alpha(\theta^*|\theta)$ is reasonably low. We discuss this issue in Sect. 3.4.

3.4   Control the Uncertainty of Decision-Making in wABC Using GPS

The control of uncertainty in the GPS-based MCMC algorithm serves two purposes: to control the error rate of making decisions (e.g., the decision of accepting/rejecting the proposed θ^*) based on GPS in the MCMC algorithm, and to provide a strategy of refining the GPS of the simulator. The main idea is to keep adding training data to the GPS at each iteration until the expected probability of making the wrong decision is less than a pre-specified threshold ξ (e.g., $\xi = 0.3$).

In particular, since $\mu_{\theta*}^{j,\dagger}$ and $\mu_{\theta}^{j,\dagger}$ are random samples from the GPS, α in Eq. (7) is a random variable. In stead of making decisions based on one α value, we produce L samples $\{\alpha^{(l)}, l = 1, \ldots, L\}$, and calculate a summary statistic ζ from it. We will accept θ^* if $u < \zeta$ and reject θ^* if $u \geq \zeta$. Here, $u \sim \text{Unif}(0, 1)$.

Now we can calculate the probability of making a mistake following the above decision rule. If $u < \zeta$, we will accept θ^*, and this will be a wrong decision if indeed $\{u > \alpha\}$, in which case we should reject θ^*. The probability that this situation appears is $1_{\{u<\zeta\}}Pr(\{u > \alpha\})$. Similarly if $u \geq \zeta$, the probability of making a wrong decision is $1_{\{u\geq\zeta\}}Pr(\{u \leq \alpha\})$. Therefore, given a value of u, the overall probability of making an error is

$$W_u(\alpha) = 1_{\{u<\zeta\}}Pr(\{u > \alpha\}) + 1_{\{u\geq\zeta\}}Pr(\{u \leq \alpha\}), \quad u \sim \text{Unif}(0, 1).$$

We can further integrate out u from the above conditional error function to obtain the marginal probability of making an error, i.e.,

$$W(\alpha) = \int_0^1 W_u(\alpha)du,$$

The above error probability $W(\alpha)$ is minimized when $\zeta = median(\alpha)$; a detailed argument can be found in the Section 3.1 of Meeds and Welling (2014) and the reference therein.

The above result enables us to control the probability of making a wrong decision in the Step 3 in Sect. 3.3 by calculating α L times, each with different samples of $\mu_{\theta*}^{j,\dagger}$ and $\mu_{\theta}^{j,\dagger}$. This calculation is very efficient since obtaining L samples from a multivariate normal distribution is fast. Based on the L samples of α, we set ζ to be the sample median of α and calculate $W(\alpha)$ numerically. If $W(\alpha) > \xi$, we will add more training points (i.e., creating a denser grid on the support of θ) and repeat Step 2–3 in Sect. 3.3 again, until $W(\alpha) \leq \xi$. We finally accept the proposed θ^* if $u < \zeta$ for a random u sampled from $\text{Unif}(0, 1)$. This completes one iteration of the MCMC. The above adaptive strategy allows us to adjust for the training points for the GPS so that the probability of making a wrong decision is controlled during each MCMC iteration.

4 The Algorithm and Parameter Settings

We describe the algorithm for the proposed wABC approach in the context of foliage echo data. Detailed steps are described in Algorithm 1. Algorithm 1 is an approximate MCMC algorithm because we have used GPS to approximate the simulator. These samples are used to approximate samples from the simulator. With GPS, we only need to call the simulator Δ times at each iteration under the condition $W(\alpha) > \xi$. As more training points are added, the GPS will become more reliable. Eventually, there will be no need to call the simulator at all during the MCMC iterations.

Algorithm 1: An MCMC algorithm for wavelet-based ABC using GPS

Input: $\mathbf{Y}$, A, Δ, θ, ε, ξ, $q(\cdot \mid \cdot)$, $\{\sigma_j^2\}$, $\pi(\theta)$, m, N, $k(\cdot, \cdot)$, the simulator.

Step 1: Perform wavelet decomposition and compression on $\mathbf{Y}$ to get $\widetilde{\mathbf{D}}_y$.

Step 2: Create a grid Θ of size A. Generate initial training points $\mathbf{X}$ from the simulator at each grid point in Θ. Perform wavelet decomposition and compression on each $\mathbf{X}$ to get $\{(\theta_i, \bar{d}_{x,i}^j), i = 1, \ldots, A\}$ for $j = 1, \ldots, J$.

Step 3: Run the following MCMC iterations.

for $i = 1$ *to* N **do**

    Propose θ^* from $q(\theta^* \mid \theta)$;

    while $W(\alpha) > \xi$ **do**

        Step 3.1: Calculate the mean and covariance for (θ^*, θ) following (5)–(6) for all j, $j = 1, \ldots, J$;

        Step 3.2: Generate L samples of $\mu_{\theta*}^{j,\dagger}$ and $\mu_\theta^{j,\dagger}$ and calculate $\{\alpha^{(l)}, l = 1, \ldots, L\}$ using equation (7);

        Step 3.3: Set $\zeta = \text{median}(\{\alpha^{(l)}, l = 1, \ldots, L\})$ and calculate the probability of making a wrong decision $W(\alpha)$;

        if $W(\alpha) > \xi$ **then**

            Add Δ grid points to Θ, generate new training data at each newly added grid point. Add these points to the existing training points;

        end

    end

    Sample $u \sim \text{Unif}(0, 1)$;

    if $u < \zeta$ **then**

        Set $\theta = \theta^*$;

    end

    Save θ;

end

Output: N posterior samples of θ.

For the numerical stability of the algorithm and the convenience of setting parameters, we recommend to rescale the compressed data $\widetilde{\mathbf{D}}_y$ and the simulated features $\widetilde{\mathbf{D}}_x$ using a common set of constants so that all values are in a similar scale (e.g., $[-1, 1]$). The scaling constants can be estimated from the observed data (e.g., using the minimum and maximum of $\mathbf{d}_y^j$ for each j). Similarly, in the GPS calculation, we recommend to scale all θ parameters to a common range (e.g., $[0, 1]$).

Parameter Settings There are two types of model parameters we need to specify in the wABC algorithm—those in the GPS and those in the MCMC algorithm. Generally speaking, we suggest to determine parameters in GPS by checking the GP prediction at some θ values, so that the resulting GP prediction is comparable with that obtained by directly sampling from the simulator. Figure 6 provides an example of such comparison. Furthermore, we suggest to tune parameters in the MCMC algorithm by controlling the expected performance of the algorithm, such as the acceptance rate of the Metropolis-hastings sampler. In what follows, we introduce some specific guidelines.

The parameter ε in Eq. (7) is a small value that controls the expected discrepancy between simulated and observed data. We suggest to set a small value (e.g., 1e−4) for ε. In the GPS MCMC algorithm, it is possible to set $\varepsilon = 0$ as done by Meeds and Welling (2014). The parameters $\{\sigma_j^2\}$ in (4) control the noise level in the GP regression. We found that these parameters may substantially influence the predictive covariance of the GPS, i.e., the covariance in (6). A reasonable way to determine $\{\sigma_j^2\}$ is to take the empirical variance of $\mathbf{d}_x^j$ (calculated across the m replicates of $\widetilde{\mathbf{D}}_x$) and average them across all grid points in Θ. The parameters in the GP kernel $k(\cdot,\cdot)$ also play important roles in determining the predictive mean and covariance of the GPS. We have used the squared exponential kernel $k_j(\theta,\theta^*) = \phi_j^2 \exp\{-||\theta-\theta^*||^2/(2\tau_j^2)\}$ for each j. In the foliage-echo data analysis, we have scaled the θ parameters to $[0,1]$ and scaled all $\bar{d}_x^j, j = 1,\ldots,J\}$ to $[-1,1]$. Under these setups, we found that setting $\phi_j \equiv 0.1$ and $\tau_j \equiv 0.4$ is a reasonable choice. In practice, we recommend the users to start with the one-parameter settings (i.e., fixing all other parameters) and plot the predictive error bar like shown in Fig. 6. This helps visualize the effect of the parameter setups. The parameters ξ, m, N, A, and Δ can be tuned based on the computation speed and the acceptance rate of the MCMC algorithm.

In general, the accuracy of the posterior estimation can be improved by increasing the sample size in data $\mathbf{Y}$, reducing the threshold ξ for the probability of making an error in the MH sampler, increasing the size of the training grid for GPS, and increasing the number of training samples m at each GP training grid.

5 The Analysis of Simulated Foliage-Echo Data

While our ultimate goal is to apply wABC on real foliage-echo data collected under experimental or natural environments, at this stage, the real data have not yet been made available. Therefore, in this analysis, we will only provide the parameter estimation result based on echoes simulated from the foliage-echo simulation model described in the Appendix. Because the true parameters are known in this simulation setup, our analysis provides the proof-of-concept for the feasibility of wABC for complex systems.

We applied the proposed wABC approach to a set of foliage-echo data simulated from the sonar-foliage simulator. The data consists of $n = 100$ echo envelope signals sampled independently from the simulator under the true parameter $(\theta_1, \theta_2, \theta_3) = (30, 0.017, 45)$. We aim to solve the inverse-problem by estimating the three underlying parameters based on the 100 echo envelopes while assuming that the domains of the parameters are $\theta_1 \in [5, 50]$, $\theta_2 \in [0.005, 0.05]$, and $\theta_3 \in [1e{-}4, 90]$.

We applied the wavelet transformation to each echo envelope using Daubechies wavelets with the maximal number of vanishing moments being 12 (i.e., db12). The number of resolution levels is set to be $J = 20$, and the boundary extension mode is set to be periodic. The wavelet decomposition transforms each echo envelope from the time domain (with 24,000 measurement points) to the wavelet domain (with 24,008 wavelet coefficients). We further applied wavelet compression by retaining $\delta_1 = 0.999$ of the total energy. This reduces the dimension of the wavelet coefficients from 24,008 to 992. We then applied MCMC with GPS using Algorithm 1. We adopted a random walk proposal by setting the proposal distribution $q(\theta^* \mid \theta)$ to be a truncated log-normal with a scale parameter 0.05. To train the GPS, we segmented the domain of $(\theta_1, \theta_2, \theta_3)$ using a $10 \times 10 \times 10$ equally-spaced grid. This gave a total of 1000 training points for the GPS. The number of repeated samples in $\mathbf{X}$ on each grid point was set to be $m = 3$. The kernel parameters for the Gaussian process kernel function were set to be $\phi_j \equiv 0.1$, $\tau_j \equiv 0.4$. The ε parameter in the MCMC-ABC was set to be $1e{-}4$ and the ξ parameter in the GPS procedure was set to be 0.3. These setups resulted in an acceptance rate of 35% in the MCMC MH sampler. We monitored the behavior of the posterior samples by checking the trace plots and the autocorrelation plots. We tested the convergence of the chains by calculating the Geweke's Z-statistics (Geweke 1992). We ran 30,000 MCMC iterations and took the first 10,000 iterations as the burn-in period. Summary statistics of the parameter estimation, including the posterior means and the 95% credible intervals (CIs), are listed in Table 1. Table 1 shows that all three CIs cover the true values of the parameters.

We further summarized the posterior distribution of parameters using 1-d and 2-d marginal kernel density estimations. In Fig. 7, we plot the heatmaps of the 2-d kernel density estimations for each pair of the parameters. The gray dots on the heatmaps are the scatter plots of the posterior samples (a total of 15,000 samples

Table 1 The posterior estimation for the three parameters in the foliage-echo data

	θ_1	θ_2	θ_3
Meaning	Density in 3-d	Mean radius	Mean orientation
Unit	Counts per m^3	Meter	Degree
Domain	[5, 50]	[0.005, 0.05]	[1e$-$4, 90]
True value	30	.017	45
Post. mean	28.45	.018	42.57
Post. CIs	[17.1, 41.9]	[.017, .026]	[10.1, 72.7]

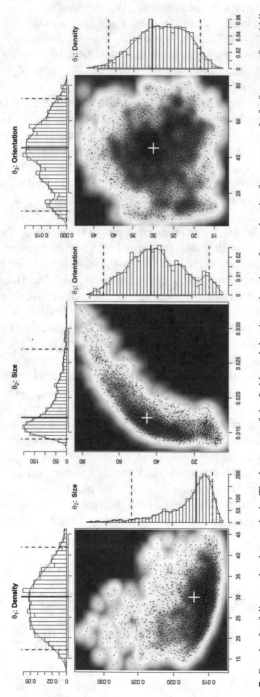

Fig. 7 Results for foliage-echo data analysis. The heatmaps of the 2-d kernel density estimations for each pair of parameters. Left: θ_1 versus θ_2; middle: θ_2 versus θ_3; right: θ_3 versus θ_1. The gray dots on the heatmaps are the scatter plots of the posterior samples. The white cross symbol on the heatmaps marks the true parameter values. The histograms on the top and the right-hand side of each heatmap are the marginal distributions (histograms superimposed by the 1-d kernel density estimations) for each parameter. The red vertical bar in each histogram indicates the location of the posterior mean, and the red dashed bars indicate the 95% credible interval

after the burnin period). The white cross sign on the heatmaps mark the true values of the parameters. The histograms on the top and right-hand side of each heatmap show the marginal distributions of the parameters (superimposed by the 1-d density estimations). The red vertical bar in each histogram indicates the location of the posterior mean, and the red dashed bars indicate the 95% credible interval.

From Fig. 7, we observe that the posterior distributions of the parameters demonstrate skewed, multi-modality shapes. In particular, the marginal distribution of the leaf size is skewed to the right, and the leaf orientation demonstrates two modes, one near 10° and the other near 40°. Furthermore, the 95% CIs for the leaf density and the orientation are fairly wide. Wide CIs indicate high uncertainty in the point estimates. These results are not a surprise, because they reflect several characteristics of the foliage-echo simulation. First, the echo signals are highly stochastic—using 100 echoes samples to recover the statistical properties of the foliages is a challenging task. Second, the multi-modal behavior of the posterior distribution reflects the non-identifiability nature of the inverse-problem, i.e., different combinations of the leaf density, size, and orientation could result in similar reflection behavior of the sound wave. Therefore, the solution to the inverse-problem is not unique. Despite these challenges, our proposed wABC still provide a comprehensive view for the distributions of the underlying parameters under a moderate number of samples—a result that is intractable if using any other existing statistical approaches. These results demonstrate the promise of solving ill-posed inverse-problems even when the data is highly stochastic and of high-dimension.

6 Discussion

We have proposed a general simulation-based approach called wABC to estimate the parameters of a complex system with functional data outputs. The proposed method relies on simulating from the complex system to estimate the parameters of interest, which avoids the difficulty of specifying the intractable likelihood. We accommodate functional data measured on a dense, high-dimensional grid by combining wavelet decomposition with compression, and achieve scalable computation using a Gaussian process surrogate to the simulator. Our inference is based on posterior samples of the underlying parameters which can be used to recover the joint distributions of all parameters.

The proposed wABC approach is generally applicable to a large family of inverse-problems associated with complex systems, such as solving differential equations based on noisy data and estimating parameters of a biological system. However, it requires a "simulator" to generate pseudo-data. The simulator needs to resemble the real system with sufficient accuracy. Otherwise, even if the wABC is tuned to perform well with simulated data, it may fail on real-word data.

While the GPS has the benefit of avoiding repeatedly calling the simulator, the computation of GP may become inefficient when the number of grid points goes beyond 1000. The main difficulty comes from the evaluation of the inverse covariance matrix in the predictive calculation, i.e., Eqs. (5)–(6). Our future work involves replacing the GPS by a local-GPS, i.e., using only a portion of the training points to predict the mean and standard deviation at (θ^*, θ). A promising strategy is to use the K-nearest neighbor approach. Similar ideas have been adopted by Gramacy and Apley (2015) and Gramacy and Haaland (2014) in GP regression.

While we have focused on systems with highly-stochastic functional outputs, the proposed framework is also suitable for deterministic systems in which the simulator yields a deterministic functional output subject to random measurement error. An example is the LIDAR data introduced in Sect. 1. In these situations, we just need to set $n = 1$ and $m = 1$ in wABC. These problems are often easier to solve than the stochastic systems considered here.

Although ABC brings substantial convenience by enabling likelihood-free inference, it is well-recognized that ABC suffers from "curse of dimensionality" when the number of parameters increases. That is, it becomes more difficult to accept a proposed parameter θ^* as the dimension of the parameter space increases (Turner and Van Zandt 2012). We adopted an MCMC algorithm in this paper, which has been proposed to attenuate the low acceptance rate issue. However, it remains generally true that a larger number of parameters is more expensive to be estimated using ABC-based approaches.

Though a real data analysis is not included in this paper, our simulation study provides a solid validation of the statistical component of the method. Given that the proposed method performs well under simulated setting, the only situation under which it will fail in a real data analysis is when the physical model (i.e., the simulator) does not describe the scenario of the real data properly. If that happens, one either adjusts the way to collect real data or modifies the physical model.

Finally, we note that it remains a future work to develop the theoretical properties of the proposed wABC approach. In particular, it is of interest to demonstrate the convergence of the MCMC to a stationary distribution, and show that the resulting stationary distribution approximates the true posterior distribution with a bounded error. These theoretical investigations may be done following the arguments/hints in Korattikara et al. (2014) and Meeds and Welling (2014).

Appendix: More Details of the Foliage-Echo Simulator

In this appendix, we provide more details about the simulation model. Let $Y(t)$ denote a random echo signal to be simulated based on the sonar scene described in Sect. 2. We will simulate $Y(t)$ discretely, i.e., simulate the vector $\mathbf{y} = (y_1, \ldots, y_v)^T$, a discretized version of $Y(t)$. Here, the sampling frequency of $\mathbf{y}$ is 400 kHz. To achieve this, we first simulate $\widehat{\mathbf{y}} = (\widehat{y}_1, \ldots, \widehat{y}_{v'})^T$, which is the Fourier transform of $\mathbf{y}$ in the frequency domain. We then apply the inverse fast Fourier transform to $\widehat{\mathbf{y}}$ to obtain $\mathbf{y}$.

Each component in $\widehat{\mathbf{y}}$ corresponds to a fixed frequency. We denote by f_k the frequency corresponding to $\widehat{y}_k$ (the kth component of $\widehat{\mathbf{y}}$). In this simulation, we mimic the frequency range of a horseshoe bat's echolocation call (Vaughan et al.

1997) and only simulate the Fourier components corresponding to frequencies in the range of $[60, 80]$ kHz. All other Fourier components are set to zero. For $f_k \in [60, 80]$ kHz, $\widehat{y}_k$ is a complex number in the form of $\widehat{y}_k = \sum_{i=1}^{s} A_{k,i} \cos(\phi_{k,i}) + j \sum_{i=1}^{s} A_{k,i} \sin(\phi_{k,i})$, where j denotes the imaginary unit, s denotes the number of leaves considered, $A_{k,i}$ is the amplitude at frequency f_k for the ith leaf, and $\phi_{k,i}$ is a phase delay parameter at f_k for the ith leaf.

The key of our simulation is the calculation of $\{(A_{k,i}, \phi_{k,i}), k = 1, \ldots, v', i = 1, \ldots, s\}$ based on the physical laws of sound transmission and reflection. This calculation is performed through four steps:

1. **Simulate the foliage scene.** From the input parameters $(\theta_1, \theta_2, \theta_3)$, simulate the total number of leaves (denoted by s_0), the radii of leaves $\{a_i\}$, the 3-d coordinates of the leaf centers $\{(x_i, y_i, z_i), i = 1, \ldots, s_0\}$, and the incident angles $\{\beta_i, i = 1, \ldots, s_0\}$ following the description in Sect. 2.
2. **Select leaves that contribute to echo.** Based on the locations of the leaves and the sonar, we calculate the sonar's beampattern gains (i.e., the spatial distribution of sound pressure) at all leaves, and filter out those leaves that have small gain values. Therefore, only leaves at locations with large enough sonar gain values are used to simulate **y**. We denote the number of leaves passing this filter by s.
3. **Calculate amplitudes.** The parameter $A_{k,i}$ represents the amplitude corresponding to the wave reflected from the ith leaf at frequency f_k. It is calculated based on the formula:

$$A_{k,i} = S(az_i, el_i, f_k, r_i) L_i(\beta_i, a_i, f_k) \frac{\lambda_k}{2\pi r_i^2}. \tag{8}$$

Below, we will explain the meaning of each factor in (8):

(a) The factor $S(az_i, el_i, f_k, r_i)$ denotes the sonar beampattern, a function that describes the spatial distribution of the power density of the emitted wave. The arguments (az_i, el_i) denote the azimuth and elevation angles of the line that connects the origin (i.e., the sonar) and the ith leaf center, and the argument r_i denotes the distance between the sonar and the ith leaf center. Here, (az_i, el_i) and r_i can be directly calculated from the leaf center coordinates (x_i, y_i, z_i). For a given sonar, $S(\cdot)$ is assumed to be known. In this study, we used a Gaussian function to approximate the sonar beampattern. The parameters of the Gaussian function are determined using empirical data. In particular, the Gaussian function parameters are determined by three variables: the beamwidth of the sonar beampattern (-3 dB), the direction that sonar faces, and the peak amplitude of the sonar beampattern.
(b) The factor $L_i(\beta_i, a_i, f_k)$ denotes the beampattern of the ith leaf, which describes the spatial distribution of the power density of the reflected wave at the ith leaf. Here, β_i is the incident angle of the ith leaf, a_i is the radius of the ith leaf, and f_k is the kth frequency. The leaf beampattern can be calculated using complicated physical equations (Bowman et al. 1987). In this study, we approximate the leaf beampattern using

$$L_i(\beta_i, a_i, f_k) = P_1(c(f_k, a_i)) \cos(P_2(c(f_k, a_i))\beta_i),$$

where $c(f_k, a_i) = 2\pi a_i f_k / v$, $v = 340$ (meters per second) denotes the speed of sound, $P_1(c(f_k, a_i)) = 0.5003c^2 + 0.6867$, and $P_2(c(f_k, a_i)) = 0.3999c^{-0.9065} + 0.9979$. The functions $P_1(\cdot)$ and $P_2(\cdot)$ are nonlinear regression functions estimated based on data obtained from numerical evaluation (Adelman et al. 2014).

(c) In the factor $\lambda_k/(2\pi r_i^2)$, r_i is the distance between the sonar and the ith leaf center, and λ_k is the wavelength of the emitted sound wave corresponding to the frequency f_k. Here, λ_k is a known constant.

4. **Calculate phase delays.** The phase delay parameters $\{\phi_{k,i}\}$ reflect the phase change at leaf i and frequency f_k due to wave propagation. After waves travel r_i meters, the phase delay becomes $2\pi r_i/\lambda_k$. As it is a round trip for the sound to travel from sonar to leaf and from leaf to sonar, the phase delay due to propagation is $4\pi r_i/\lambda_k$. Another part that contributes to the phase delay is the phase shift after the wave strikes the leaf. The phase shift depends on the frequency f_k, the leaf radius a_i, and the incident angle β_i. To make the computation efficient, we estimate the phase shift by fitting a nonlinear regression based on data obtained from numerical evaluation (Adelman et al. 2014), which gives

$$\text{Phase\_shift}(f_k, a_i, \beta_i) = \text{erf}(\text{PA}(c(f_k, a_i))(1.57 - \beta_i)) - 2.6343,$$

where $\text{erf}(x) = \frac{2}{\sqrt{\pi}} \int_0^x e^{-t^2} dt$, $\text{PA}(c(f_k, a_i)) = 0.9824c(f_k, a_i)^{0.3523} - 0.9459$, and $c(f_k, a_i) = 2\pi a_i f_k / v$. Based on these results, the phase delay can be calculated by

$$\phi_{k,i} = -\frac{4\pi r_i}{\lambda_k} - \text{Phase\_shift}(f_k, a_i, \beta_i) \tag{9}$$

Steps 1–4 provide the values of $\{(A_{k,i}, \phi_{k,i})\}$, based on which we can calculate the frequency domain vector $\widehat{\mathbf{y}}$. The final time domain signal $\mathbf{y}$ is calculated by using the inverse fast Fourier transform. Before applying the transform, we also applied a Hann window function to weight $\widehat{\mathbf{y}}$, which helps minimize the signal side lobes (unwanted ripples) in the resulting time domain signal.

References

Adelman, R., Gumerov, N. A., & Duraiswami, R. (2014). Software for computing the spheroidal wave functions using arbitrary precision arithmetic. CoRR. http://arxiv.org/abs/1408.0074
Bowman, J., Senior, T., & Uslenghi, P. (1987). *Electromagnetic and acoustic scattering by simple shapes*. New York: Hemisphere Publishing Corporation.

Cardot, H. (2005). Nonparametric regression for functional responses with application to conditional functional principle component analysis. http://www.lsp.ups-tlse.fr/Recherche/Publications/2005/car01.pdf

Chiou, J., Müller, H., & Wang, J. (2003). Functional quasi-likelihood regression models with smooth random effects. *Journal of the Royal Statistical Society: Series B (Statistical Methodology)*, *65*, 405–423.

Didelot, X., Everitt, R. G., Johansen, A. M., & Lawson, D. J. (2011). Likelihood-free estimation of model evidence. *Bayesian Analysis, 6*(1), 49–76. https://doi.org/10.1214/11-BA602

Ferraty, F., & Vieu, P. (2006). *Nonparametric functional data analysis*. New York, Springer.

Geweke, J. (1992). Evaluating the accuracy of sampling-based approaches to the calculation of posterior moments. *Bayesian Statistics, 4*, 169–193.

Gramacy, R. B., & Apley, D. W. (2015). Local gaussian process approximation for large computer experiments. *Journal of Computational and Graphical Statistics, 24*(2), 561–578.

Gramacy, R. B., & Haaland, B. (2014). Speeding up neighborhood search in local Gaussian process prediction. ArXiv e-prints.

Horváth, L., & Kokoszka, P. (2012). *Inference for functional data with applications*. New York: Springer.

Korattikara, A. B., Chen, Y., & Welling, M. (2014). Austerity in MCMC land: Cutting the Metropolis-Hastings budget. In *Proceedings of the 31st International Conference on Machine Learning, Cycle 1, JMLR Proceedings* (Vol. 32, pp. 181–189). JMLR.org.

Lehmann, E. L., & Casella, G. (1998). *Theory of point estimation* (2nd ed.). New York: Springer.

Lu, T., Liang, H., Li, H., & Wu, H. (2011). High dimensional odes coupled with mixed-effects modeling techniques for dynamic gene regulatory network identification. *Journal of the American Statistical Association, 106*(496), 1242–1258.

Marin, J. M., Pudlo, P., Robert, C. P. R., & Ryder, R. J. (2012). Approximate Bayesian computational methods. *Statistics and Computing, 22*, 1167–1180.

Meeds, E., & Welling, M. (2014). GPS-ABC: Gaussian process surrogate approximate Bayesian computation. In *Proceedings of the 30th Conference on Uncertainty in Artificial Intelligence (UAI)*.

Morris, J. S. (2015). Functional regression. *Annual Review of Statistics and Its Application, 2*, 321–359.

Pritchard, J.K., Seielstad, M. T., Perez-Lezaun, A., Feldman, M. W. (1999). Population growth of human Y chromosomes: A study of y chromosome microsatellites. *Molecular Biology and Evolution, 16*, 1791–1798.

Ramsay, J. O., & Li, X. (1998). Curve registration. *Journal of the Royal Statistical Society: Series B (Statistical Methodology), 60*(2), 351–363.

Ramsay, J. O., & Silverman, B. W. (1997). *Functional data analysis*. New York: Springer.

Ramsay, J. O., Hooker, G., Campbell, D., & Cao, J. (2007). Parameter estimation for differential equations: A generalized smoothing approach. *Journal of the Royal Statistical Society: Series B (Statistical Methodology), 69*(5), 741–796.

Rice, J. A., & Silverman, B. W. (1991). Estimating the mean and covariance structure nonparametrically when the data are curves. *Journal of the Royal Statistical Society: Series B (Statistical Methodology), 53*, 233–243.

Sadegh, M., & Vrugt, J. A. (2014). Approximate Bayesian computation using Markov chain monte carlo simulation: Dream(abc). *Water Resources Research, 50*(8), 6767–6787. https://doi.org/10.1002/2014WR015386

Sanders, J., & Kandrot, E. (2010). *CUDA by example: An introduction to general-purpose GPU programming* (1st ed.). Boston, MA: Addison-Wesley Professional.

Scheipl, F., Staicu, A. M., & Greven, S. (2014). Functional additive mixed models. *Journal of Computational and Graphical Statistics, 24*, 477–501.

Tang, R., & Müller, H. G. (2008). Pairwise curve synchronization for functional data. *Biometrika, 95*(4), 875.

Turner, B. M., & Van Zandt, T. (2012). A tutorial on approximate Bayesian computation. *Journal of Mathematical Psychology, 56*, 69–85.

Vanderelst, D., Steckel, J., Boen, A., Peremans, H., & Holderied, M. W. (2016). Place recognition using batlike sonar. *eLife, 5*, e14188. https://doi.org/10.7554/eLife.14188

Vaughan, N., Jones, G., & Harris, S. (1997). Identification of british bat species by multivariate analysis of echolocation call parameters. *Bioacoustics, 7*(3), 189–207.

Wang, J.-L., Chiou, J.-M., & MÏler, H. (2016). Functional data analysis. *Annual Review of Statistics and Its Application, 3*, 257–295.

Wegmann, D., Leuenberger, C., & Excoffier, L. (2009). Efficient approximate Bayesian computation coupled with markov chain monte carlo without likelihood. *Genetics, 182*(4), 1207–1218. https://doi.org/10.1534/genetics.109.102509

Wikipedia (2017). Sonar — Wikipedia, the free encyclopedia. https://en.wikipedia.org/wiki/Sonar. Accessed 20 May 2017.

Xun, X., Cao, J., Mallick, B., Maity, A., & Carroll, R. J. (2013). Parameter estimation of partial differential equation models. *Journal of the American Statistical Association, 108*(503), 1009–1020.

Yang, J., Zhu, H., Choi, T., & Cox, D. D. (2016). Smoothing and mean-covariance estimation of functional data with a Bayesian hierarchical model. *Bayesian Analysis, 11*(3), 649–670.

Yao, F., Müller, H. G., & Wang, J. L. (2005). Functional data analysis for sparse longitudinal data. *Journal of the American Statistical Association, 100*, 577–590.

Zhang, X., Cao, J., & Carroll, R. J. (2017). Estimating varying coefficients for partial differential equation models. *Biometrics, 73*(3), 949–959. ISSN: 1541–0420. http://dx.doi.org/10.1111/biom.12646

Zhu, H., Brown, P. J., & Morris, J. S. (2011). Robust, adaptive functional regression in functional mixed model framework. *Journal of the American Statistical Association, 495*, 1167–1179.

A Maximum Likelihood Approach for Non-invasive Cancer Diagnosis Using Methylation Profiling of Cell-Free DNA from Blood

Carol K. Sun and Wenyuan Li

1 Introduction

Cancer is a common human disease with over one million people getting cancer every year in US alone. To combat cancer, President Obama announced the National Cancer Moonshot Initiative during his 2016 State of Union address and Vice President Biden led the initiative. One of the objectives of the initiative is to improve cancer detection tools that can make cancer detection as simple as getting blood drawn.

A variety of different approaches have been developed for cancer detection including mammograms and MRI for breast cancer; sigmoidoscopy, colonoscopy and CT for colon and rectal cancer; etc. These tests are usually invasive and expensive. Therefore, new cancer detection methods are urgently needed.

It was discovered that tumor-derived DNA is present in blood of cancer patients (Schwarzenbach et al. 2011). This fundamental discovery led to the use of blood sample for the detection of cancer (Bettegowda et al. 2014; Chan et al. 2013; Leary et al. 2012; Siravegna and Bardelli 2014). In these studies, chromosomal alterations such as copy number variation and genome rearrangements were used for cancer detection. Oesper et al. (2013) developed a statistical method to estimate the fraction of different cell types based on copy number variations. However, such methods usually require deep sequencing to accurately estimate chromosomal aberrations.

C.K. Sun (✉)
Oak Park High School, Oak Park, CA, USA
e-mail: carolsun5@gmail.com

W. Li (✉)
Department of Pathology and Laboratory Medicine, University of California at Los Angeles,
Los Angeles, CA, USA
e-mail: WenyuanLi@mednet.ucla.edu

© Springer International Publishing AG 2017
D.-G. Chen et al. (eds.), *New Advances in Statistics and Data Science*,
ICSA Book Series in Statistics, https://doi.org/10.1007/978-3-319-69416-0_10

DNA methylation is an epigenetic modification that occurs by adding a methyl group to the $5'$ carbon cytosine ring, producing 5-methylcytosine. DNA methylation is primarily found in cytosine-guanine dinucleotides (CpGs). CpG sites can be found throughout the genome, but more frequently at small stretches, called CpG islands. These islands are usually located in or near the promoter regions of genes. Therefore, methylation can effectively inhibit transcription due to the placement of the CpG islands. Hypermethylation may silence important growth regulators, such as tumor suppressor genes, and hypomethylation may affect oncogenes, resulting in cancer (Sharma et al. 2010). These methylated DNA can be released to blood and are called circulating cell-free DNA (cfDNA). Therefore, blood of a cancer patient contains a mixture of normal and tumor-derived cfDNA. Zheng et al. (2014) developed a mixture model for methylation profiles of tumor samples and an expectation-maximization (EM) algorithm to estimate minor and major cell population components and their fraction in each genomic region. However, they did not use methylation profiles of different cell population components of many individuals as given in the TCGA (The Cancer Genome Atlas at https://cancergenome.nih.gov/).

Many factors affect DNA methylation patterns including genetics, diet, life style, age, gender, cell states, etc. (Wu et al. 2015). In this paper, we concentrate on regions with different methylation patterns between normal and tumor cells. In particular, the DNA methylation patterns for tumor cells and normal cells are different in many regions along the human genome. Therefore, the cfDNA methylation can be used to distinguish between cancer patients and healthy individuals (Chan et al. 2013; Zheng et al. 2014). However, cfDNA extracted from blood contains DNA released from both healthy and tumor DNA. Usually the fraction of tumor-derived cfDNA is low, making it challenging to separate the tumor-derived cfDNA from the normal cfDNA. Also, the proportion of tumor-derived cfDNA in the blood varies among the patients, adding an additional component of complexity into the problem.

In this study, we develop a novel computational method to infer the composition of cfDNA in blood samples using the genome wide DNA methylation data and to make stable diagnostic cancer prediction. Given the blood cfDNA sample of an individual with unknown cancer status, we measure the methylation levels on a set of CpG sites distributed across the whole genome. We investigate the composition of the cfDNA released from healthy and tumor cells and estimate the proportion of the normal and tumor cfDNA in a new blood sample. To do this, we use methylation sequencing data of blood samples to measure the methylation level at each CpG site. We first develop a probabilistic model for the observed counts of both total and methylated cytosines at each CpG site. We then use a maximum likelihood estimation (MLE) and an efficient computational method to estimate the fraction of tumor-derived cfDNA in the blood samples as well as the methylation patterns of the normal and tumor cells for the particular individuals. The accuracy of estimation depends on two parameters: sequencing depth and the fraction of tumor-derived cfDNA within the blood samples. The sequencing depth is the average number of reads covering a CpG site. We study the effect of these parameters on the accuracy of the estimated fraction of tumor-derived cfDNA using simulation data. We also apply our method to estimate the fraction of liver tumor-derived cfDNA in 24 normal individuals and 24 liver cancer patients to see if our method can predict cancer status. It is shown that the estimated fractions of tumor-derived cfDNA among the liver cancer patients are generally larger than that of the normal individuals. Using the estimated fraction of tumor-derived cfDNA in the blood for cancer detection, the prediction accuracy is as high as 94%. Finally, we study the change of fraction of tumor-derived cfDNA before and after surgery for two liver cancer patients, indicating that the estimated fraction of tumor-derived cfDNA can be used to predict patient survival. Therefore, our method is promising for cancer diagnosis and for predicting survival.

2   Methods

We consider the cfDNA in a patient coming from two sources: normal cells and tumor cells. To estimate the proportion of tumor-derived cfDNA in the mixture, we need to model the methylation profiles in the two cell types. Figure 1 shows the schema of our procedures based on sequencing techniques.

2.1   Model the Methylation Probabilities

We use liver cancer as an example. The method developed in the paper can also be applied for the analysis of other cancer types that have preliminary data on the distribution of methylation values at each CpG site or CpG-rich region. For our study, the methylation data of liver cancerous cells and normal liver cells from TCGA are used. In TCGA, 377 liver cancer samples and 50 normal liver samples from some patients have their DNA methylation levels measured by Infinium HumanMethylation450 microarray.

The methylation level of a CpG site or a CpG-rich region is represented by the β-value (denoted as x) that is defined as:

$$x = \frac{M}{U + M}, \tag{1}$$

where U and M are the numbers of unmethylated and methylated cytosines at the CpG site (or CpG-rich region), respectively. That is, the β-value is the probability that a copy of DNA is methylated at the particular site or region. Multiple experimental platforms have been used to measure methylation levels including microarray technologies and methylation generation sequencing. For the microarray platform, the intensities measured by unmethylated and methylated probes are used for the calculation of β-values. The microarray techniques only measure β-values at single CpG sites with low cost, and cannot yield information on the sequences

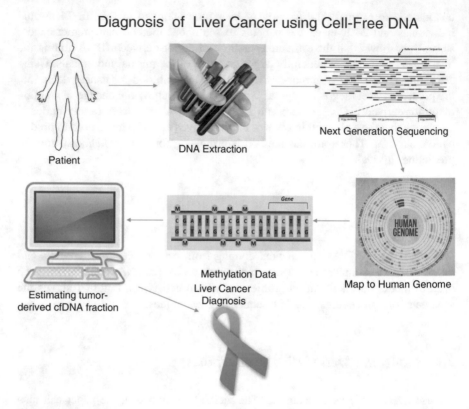

Fig. 1 Schema of our cancer diagnosis method based on NGS. For a given patient, blood samples are drawn from the patient and DNA samples are extracted. The DNA samples are sequenced using methylation sequencing technique and the sequencing reads are mapped to the human genome to identify methylation patterns. Based on the methylation patterns, the fraction of tumor-derived cfDNA is estimated and a diagnosis is given based on the estimated fraction of tumor-derived cfDNA

with methylated/unmethylated CpG sites; while bisulfite sequencing techniques can yield the highest resolution of DNA methylation data at the DNA sequence level, but currently at high cost. Please refer to a recent review (Yong et al. 2016) for details. However, due to the lack of bisulfite sequencing data of tumors, we can only use the array data of tumors that have a large number of samples in the massive TCGA database, for estimating the distribution of β-values. As shown in a recent study (Titus et al. 2016), there is a high correlation of methylation measurements between array and sequencing data collected from matched TCGA tumor samples. In this work, we therefore used a large amount of microarray data to model the distribution of β-values in normal and tumor samples, and used sequencing data for the patient's plasma cfDNA samples. With the development of high throughput sequencing technologies, a very large number of methylation sequencing data for tumor sample sequences can be generated cheaply and efficiently. With sequencing, it is possible to count the numbers of methylated and unmethylated sequences at each CpG site and it is possible to investigate the variation of the estimated β-values.

For a given CpG site (or CpG-rich region), there is variation of β-values among the normal samples as well as tumors. We assume that the β-values of each site/region follow a beta distribution, in order to model the biological variation of a sample type among individuals. We use beta distribution because it is flexible and is frequently used to model fraction data. We also plot the histograms of the β-values based on the TCGA data which validate the beta distribution assumption. Specifically, the β-values of a CpG site/region s in the normal individuals follow a beta distribution Beta(α_{s1}, β_{s1}). Similarly, the β-values of a CpG site/region s in the tumor cells follow another beta distribution Beta(α_{s2}, β_{s2}). These parameters are separately estimated using moment estimators for normal and tumor samples based on the β-values of each site/region measured. Specifically, for CpG site/region s, we first calculate the sample mean $\hat{m}$ and variance $\hat{\sigma}^2$ of the β-values of the normal plasma samples and liver tumor samples, respectively. We then let the theoretical mean and variance of the beta distribution equal to $\hat{m}$ and variance $\hat{\sigma}^2$, respectively. Finally, the parameters can be estimated.

2.2 Estimate the Composition of Tumor-Derived cfDNA Using Methylation Data

For each CpG site/region s, let n_s be the total number of cytosines and m_s be the number of methylated cytosines. Let two vectors $\vec{n} = (n_s)_{N \times 1}$ and $\vec{m} = (m_s)_{N \times 1}$ denote these cytosine counts for all N CpG sites (or CpG-rich regions). Our objective is to estimate the fraction of tumor-derived cfDNA and the methylation profiles of the normal plasma and the tumor of the particular patient.

We model the probability $P(n_s, m_s | [X \vec{\lambda}]_s)$ with two sets of parameters: (1) a methylation level matrix $X = (x_{sj})_{N \times 2}$, where $x_{sj} \in [0, 1]$ is the β-value of CpG site s in the j-th sample type, $j = 1$ for the normal plasma and $j = 2$ for the tumor as above; and (2) a genome mixing vector $\vec{\lambda} = [\lambda_1, \lambda_2]'$ where λ_j is the fraction of cfDNA from the j-th sample type such that $\lambda_2 = p$ and $\lambda_1 + \lambda_2 = 1$. We aim to estimate the fractions of the tumor cells p and the β-values across all the CpG sites/regions for both normal and cancerous cells $x_{sj}, s = 1, 2, \cdots, N; j = 1, 2$ for the particular individuals with a total of $2N + 1$ parameters.

This problem can be formulated as finding the underlying matrix X and genome mixing vector $\vec{\lambda}$ that maximize the joint probability $P(\vec{m}, \vec{n}, \vec{\lambda}, X)$ that can be expressed as:

$$P(\vec{m}, \vec{n}, X | \vec{\lambda}) = P(X)P(\vec{m}, \vec{n} | X, \vec{\lambda}) = \prod_{s=1}^{N} \prod_{j=1}^{2} P(x_{sj}) \prod_{s=1}^{N} P(m_s, n_s | [X \vec{\lambda}]_s),$$

$$(2)$$

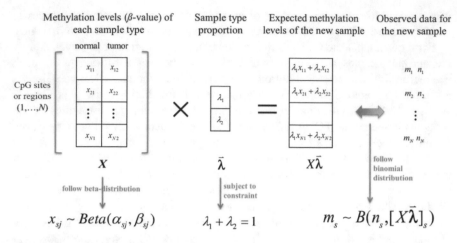

Fig. 2 Mathematical formulation of the problem

where $P(x_{sj})$ can be calculated by the beta distribution estimated from the methylation data from TCGA, that is, based on the TCGA data, we can estimate α_{sj} and β_{sj} using the moment estimator, and $P(m_s, n_s|[X\vec{\lambda}]_s)$ can be obtained by the fact that m_s follows the binomial distribution $\text{Bin}(n_s, [X\vec{\lambda}]_s)$, where $[X\vec{\lambda}]_s$ is the expected methylation level (β-value) for the CpG site/region s in the new blood sample. Figure 2 shows the details of this formulation.

Specifically, the negative logarithm of $P(\vec{m}, \vec{n}, \vec{\lambda}, X)$ can be represented as follows,

$$-\log(P(\vec{m}, \vec{n}, \vec{\lambda}, X))$$

$$= -\log(P(X)) - \log(P(\vec{m}, \vec{n}|X, \vec{\lambda}))$$

$$= \sum_{s=1}^{N}\sum_{j=1}^{2}\left[\log(B(\alpha_{sj}, \beta_{sj})) - (\alpha_{sj}-1)\log(x_{sj}) - (\beta_{sj}-1)\log(1-x_{sj})\right]$$

$$- \sum_{s=1}^{N}\left[\log\binom{n_s}{m_s} + m_s\log([X\vec{\lambda}]_s) + (n_s - m_s)\log([X\vec{\lambda}]_s)\right], \tag{3}$$

where $B(\cdot, \cdot)$ indicates the beta function. Since there are $2N + 1$ parameters, finding the optimal point is challenging. Therefore, we employ the nonlinear optimization "interior-point algorithm" (Byrd et al. 1999) to minimize $-\log(P(m, n, \lambda, X))$ in Eq. (3), subject to the constraint $\lambda_1 + \lambda_2 = 1$ and $\lambda_1 > 0, \lambda_2 = p > 0$. The interior-point algorithm of Byrd et al. (1999) is based on two major techniques: sequential quadratic programming and the trust region technique. The former is used to deal with nonlinearity in the constraints and the latter is used to uniformly handle both convex and non-convex optimizations. Due to their efficient applications of these techniques, the algorithm is fast and also more likely to find the optimal points. In addition, because the Hessian matrix of Eq. (3) is very sparse, this algorithm can quickly converge to the solution. In addition, the algorithm may converge to multiple points and we run the program multiple times (1000 times in our study) and choose the median of all the outputs as the final estimates for X and p.

2.3 Simulate the Methylation Sequencing Data of Plasma cfDNA Samples

We carry out simulation studies to investigate the estimation accuracy under different settings of sequencing depth and fraction of tumor-derived cfDNA in the blood. In the simulation study, we generate the data at the level of CpG sites. The conclusions will apply to the data measured at the level of CpG-rich regions. Sequencing depth is defined as the average number of reads covering a CpG site. If the sequencing depth is low, the number of reads covering a CpG site is low resulting in an inaccurate estimation of the fraction of tumor-derived cfDNA in the blood. Similarly, when the fraction of tumor-derived cfDNA in the blood is low, it is difficult to sample reads from the tumor-derived cfDNA resulting in the decrease of estimation accuracy. In this study, we want to quantify such reduction in estimation accuracy due to changes in sequencing depth and in the fraction of tumor-derived cfDNA in the blood.

We assume that every piece of genomic DNA in a cell has the same opportunity to be released into the circulating system when the cell undergoes apoptosis or necrosis. Therefore, the cfDNA in the blood of a patient can be modelled as a combination of normal cfDNA and tumor-derived cfDNA mixed at the same ratio over all the genomic regions.

We simulate the methylation patterns of cfDNA by extracting methylation data from randomly picked samples, one from normal set and one from tumor set, respectively. Then we mix them at a given ratio to generate a simulated plasma sample. We use a large number of TCGA liver tumor samples for the tumor set and a large number of TCGA normal liver samples for the normal set. Given a CpG site, suppose its average methylation levels in normal and tumor samples are x_0 and x_1, respectively. If the proportion of tumor-derived cfDNA in the blood is p, then the proportion of normal cfDNA in blood is $1 - p$. In the blood sample, using the law of total probability, a read is methylated with probability $x_B = p \times x_1 + (1-p) \times x_0$. The proportion p is given as a parameter in the data simulation procedure and the expected β-value in blood is estimated as x_B. We simulate the experimental process of the reduced representation bisulfite sequencing (RRBS) (Meissner et al. 2005) on the blood sample to measure the methylation patterns. We further simulate the variation introduced by the sequencing technique. With the methylation sequencing technique, the reads are randomly sampled from the genome and, thus, the number of reads covering each position is not constant. Instead, it is a random variable. When the sequencing depth is D, which is given as a parameter as well, the number of reads covering a CpG site follows a Poisson distribution with mean D. Finally, we simulate the number of methylated and unmethylated reads. Suppose the actual reads coverage of this CpG site is n and its methylation level in blood is the β-value x_B. The number of methylated reads m from this site is generated from the binomial distribution $\text{Bin}(n, x_B)$.

We generate a set of simulated RRBS sequencing data with tumor-derived DNA proportion, p, and average sequencing depth, D, both of which are the parameters of this data simulation process. For each combination of the parameters, 200 plasma cfDNA samples are randomly simulated.

For each combination of sequencing depth D and fraction of tumor-derived cfDNA p, a total of $R = 200$ estimates for the fraction of tumor-derived DNA are obtained. We plot the histogram of the estimates. We also calculate the mean, median, root-mean-square-error (RMSE), and the relative error of the estimated fraction of tumor-derived cfDNA. Let $\hat{p}_i$ be the estimated fraction of tumor-derived cfDNA in the i-th individual and $\hat{m}$ be the mean of $\hat{p}_i$, $i = 1, 2, \cdots, 200$. The RMSE is defined as

$$\text{RMSE} = \sqrt{\frac{\sum_{i=1}^{200} (\hat{p}_i - p)^2}{200}},$$

and the relative error is defined as $RMSE/\hat{m}$.

2.4 Cancer Prediction Using Estimated Fraction of Tumor-Derived cfDNA and Evaluation Criteria

We can use the estimated fraction of tumor-derived cfDNA to predict cancer status. For a given threshold, individuals with estimated fraction of tumor-derived cfDNA above the threshold are predicted as having cancer and those with estimated fraction of tumor-derived cfDNA below the threshold are predicted as not having cancer. The false positive rate (FPR) is the fraction of normal individuals who are predicted as having cancer. The true positive rate (TPR) is the fraction of liver cancer patients who are predicted as having liver cancer. By changing the threshold, we can obtain the relationship between FPR and TPR. The receiver operating characteristic (ROC) curve shows the relationship between FPR and TPR. The area under the ROC curve (AUC) is used to evaluate the prediction method. Another evaluation criterion is the prediction accuracy that is defined as the fraction of correct predictions over the total number of individuals.

We also use the Wilcoxon-Mann–Whitney (WMW) statistic (Samuels et al. 2012) to test if the predicted fractions of tumor-derived cfDNA in cancer patients are higher than that in normal individuals.

2.5   Applications to Real Data

In addition to simulated data, we also apply our method to estimate the fractions of tumor-derived cfDNA from blood samples of 24 normal individuals and 24 liver cancer patients. We predict liver cancer status of the individuals based on the estimated fractions of tumor-derived cfDNA in the blood samples of the individuals. The usefulness of our method is evaluated using accuracy, receiver operating characteristic (ROC) curve, and the Wilcoxon-Mann–Whitney (WMW) statistic (Samuels et al. 2012) to test if the fractions of tumor-derived cfDNA in liver cancer patients are higher than that in normal individuals. Further, we estimate the fractions of tumor-derived cfDNA from blood samples of two liver cancer patients before and at several time points after surgery. The data are obtained from Chan et al. (2013).

3   Results

In this section, we first present the simulation results on the accuracy of the estimated fraction of tumor-derived cfDNA for different values of sequencing depth D and fraction of tumor-derived cfDNA p. Then we present the results based on the blood samples of normal individuals and liver cancer patients. Finally, we present the results based on the blood samples of two liver cancer patients before surgery and several times after surgery.

3.1   Estimation Accuracy Increases with Sequencing Depth and Fraction of Tumor-Derived cfDNA in Simulation Data

We simulate the blood methylation data of 200 individuals based on the procedures in Sect. 2.3 for given values of the fraction of tumor-derived cfDNA $p = (0, 0.01, 0.05, 0.1, 0.2, 0.3)$ and sequencing depth $D = (5, 10, 20, 50)$. We then use the estimation method described in Sect. 2.2 to estimate the fraction of tumor-derived cfDNA based on the methylation sequencing data resulting in 200 estimates for each pair of (p, D). Figure 3 shows the histograms of the estimated fractions of tumor-derived cfDNA for some values of p and sequencing depth D.

Looking down the columns, the fraction is fixed and the depth is the independent variable. For example, the first column shows the case of $p = 0.01$. The mode of the histogram is 0.028 at depth 5, 0.021 at depth 10, and 0.015 at depth 20. As the sequencing depth increases, the mode becomes close to the true fraction. The same observation holds for other values of p.

Looking across the rows, the depth is fixed and the fraction of tumor-derived cfDNA becomes the independent variable. At depth 5, the modes of the histograms are 0.028, 0.139, and 0.265 when the fractions of cancer cells are 0.01, 0.1, and

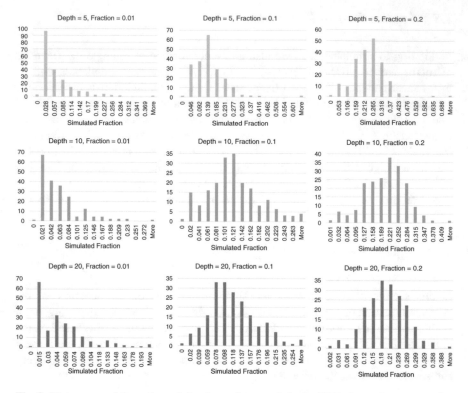

Fig. 3 Histograms of the estimated fractions of tumor-derived cfDNA for various sequencing depths $D = (5, 10, 20)$ when the true fraction p is 0.01, 0.1 and 0.2, respectively

0.2, respectfully. As the fraction of tumor-derived cfDNA increases, the mode also increases. This observation also holds for all the other depths.

Table 1 shows the median, mean, root-mean-square-error (RMSE), and the relative error (RE) of the estimated fraction of tumor-derived cfDNA for different values of true fraction of tumor-derived cfDNA p and sequencing depth D. The table shows that when the fraction of tumor-derived cfDNA is small (for example, $p = 0.01$), the median of the estimated fraction is between 0.03 and 0.04. The relative error can be as high as 120%. These results indicate the difficulties of estimating the fraction of tumor-derived cfDNA when this fraction is low. More accurate methods are needed to estimate the fraction of tumor-derived cfDNA when the fraction is low.

On the other hand, when the fraction of tumor-derived cfDNA is large ($p = 0.3$), the median and mean of the estimated fraction are close to the true fraction. For a given fraction, the root-mean-square error and the relative error decrease as the sequencing depth increases. When the sequencing depth is at least 10, the relative error is less than 43%, showing that the accuracy stabilizes when the sequencing depth is above 10.

Table 1 The median, mean, root-mean-square-error (RMSE), and the relative error (RE) of the estimated fraction of tumor-derived cfDNA for different values of true fraction of tumor-derived cfDNA p and sequencing depth D

Fraction (p)	Depth (D)	Median	Mean	RMSE (%)	RE (%)
0	5	0.018	0.043	7.5	175
0	10	0.030	0.043	6.4	150
0	20	0.027	0.040	5.8	145
0	50	0.026	0.035	5.1	145
0.01	5	0.030	0.048	7.3	152
0.01	10	0.040	0.049	6.2	128
0.01	20	0.036	0.044	5.6	125
0.01	50	0.033	0.040	5.0	123
0.05	5	0.066	0.078	7.4	95
0.05	10	0.065	0.073	5.8	80
0.05	20	0.065	0.071	5.3	75
0.05	50	0.059	0.065	4.4	67
0.1	5	0.117	0.119	8.4	70
0.1	10	0.103	0.109	6.2	57
0.1	20	0.101	0.107	5.4	51
0.1	50	0.093	0.096	5.0	52
0.2	5	0.215	0.210	9.8	46
0.2	10	0.200	0.189	7.5	40
0.2	20	0.181	0.182	7.2	39
0.2	50	0.166	0.176	7.8	44

3.2 Estimated Fraction of Tumor-Derived cfDNA in Real Blood Samples Can Predict Normal from Liver Cancer Patients

We download the bisulfite sequencing data of cfDNA from blood samples of 24 normal individuals and 24 liver cancer patients from Chan et al. (2013). We then calculate the methylation fraction of CpG-rich regions from the whole-genome bisulfite sequencing of these samples, because the very low coverage of the sequencing data can allow us to reliably calculate the methylation level at CpG-rich region, not at individual CpG sites. Using our algorithm, we calculate the estimated fraction of tumor-derived cfDNA for each real blood sample. The resulting fractions are given in Table 2 and the corresponding histograms and scatter plots are given in Fig. 4.

It is clear from Table 2 and Fig. 4 that the estimated fractions of tumor-derived cfDNA in the blood of liver cancer patients are generally higher than that of the normal individuals. Twenty-two out of the 24 normal individuals have estimated fraction less than 4%, while 23 of the 24 liver cancer patients have estimated fraction at least 4%. Therefore, if we use 4% as a threshold of the estimated fraction for

Table 2 The estimated fractions (%) of tumor-derived cfDNA in the blood samples of 24 normal individuals and 24 liver cancer patients

Normal			Cancer		
0.8	2.2	3.2	3.2	5.8	16.4
1.3	2.4	3.2	4.0	5.8	16.8
1.4	2.4	3.4	4.2	7.0	17.5
1.5	2.5	3.6	4.4	7.2	17.9
1.6	2.7	3.7	4.8	7.5	18.4
2.1	2.7	3.7	4.9	7.8	18.5
2.1	2.8	4.4	5.7	8.1	22.2
2.1	3.1	8.6	5.8	16.0	29.4

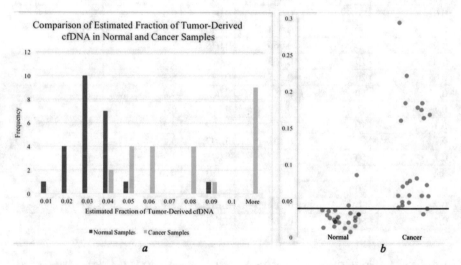

Fig. 4 The (**a**) histograms and (**b**) scatter plots of the estimated fractions of tumor-derived cfDNA in the blood samples of 24 normal and 24 liver cancer patients. The line in (**b**) is the threshold $y = 0.04$. The estimated fractions of tumor-derived cfDNA in liver cancer patients are generally higher than that in the normal individuals

predicting liver cancer status, the prediction accuracy is 45/48 = 94%. Only 2 out of the 24 normal individuals are predicted as having liver cancer, and only 1 out of the 24 liver cancer patients is predicted as normal.

We also use receiver operating characteristic (ROC) curve to evaluate our method as described in Sect. 2.4. For our study, the ROC curve is shown in Fig. 5, and the area under the ROC curve (AUC) is 0.96, again indicating very high prediction accuracy.

In addition, we also use the Wilcoxon-Mann–Whitney statistic to test if the estimated fractions of tumor-derived cfDNA in the blood of liver cancer patients are higher than that for the normal individuals. The resulting statistic is $W = 555.5$ and the p-value is 2.576×10^{-8}, thus strongly against the null hypothesis.

Fig. 5 The ROC curve for predicting liver cancer status based on the estimated fraction of liver tumor-derived cfDNA

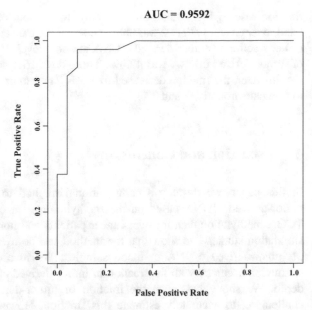

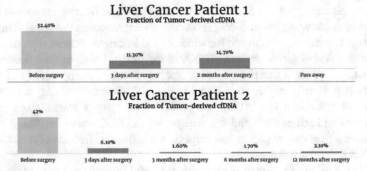

Fig. 6 Fractions of tumor-derived cfDNA in two liver cancer patients before and after surgery. The estimated fraction of tumor-derived cfDNA is significantly decreased after surgery. Data is obtained from Chan et al. (2013)

3.3 The Fractions of Tumor-Derived cfDNA in the Blood of Liver Cancer Patients Are Significantly Decreased After Surgery

We next study the change of tumor-derived cfDNA fraction in the blood samples of liver cancer patients after surgery. Figure 6 shows the results based on two individuals. We can see from the bar graphs that the fraction of tumor-derived cfDNA is significantly reduced after surgery. In liver cancer patient 1, the fraction of tumor-derived cfDNA is 52.4% before surgery. Three days after the surgery, the fraction has significantly decreased to 11.3%. Two months after surgery, the fraction rose to 14.7% and, unfortunately, the patient passed away. On the other hand, liver cancer patient 2 was able to combat the cancer and was able to lower his or her fraction of tumor-derived cfDNA at a low level. Before surgery, the fraction of tumor-derived cfDNA was 42.0%. Three days after surgery, it was 6.1% and 3 months later, the fraction decreased to 1.6%. The tumor-derived cfDNA continued to fluctuate around 1% and 2%.

4   Discussion and Conclusions

In this paper, we develop a computational method to estimate the fraction of tumor-derived cfDNA based on the methylation data of blood samples and the TCGA methylation data for liver cancer patients and normal individuals. Through simulation studies, we show that the method can be used to estimate the fraction of tumor-derived cfDNA in blood samples. We investigate the relationship of estimation accuracy with the fraction of tumor-derived cfDNA and the sequencing depth. We show that when the fraction of tumor-derived cfDNA is low, it is challenging to accurately estimate this fraction. However, when the fraction is relatively high (e.g. $p \geq 0.05$), the mode of the estimated fraction is close to the true fraction at sequencing depth 5–50. The accuracy increases as the sequencing depth increases. The mean, median and the mode of the estimated fractions increases with the true fraction of tumor-derived cfDNA in the blood. Using our method in a real-life situation, we show that the estimated fraction of tumor-derived cfDNA in cancer patients is generally higher than that in normal individuals. Using the estimated fraction of tumor-derived cfDNA to predict liver cancer status, the prediction accuracy is as high as 94% and the area under the ROC curve is as high as 96%. Also, after a liver cancer patient has surgery, the estimated fraction of tumor-derived cfDNA is drastically decreased.

We use a relatively simple mathematical model to study the methylation levels of blood samples. However, the blood is a complex mixture of different cell types, making it difficult to accurately model the methylation levels. As we learn more about the methylation levels of different cell types, we can incorporate the knowledge into our model for estimating the fraction of tumor-derived cfDNA for cancer detection. In our model, we assumed that the fraction of tumor-derived cfDNA p is a constant across the different CpG sites. It is possible that the probability of shedding tumor-derived cfDNA is genomic region dependent and varies along the genome. Under this assumption, we may model p as a random variable and a Bayesian approach can be used to estimate the fraction of tumor-derived cfDNA (Wu et al. 2015). In this study, we concentrate on the detection of just one cancer type, i.e. liver cancer. How to extend our model to the detection of multiple different cancer types is an important problem for further study.

In conclusion, our method can potentially be used to estimate the fraction of tumor-derived cfDNA for cancer detection. More studies are needed to accurately estimate the presence of tumor-derived cfDNA when the fraction is low.

Acknowledgements We would like to thank Professor Jasmine Xianghong Zhou at UCLA for the inspiration for this project and for supervision. We are grateful for her patience explaining methylation and its relationship to cancer and for editing the manuscript. This project would not have been finished without her constant encouragement. The authors greatly acknowledge Dr. Yuk Ming Dennis Lo and his circulating nucleic acids research group in the Chinese University of Hong Kong for his cfDNA data (Chan et al. 2013).

References

Bettegowda, C., Sausen, M., Leary, R. J., Kinde, I., Wang, Y. X., Agrawal, N., et al. (2014). Detection of circulating tumor DNA in early-and late-stage human malignancies. *Science Translational Medicine, 6,* 224.

Byrd, R. H., Hribar, M. E., & Nocedal, J. (1999). An interior point algorithm for large-scale nonlinear programming. *SIAM Journal on Optimization, 9,* 877–900.

Chan, K. C. A., Jiang, P. Y., Chan, C. W. M., Sun, K., Wong, J., Hui, E. P., et al. (2013). Noninvasive detection of cancer-associated genome-wide hypomethylation and copy number aberrations by plasma DNA bisulfite sequencing. *Proceedings of the National Academy of Sciences, 110,* 18761–18768.

Leary, R. J., Sausen, M., Kinde, I., Papadopoulos, N., Carpten, J. D., Craig, D., et al. (2012). Detection of chromosomal alterations in the circulation of cancer patients with whole-genome sequencing. *Science Translational Medicine, 4,* 162.

Meissner, A. Gnirke, A., Bell, G. W., Ramsahoye, B., Lander, E. S. & Jaenisch, R. (2005). Reduced representation bisulfite sequencing for comparative high-resolution DNA methylation analysis. *Nucleic Acids Research, 33,* 5868–5877.

Oesper, L., Mahmoody, A., & Raphael, B. J. (2013). THetA: Inferring intra-tumor heterogeneity from high-throughput DNA sequencing data. *Genome Biology, 14,* R80.

Samuels, M. L., Jeffrey, A. W., & Andrew, S. (2012). *Statistics for the life sciences.* London: Pearson Education.

Schwarzenbach, H., Hoon, D. S. B., & Pantel, K. (2011). Cell-free nucleic acids as biomarkers in cancer patients. *Nature Reviews Cancer, 11,* 426–437.

Sharma, S., Kelly, T. K., & Jones, P. A. (2010). Epigenetics in cancer. *Carcinogenesis, 31*(1), 27–36.

Siravegna, G., & Bardelli, A. (2014). Genotyping cell-free tumor DNA in the blood to detect residual disease and drug resistance. *Genome Biology, 15,* 449.

Titus, A. J., Houseman, E. A., Johnson, K. C., & Christensen, B. C. (2016). methyLiftover: Cross-platform DNA methylation data integration. *Bioinformatics, 32*(16), 2517–2519.

Wu, X. W., Sun, M. A., Zhu, H. X., & Xie, H. H. (2015). Nonparametric Bayesian clustering to detect bipolar methylated genomic loci. *BMC Bioinformatics, 16*(1), 11.

Yong, W. S., Hsu, F. M., & Chen, P. Y. (2016). Profiling genome-wide DNA methylation. *Epigenetics & Chromatin, 9*(1), 26.

Zheng, X. Q., Zhao, Q., Wu, H. J., Li, W., Wang, H. Y., and Meyer, C. A., et al. (2014). MethylPurify: Tumor purity deconvolution and differential methylation detection from single tumor DNA methylomes. *Genome Biology, 15,* 419.

Part III
Clinical Trials, Statistical Shape Analysis and Applications

A Simple and Efficient Statistical Approach for Designing an Early Phase II Clinical Trial: Ordinal Linear Contrast Test

Yaohua Zhang, Qiqi Deng, Susan Wang, and Naitee Ting

1 Introduction

In the drug development process, a candidate compound goes through a stringent series of tests to assess its toxicity, pharmacokinetics, efficacy, and safety before being released to the market. After the initial safety assessment in humans, a proof of concept together with dose-response experiment is conducted in which several doses of the compound are administered to separate groups of experiment units. A good understanding and characterization of the dose response relationship is an important step in the investigation of a new compound. The importance and challenges in designing and analyzing dose-response trials can be found in the ICHE4 (1994) guidance document.

There are usually three phases in clinical studies prior to a registration. Generally speaking, the objective of Phase I is to find the upper end of a dose range that will not cause some undesirable effect. Different from Phase I, the intent of Phase II is to show drug effect (proof of concept) and to estimate the lower end of dose range that will demonstrate some desirable effect. Therefore, a critical component of this entire process is the dose and/or dose range selected for further confirmation in phase III studies. In this manuscript, we address methods employed in an early Phase II.

Y. Zhang
Department of Statistics, University of Connecticut, Storrs, CT, USA
e-mail: yaohua.zhang@uconn.edu

Q. Deng • S. Wang • N. Ting (✉)
Boehringer-Ingelheim Pharmaceuticals, Inc., 900 Ridgebury Rd, Ridgefield, CT, USA
e-mail: qiqi.deng@boehringer-ingelheim.com; susan.wang@boehringer-ingelheim.com; naitee.ting@boehringer-ingelheim.com

© Springer International Publishing AG 2017
D.-G. Chen et al. (eds.), *New Advances in Statistics and Data Science*,
ICSA Book Series in Statistics, https://doi.org/10.1007/978-3-319-69416-0_11

Searching for an adequate dose has been extensively studied by researchers in history. Williams (1971,1972) proposed one of the first dose-finding procedures. William's procedure is based on finding the difference between lowest response dose and placebo. Ruberg (1989) proposed some procedures based on selected contrasts of the sample means at different doses. In 2004, the Food and Drug Administration (FDA) released a White Paper entitled "Stagnation/Innovation: Challenge and Opportunity on the Critical Path to New Medical Products." This white paper triggered many activities across pharmaceutical industry to enhance current dose finding practices. For example, Pharmaceutical Research and Manufacturers of America (PhRMA) has organized a working group on "Adaptive Dose Ranging Studies" to offer recommendations to address the problem of inadequate dose response information.

One very useful, yet not necessarily popular method to prove the concept is the application of ordinal linear contrast test (OLCT). This approach has been successfully implemented in designing early Phase II clinical trials (Ting 2009), and has been proposed for more general applications (Wang and Ting 2012). This technique, referred to "linear contrast test", or "trend test" previously is straightforward. The objective of this article is to encourage more practitioners to apply OLCT in solving real world problems. The popular method nowadays is MCP-Mod, but it is rather complicated. In practice, a useful statistical method should be simple so that it can be easily accepted by non-statisticians. Also it is less likely to cause errors by inexperienced statisticians.

Bretz et al. (2005) put forward MCP-Mod, a combination of multiple comparisons and modeling techniques. It received a positive Committee for Medical Products for Human Use (CHMP) qualification opinion in January 2014 as an efficient statistical methodology for model-based design and analysis of Phase II dose finding studies under model uncertainty. Unfortunately, MCP-Mod has led to confusions due to the high thresholds of complete understanding this methodology, the requirement of excessive assumptions, and the difficulties in use of the software.

This article compares OLCT with MCP-Mod, and two other methods in designing early Phase II clinical trials. It is organized as follows. Section 2 presents some necessary notations and assumptions. Each of the statistical method is introduced in Sect. 3. In Sect. 4, we discussed issues relating to dose spacing of a trial design. In Sect. 5, we compared the performance of each method from a power perspective. Section 6 provides conclusion and discussion.

2 Notation and Assumptions

We start this section by introducing some notations and model setups throughout this article.

2.1 Model Description

Continuous data Y is observed for a set of groups of patients corresponding to a set of increasing dose levels $d_0, d_1, d_2, \cdots, d_k$, where d_0 corresponds to the placebo control. Under a one-way layout setting in which n_i experiment units are tested at dose level d_i, $i = 0, 1, 2, \cdots, k$. We assume that all observations Y_{it}, $t = 1, 2, \cdots, n_i$ are mutually independent, then a general model for Y_{it} is defined as

$$Y_{it} = f(d_i, \boldsymbol{\theta}) + \varepsilon_{it}, \tag{1}$$

where $f(.)$ denotes the mean response at dose d_i for some dose-response model $f(d, \boldsymbol{\theta})$ and $\boldsymbol{\theta}$ refers to the vector of model parameters. Let ε_{it} be independent and identically distributed Gaussian noise with mean zero and variance σ^2 (we assume equal variance in this article). For the purpose of detecting an overall trend, we rewrite Eq. (1) in the format of a usual one-way analysis of variance (ANOVA) model,

$$Y_{it} = \mu_{d_i} + \varepsilon_{it} \tag{2}$$

where $\mu_{d_i} = f(d_i, \boldsymbol{\theta})$. Let $\bar{Y}_{i.} \sim N(\mu_{d_i}, \sigma^2/n_i)$ be an estimator of μ_{d_i}, and let $s^2 \sim$ Gamma$(v/2, 2\sigma^2/v)$ be an estimator of σ^2, independent of $\bar{Y}_{i.}$. Here $v = \sum_{i=0}^{k} n_i - (k+1)$ is the degree of freedom. Without losing generality, in this article, we restrict to the case where $n_0 = n_1 = \cdots = n_k = n$ and hence only focus on a balanced clinical trial, although unbalanced trial can be handled in a similar manner.

2.2 Monotonicity

A typical proof of concept (PoC) study which demonstrates a feasible proposal via comparing the maximum tolerated dose (MTD) of test product with a placebo control is based on monotonicity assumption. In other words, the hidden justification of choosing the highest tolerable dose for proof of concept is that this dose offers the best possible efficacy among all of the candidate doses. However, the underlying is if it is reasonable to assume a monotonic efficacy dose-response relationship.

Regarding product safety, it is generally believed that the safety issues (adverse events, lab abnormalities etc.) increase as doses increase. This is why MTD serves as an anchor of the upper end of dose range to be studied. The reason behind such a belief or such an assumption is that every medicinal product is toxic. If a product could cure a disease, or improve a particular health condition, it must have changed the biological system in human body. If the product changes the biological system, it could cause problems to the human body. Hence by increasing the amount of exposure, it is expected that the potential safety problems could increase, resulting in a monotonicity assumption.

In most of the therapeutic areas, this monotonicity assumption is also applicable to product efficacy. If the medicinal product helps improve health conditions, then more of such a product would improve the health condition more efficiently. For example, if a product is developed to reduce pain, then it is expected that more of such a product in the body could translate to more pain reduction for the patient who suffers from pain. This idea is applicable in most of therapeutic areas. Hence unless it is proven, the generally accepted assumption is that as doses increase, efficacy responses increase. Monotonicity assumption for efficacy can be expressed mathematically as

$$\mu_{d_0} \leq \mu_{d_1} \leq \mu_{d_2} \leq \cdots \leq \mu_{d_k}.$$

In practice, most of the cases, we will see monotonic data. Our OLCT method is built on this monotonicity assumption.

2.3 Family-Wise Error Rate

When multiple doses are compared, there is a multiple hypothesis testing problem. Thus it is necessary to require control of the family-wise error rate (FWER). FWER is defined as the probability of observing at least one null hypothesis rejected. Thus, by assuring FWER is less than or equal to α, the probability of making type I error in the family is controlled at level α. Here family is defined by Hochberg and Tamhane (2009) as "any collection of inferences for which it is meaningful to take into account some combined measure of error".

3 Statistical Methods

3.1 Ordinal Linear Contrast Test

Using contrasts to analyze clinical trial data is a common practice. OLCT is not a new method. It originated from the linear contrast test, and is generally referred to the trend test in the literature (Ting 2009; Wang and Ting 2012). Assumptions for applying OLCT are correct maximum tolerated dose (MTD) and monotonicity in efficacy. It should be noted that mild violation of monotonicity assumption will not affect the performance of OLCT. We provide a detailed discussion regarding some mis-perceptions and issues related to OLCT in Sect. 5.7. An OLCT can be expressed in terms of an ordinal linear contrast with statistical hypotheses as

$$H_0 : a_0\mu_0 + a_1\mu_1 + \cdots a_k\mu_k = 0 \quad \text{versus} \quad H_a : a_0\mu_0 + a_1\mu_1 + \cdots a_k\mu_k > 0$$

Table 1 Coefficients to be used in contrast for the trend test

# of doses	Placebo	Lowest dose	Medium doses				Highest dose
2	−1	0					1
3	−3	−1	1				3
4	−2	−1	0	1			2
5	−5	−3	−1	1	3		5
6	−3	−2	−1	0	1	2	3

where a_i's subject to $\sum_{i=0}^{k} a_i = 0$ and the difference between two consecutive a_i's is a constant (equally spaced contrasts). The corresponding t statistic is given by

$$t = \frac{\sum_{i=0}^{k} a_i \bar{Y}_{i.}}{s\sqrt{\sum_{i=0}^{k} a_i^2/n}} \sim t_v$$

where s is the square root value of s^2 defined in Sect. 2.1. The critical values of the test depend on a t distribution with degree of freedom v. For trials with different number of dose groups, the associated contrast coefficients (a_i) are listed in Table 1.

As an example, assume a phase II trial has included three doses of test drug and a placebo arm. The null and alternative hypotheses for OLCT can be written as

$$H_0 : -3\mu_{d_0} - \mu_{d_1} + \mu_{d_2} + 3\mu_{d_3} = 0 \quad \text{versus} \quad H_a : -3\mu_{d_0} - \mu_{d_1} + \mu_{d_2} + 3\mu_{d_3} > 0$$

where $\mu_{d_0}, \mu_{d_1}, \mu_{d_2}$, and μ_{d_3} represent the mean response of placebo, low dose, medium dose and high dose, respectively. Coefficients associated with this contrast are −3, −1, 1, and 3. For balanced clinical trials, these coefficients are the optimal contrast when the dose response curve follows a linear function, and the doses are equally spaced, such as 0, 10, 20, and 30 mg.

3.2 MCP-Mod

Prior to the MCP-Mod approach (Bretz et al. 2005), dose-response studies were designed and analyzed from two different angles of thinking: multiple comparison procedures (MCP) and modeling procedures. The MCP adjustment was applied to pairwise comparison hypotheses test of each dose against placebo or to certain pre-defined contrast(s). On the other hand, the use of a dose-response model is to help estimate parameters associated with a given dose-response relationship. Hence MCP represents the hypothesis testing feature of dose-ranging trials, while modeling procedure reflects the estimation thinking about the dose-response relationships.

MCP-Mod combines these two different ways of thinking into a unified procedure. It employs MCP to select models from candidate models first. After a model
is selected, a modeling procedure is used to estimate the dose-response relationship.
To formalize the idea, we assume that a set $\mathbb{M}$ of M parameterized candidate models
is given, with corresponding model functions $f_m(d_i, \boldsymbol{\theta}_m), i = 0, 1, 2, \cdots, k; m =$
$1, 2, \cdots, M$ and prior guesses for the parameters of the standardized models $\boldsymbol{\theta}_m^0$.
Each of the dose response curve in the candidate set is then tested using a single
contrast test, with contrast coefficients chosen to maximize the power of the contrast
tests introduced further below. The single contrast test for detecting the mth model
curve is defined by

$$T_m = \frac{\sum_{i=1}^{k} c_{mi} \bar{Y}_{i.}}{s\sqrt{\sum_{i=1}^{k} c_{mi}^2/n_i}}, \quad m = 1, 2, \cdots, M \tag{3}$$

where s is the square root value of s^2 defined in Sect. 2.1, and $c_m =$
$(c_{m1}, c_{m2}, \cdots, c_{mk})'$ is the optimal contrast vector for model $f_m(d_i, \boldsymbol{\theta}_m)$, subject
to $\sum_{i=1}^{k} c_{mi} = 0$. Let $\boldsymbol{\mu} = (\mu_{d_1}, \mu_{d_2}, \cdots, \mu_{d_k})'$ denote the true response means at
each dose level, the associated null hypotheses to be tested are

$$H_{0m} : c_m \boldsymbol{\mu} = 0 \quad \text{versus} \quad H_{am} : c_m \boldsymbol{\mu} > 0$$

Let N be the total number of observations and k to be the number of treatment
arms. Under the assumption of model (2) and null hypothesis, T_m follows central
t-distribution with degree freedom $v = N - k$. The final decision of a significant
dose-response curve or a model from the candidate set is based on the maximum
contrast test statistics $T_{\max} = \max\{T_1, T_2, \cdots, T_m\}$. Proof of concept (PoC) can
hence be established if $T_{\max} > q$, where q is an appropriate critical value. Details
of how to compute q and account for FWER are discussed in Bretz et al. (2005) and
Hochberg and Tamhane (2009). Once a dose-response curve has been selected, one
can proceed to estimate the target dose of interest.

3.3   ANOVA F Test

The classical ANOVA F test is designed to detect any pattern of differential response
among several dose levels by comparing the variation among replicated samples
within and between dose levels. Consider a model setting described in Sect. 2.1, the
hypotheses are

$$H_0 : \mu_0 = \mu_1 = \cdots = \mu_k \quad \text{versus} \quad H_a : \text{means are not all equal}$$

To assess whether any of the arms is on average different versus the null hypothesis
that all arms yield the same mean response, we employed the F statistic

$$F = \frac{\sum_{i=1}^{k} n_i (\bar{Y}_{i.} - \bar{Y}_{..})^2 / (k-1)}{\sum_{i=1}^{k} \sum_{t=1}^{n_i} (Y_{it} - \bar{Y}_{i.})^2 / v}$$

This F statistic follows a $F_{k-1,N-k}$ distribution under null hypothesis. The null hypothesis is rejected if observed F value is greater than $F_{k-1,N-k,\alpha}$ for a given probability type I error α.

3.4 MaxT Test

To establish PoC, it seems intuitive to consider the Maximum t test (MaxT) which is a simple and powerful approach. MaxT test is inspired by Dunnett (1955). By computing a Student's t statistic for each comparison of the active dose versus the control (placebo), several two-sample inferences emanate. Instead of calculating the $100(1-\alpha)\%$ simultaneous confidence intervals on each two-sample inference, as in Dunnett's method, decision on PoC can be made by testing the maximum value of the t statistics. To formalize the idea, we consider the model setting described in Sect. 2.1. The hypotheses of interest are

$$H_0 : \mu_0 = \mu_1 = \cdots = \mu_k \quad \text{versus} \quad H_a : \mu_0 < \mu_i, \quad i = 1, 2, \cdots, k$$

Once the data are available from a trial, the Student's t statistics $t_1, t_2, \cdots, t_k$ can be calculated. Each t statistic is defined as $t_i = (\hat{\mu}_i - \hat{\mu}_0) \sqrt{n/2}/\sigma$. The final detection of a significant PoC is based on the maximum t value among all the statistics $T_{\max} = \max\{t_1, t_2, \cdots, t_k\}$. When σ is known, $\{t_1, t_2, \cdots, t_k\}$ follows a multivariate normal distribution with correlation matrix specified as $V = (v_{ij})$, where off diagonal $v_{ij} = 1/2$ if a balanced clinical trial is considered. Multiplicity adjusted critical values and p-values can be calculated using the identity of the set $\{T_{\max} < q_{1-\alpha}\} = \{t_1 < q_{1-\alpha}, t_2 < q_{1-\alpha}, \cdots, t_k < q_{1-\alpha}\}$, where $q_{1-\alpha}$ is the multiplicity adjusted critical value from a multivariate t distribution. Further, the statistical power to reject the null hypothesis is estimated by using

$$P(T_{\max} \geq q_{1-\alpha}\}|H_a) = 1 - P(t_1 < q_{1-\alpha}, t_2 < q_{1-\alpha}, \cdots, t_k < q_{1-\alpha} \,|H_a)$$

4 Dose Ranging

In non-adaptive design practice, usually the first dose ranging study covers a wide dose range, and then the next dose ranging study will be designed with a narrower dose range and tease out the target doses to be assessed in Phase III. Dose range in a clinical trial design is defined as the ratio of the highest dose divided by the lowest dose included in the design. For example, if the doses in trial A are placebo, 20, 40, and 80 mg, then the dose range is 4 (= 80/20). If the doses in trial B are placebo, 0.1, 1 and 10 mg, then the dose range is 100 (= 10/0.1). Although the doses used in trial A are higher than doses used in trial B, trial B has in fact a much wider dose range (25 times wider than trial A). It is critical to cover a wide dose range in the first dose ranging study. Inappropriate selection of dose range may result in failure of finding the appropriate doses and delay the phase III program and the time to market launch.

A poorly designed trial with inadequate dose range and poor spacing can not be salvaged by any sophisticated analytical methods. It is now a common agreement between regulators and industry that the narrow dose range and inadequate dose finding is among the top contributors for the high phase III failure rate. Mullard (2015) summarized the top-line message from EMA dose finding workshop in London on Dec 2014, and pointed out the pairwise comparison as a traditional way to design dose ranging trials is inadequate for dose-finding. The problem of pairwise comparison was further illustrated by a real-world example from Pfizer where the company needed to run three trials using this design over many years to chart the dose-response curve of a drug. One major drawback for pairwise comparison is that multiplicity adjustment is often needed.

By adjusting the alpha for multiplicity issue, the sample size for each arm is further increased to maintain the same level of overall type I error, which reduces the possibility of exploring more doses under restricted resources. With a small modification by only including highest doses versus placebo as PoC test, multiplicity issue can be resolved. This type of design is simple yet quite efficient when there are 2–3 test doses. Actually, it resembles the traditional wisdom of PoC (with only MTD versus Placebo) followed by dose ranging. It also presents the extreme cases that all weights in a contrast are allocated to the two ends. However, this design did not use all available data for doses in the middle and, moreover, tends to be less powerful than OLCT or MCP-Mod when there are four or more doses.

From the discussion above, it can be seen that the method for designing dose ranging trials and the choice of doses are somehow related to each other. The design should respect the doses selected and also in return influence the decision on the doses to be chosen. We recommend using binary dose spacing (BDS) proposed by Hamlett et al. (2002) to help OLCT reaching its full potential. Over the years, BDS has been successfully applied in many dose ranging designs together with OLCT (Ting 2009; Wang and Ting 2012). For example, let there be m test doses in addition to placebo, then the test doses can be given $d_1 = 1/2^m, d_2 = 3/2^m, d_3 = 3/2^{m-1}, d_4 = 3/2^{m-2}, \cdots, d_m = 3/2^2$ (suppose the highest dose is 1 mg). BDS design has numerous variations. It should be viewed as guidance for dose spacing, since it specifies ranges to select each dose. This flexibility is highly desired in practice due to the limitation in formulation. BDS is based on the same two assumptions with OLCT: knowledge of MTD and non-decreasing dose-response relationship.

In addition to BDS, other algorithms could be useful, e.g., log dose spacing, Fibonacci series, modified Fibonacci series approach (Penel and Kramar 2012), and the approach suggested by Quinlan and Krams (2006). However, it is important to note that most of these methods propose dose spacing from lower doses to higher doses. In practice, dose spacing should be considered starting with MTD and then move down to lower doses. Hence when applying any of these algorithms, the dose allocation would be reversed (from high to low, instead of from low to high). The common idea behind all those approaches is allocation of wider spacing with higher dose range and narrower spacing with lower range. Thus these dose arrangement could help users identify doses which are below MED. This is even more important than what methods to be used for hypothesis testing itself.

5 Method Comparisons

Comparisons of the four methods mentioned above are based on a simulation study. Four dose levels are compared to the zero dose level (placebo) in a balanced clinical trial. Suppose that the dose levels are as follow Assume the standard deviation of each arm is 0.67 and maximum response is 0.36. With ensuring power to be 0.8, we try to find the sample size required for each method. FWER is controlled at $\alpha = 0.025$ (one-sided test). Throughout this section, we employ Emax1 as an example to demonstrate the model setup. Sample size calculation for the other models follows the same logic (Table 2).

5.1 OLCT Approach

The dose-response data described by Emax1 is $\hat{y} = (0.0000, 0.0990, 0.1980, 0.3046, 0.3600)$. The contrast is chosen as $a = (-2, -1, 0, 1, 2)$ according to Table 1. Based on the t test described in Sect. 3.1, we could compute the total sample size N by solving the following equation

$$0.8 = P(F(1, N - 5, \lambda) \geq F_{1, N-1, 0.95})$$

where λ is calculated as

$$\lambda = N \frac{(\sum_{i=1}^{5} a_i \bar{Y}_{i.})^2}{\sigma^2 \sum_{i=1}^{5} a_i}$$

Table 2 Dose setup

D_0	D_1	D_2	D_3	D_4
0 mg	1 mg	3 mg	10 mg	30 mg

5.2 MCP-Mod Approach

We start with a set of potential models for the description of the dose-response data. From this candidate set, we select the "best" model if there is any. Proof of concept is based on whether there is one or more "best" model(s) or not. To best describe the dose-response data, we chose five candidate models as follows:

Figure 1 is the graphical display of the five potential models. The sample size required for each potential model is then calculated using an R function samSize in the package MCPMod. To make comparison simpler, our calculations for other procedures are all based on these five models (Table 3).

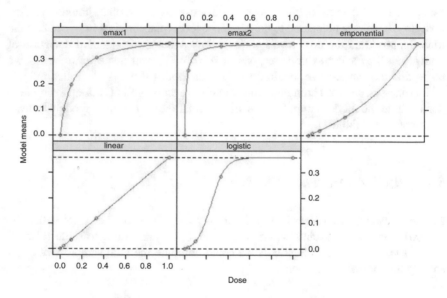

Fig. 1 Five potential models (open dots)

Table 3 Model specification

Model	Specification of θ			
Logistic	$E_0 = -0.009$	$E_{max} = 0.368$	$ED_{50} = 0.243$	$\delta = 0.065$
Emax1	$E_0 = 0$	$E_{max} = 0.396$	$ED_{50} = 0.100$	
Emax2	$E_0 = 0$	$E_{max} = 0.365$	$ED_{50} = 0.014$	
Linear	$E_0 = 0$			$\delta = 0.360$
Exponential	$E_0 = 0$	$E_1 = 0.128$		$\delta = 0.748$

5.3   ANOVA Approach

It is known that when the alternative hypothesis (not all μ_i equals 0) is true, the F-statistic which we compute to test the null hypothesis follows a non-central F distribution. The non-centrality parameter is defined as

$$\lambda = N \frac{\sum_{i=1}^{5}(\bar{Y}_{i.} - \bar{Y}_{..})^2}{\sigma^2}.$$

Then we can get the sample size (N) by solving the following equation

$$0.8 = P(F(1, N-5, \lambda) \geq F_{1,N-5,0.95})$$

5.4   MaxT Approach

The standard deviation and covariance of t-statistic are

$$var(\hat{Y}_l - \hat{Y}_1) = \frac{\sigma^2}{n} + \frac{\sigma^2}{n} = \frac{2\sigma^2}{n}$$

$$cov(\hat{Y}_l - \hat{Y}_1, \hat{Y}_l - \hat{Y}_1) = var(\hat{Y}_1) = \frac{\sigma^2}{n}$$

The correlation coefficient is then calculated as

$$\rho = \frac{\sigma^2/n}{2\sigma^2/n} = \frac{1}{2}$$

Therefore we can get the variance-covariance matrix

$$\Sigma = \begin{bmatrix} 1 & 0.5 & 0.5 & 0.5 \\ 0.5 & 1 & 0.5 & 0.5 \\ 0.5 & 0.5 & 1 & 0.5 \\ 0.5 & 0.5 & 0.5 & 1 \end{bmatrix}$$

Given σ is known, $(t_1, t_2, t_3, t_4) \sim MVN_4(\hat{\boldsymbol{\mu}}^\star, \Sigma)$ (e.g. $\hat{\boldsymbol{\mu}}^\star = (\hat{y}_2 - \hat{y}_1, \hat{y}_3 - \hat{y}_1, \hat{y}_4 - \hat{y}_1, \hat{y}_5 - \hat{y}_1) = (0.0990, 0.1980, 0.3046, 0.3600)$ under Emax1). Sample size is estimated by iteratively solving the power function described in Sect. 3.4. The algorithm is implemented in R and codes to produce Table 4 are available upon request.

5.5   Comparisons

Table 4 displays the sample size calculation for each model and each statistical
method. All calculation are based on one-sided type I error of 0.025, 80% of power,
maximum treatment difference of 0.36 and common standard deviation of 0.67. In
this study, it is clear that MCP-Mod and OLCT in general perform better than the
other two for the selected dose response relationships. When dose-response curves
are logistic and Emax1, OLCT performs better than MCP-Mod. While for the other
cases, MCP-Mod requires smaller sample size than OLCT does. In the setting where
MCP-Mod reaches its full potential in the sense that the true model including the
right guesstimates of model parameters are included in the candidate set, OLCT
leads to only three additional patients per arm, which is often considered comparable
in practice.

ANOVA F test is effective in detecting extreme curves, such as when expected
mean responses increase sharply either at lower dose or at higher dose. For gradual
increase over doses, such as the case in Emax1 and linear models, the ANOVA F
test will require larger sample size.

MaxT test requires smaller sample size only when a plateau is reached sharply
in the dose response. This is logical if we consider the power calculation formula in
Sect. 3.4. To get a larger power, each t statistic (active dose versus placebo) must be
close to its critical value.

The comparison between MCP-Mod and OLCT in Table 4 represents the ideal
scenario for MCP-Mod that the actual dose response curves are completely covered
in the candidate set by the MCP-Mod approach. This is hardly the case in practice.
To evaluate the performance when the true model is not covered in the candidate set,
we compare power of a given sample size through simulations. The comparison of
power is more straightforward than sample size under this setting because the later
one for MCP-Mod requires binary search. As a start, Table 5 presented the power
with 55 patients per arm for MCP-Mod and OLCT when the true model is included
in candidate sets (OLCT vs MCP-Mod1). When the true model is excluded from the
candidate set in a leave-one-out fashion (MCP-Mod3), the comparisons are made in
Table 6. This is done through 10,000 simulations.

Table 4 Sample size per arm calculation

Model	Mean responses					ANOVA F	MCP-Mod	MaxT	OLCT
Logistic	0	0.0055	0.0283	0.2863	0.3600	46	35	67	35
Emax1	0	0.0990	0.1980	0.3046	0.3600	63	47	64	41
Emax2	0	0.2556	0.3046	0.3501	0.3600	61	48	51	53
Linear	0	0.0120	0.0360	0.1200	0.3600	61	46	76	52
Exponential	0	0.0058	0.0183	0.0720	0.3600	59	46	77	57
Average						58	44.4	67	47.6

Table 5 Power with 55 patients per arm when true model is included in MCP-Mod

Model	Mean responses					OLCT	MCP-Mod1	MCP-Mod2
Logistic	0	0.0055	0.0283	0.2863	0.3600	0.94	0.95	0.93
Emax1	0	0.0990	0.1980	0.3046	0.3600	0.90	0.87	0.83
Emax2	0	0.2556	0.3046	0.3501	0.3600	0.81	0.86	0.83
Linear	0	0.0120	0.0360	0.1200	0.3600	0.83	0.87	0.84
Exponential	0	0.0058	0.0183	0.0720	0.3600	0.79	0.88	0.85
Average						0.85	0.88	0.84

MCP-Mod1: included only the candidate models described in Table 3. MCP-Mod2: included two U shaped curve, in addition to the five candidate models

Table 6 Power with 55 patients per arm when true model is not included in MCP-Mod

Model	Mean responses					OLCT	MCP-Mod3	MCP-Mod4
Logistic	0	0.0055	0.0283	0.2863	0.3600	0.95	0.94	0.91
Emax1	0	0.0990	0.1980	0.3046	0.3600	0.90	0.86	0.75
Emax2	0	0.2556	0.3046	0.3501	0.3600	0.82	0.75	0.75
Linear	0	0.0120	0.0360	0.1200	0.3600	0.80	0.87	0.80
Exponential	0	0.0058	0.0183	0.0720	0.3600	0.77	0.87	0.81
Average						0.85	0.86	0.80

MCP-Mod3: included the other four curves, but not the true curve. MCP-Mod4: included the other four curves and two additional U shaped curve, but not the true curve

Including or excluding the candidate model will not change the power for OLCT, but the power for MCP-Mod tends to decrease when the true candidate model is not included. As mentioned above, MCP-Mod is fairly robust, and there is no major reduction in power when the true model is not covered, as long as there is another model in the candidate set that is reasonably close to the true model. However, the small advantages of MCP-Mod1 over OLCT observed in Table 5 diminish. In practice, the true difference between the two methods is likely to be between Tables 5 and 6. As a consequence, the performance can be really close, and the difference can be considered negligible.

The comparison between MCP-Mod3 and MCP-Mod1 showed the effect of missing the true model in candidate set. On the other hand, MCP-Mod2 showed the effect of including unrealistic model into the candidate set. In MCP-Mod3, two additional non-monotonic U-shaped curves are included in the candidate set (BetaMod and quadratic in Fig. 2), on top of the five curves including the true model. In this case, the average power of MCP-Mod is reduced and is slightly below OLCT. This reduction become more apparent in MCP-Mod4 if the true model is not covered in candidate set. This example illustrated how the performance of MCP-Mod can vary for different set up of candidate models. When set up appropriately, MCP-Mod provide small improvement over OLCT; otherwise it can be worse than OLCT. The setup requires thoughtful consideration and thorough discussion with other team members like clinician and pharmacologist. Careful thinking and justification are required in considering such a collection of models.

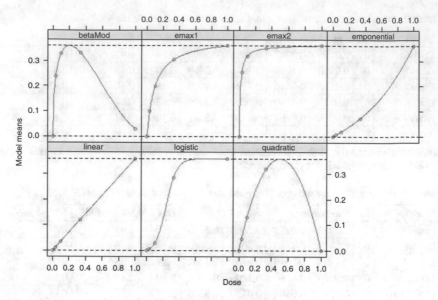

Fig. 2 Five potential models and two non-monotonic models (open dots)

In fact, both OLCT and MCP-Mod use contrasts to test a weighted average of the treatment effects. Estimation of the treatment effects can be obtained using any statistical methods that are appropriate for the endpoints and trial designs, including methods that can adjust for covariates. In practice, people may include covariates to increase the estimation precision. Detailed information and examples for using MCP-Mod are provided in Pinheiro et al. (2014). The idea behind using OLCT is similar but instead a rank-based contrast is used. It should be noted that when there is no treatment by covariate interaction considered, different covariates will only lead to a shift on treatment effect, and has no impact on the dose response relationship. It becomes complex, however, if the inclusion of covariates is to explore their impact on dose response curves (e.g. exploring the impact of covariates on the maximum effect that can be achieved in an Emax model, or the impact on slopes of the dose response curve). This type of analysis is outside the scope of this article.

5.6   When to Use MCP-Mod and When Not?

MCP-Mod is a big step forward from using a specific model to design dose-ranging trials. MCP-Mod allows multiple potential models to be explored at the design stage. These models can cover a variety of potential shapes of dose-response relationships. Although there is still a need to pre-specify some of the parameters associated with the models, research showed that the loss in power from misspecification is often acceptable for a reasonable candidate set. Also, the loss of power due to multiplicity adjustment with many models in the candidate set is small. These features make MCP-Mod a robust approach. Generally speaking, at the PoC stage, MCP-Mod performs well and researchers can consider it a safe tool to help design the trial.

A few problems were found while we were studying the MCP-Mod. Errors occur frequently when we used the R package MCPMod. For example, we encountered convergence issues in as many as 50% of simulation runs, with warning messages that at least one model failed to converge. Although this only has true impact on modeling step, it can be bothersome for some people in this highly regulated environment. A clear understanding of MCP-Mod can be challenging, in particular to non-statisticians. Thus obtaining agreement on the candidate set of models can be difficult and time-consuming. It requires competence from all trial team members for implementations. On the other hand, OLCT is easily understood by statistician and non-statisticians. Its implementation is easy and straightforward.

In fact, MCP-Mod method is a combination of contrast test and MaxT. As stated in Sect. 5.1, the first step of MCP-Mod is to find an optimal contrast for each candidate model. When a candidate model gives equally spaced response, the optimal contrast approximately equals the contrast employed in OLCT. However, if a candidate model has an "extreme" shape (e.g., Emax2 in Fig. 1), MCP-Mod will find a contrast which can mediate the effect of extremeness. The second step of MCP-Mod is to carry out a univariate t test where the test statistic is the maximum of contrast test statistics. As stated above, MaxT performs well when one curve has a sharp increase either at the beginning or in the end. Therefore, as long as there is such a candidate model, it is highly possible that we have PoC. This explains the results showed in Tables 5 and 6. That is when the true model is not included in the candidate set, the power of MCP-Mod decreases.

5.7   When to Use OLCT and When Not?

The two assumptions required for OLCT are correct maximum tolerated dose (MTD) and monotonicity in efficacy. When the two assumptions are true, use of OLCT for PoC is very powerful, because all of the experiment-wise Type I error can be allocated to a single degree of freedom test and this avoids the multiple comparison adjustment. Moreover, it is simple and easy so that people can fully understand it. Although monotonicity assumption is crucial for OLCT, it is quite robust to mild violation where there may be a small drop in the highest dose. This can happen when the endpoint is affected by safety. For example, in binary endpoint analysis, patients who drop out early due to adverse events can be considered as failure. OLCT handled this type of mild non-monotonicity quite well. For example, when mean response is (0, 0.024, 0.08, 0.24, 0.48, 0.96) with standard deviation of 1 for placebo and five test doses from low to high, OLCT under two-sided alpha of 0.2 yields 0.87 power with 10 patients each arm. In contrast, for mild non-monotonic dose response of (0, 0.008, 0.096, 0.48, 0.96, 0.8), OLCT yields 0.93

power with same number of patients under the same MCID. This is due to the fact that it integrates the treatment difference for doses in the middle, which helps to reduce sample size.

There are some mis-perceptions that ordinal linear contrast test should only be used when the dose response curve is linear. It is not true. With equal spacing dose and sample allocation, the contrasts OLCT uses are optimal under a straight line. But when doses are not equally spaced as suggested in binary spacing from Hamlett et al. (2002), optimal contrasts will occur under a different curve that may not have an easy mathematic form. In this case, the contrasts are still optimal. For example, OLCT provides close to optimal contrast for Emax1 instead of Linear in the example we provided, and it works well under logistic model. In practice, for a dose ranging study, what really matters are the responses from selected doses, instead of the underlying shape of the curves. Dose ranging study should be designed in a way that the lowest dose is likely to be in the sub-therapeutic range, and is clearly inferior to higher doses, so that the lower limit of dose range can be established. An ascending response by dose groups is a desired outcome in dose ranging trial and is reflected in OLCT method. The authors recommend using BDS to help reach this goal, and thus the full potential of OLCT method can be realized.

Although monotonicity can be assumed in general as stated above and OLCT works for mild non-monotonic dose response curves, when serious inverse U shape cannot be comfortably excluded by the study team, for example in CNS trials or biological therapy in some disease areas, OLCT may not be appropriate, and methods like MCP-Mod is still a preferred choice.

5.8   Limitations of ANOVA F Test

Although ANOVA F test is widely used, several limitations are discovered. First, Brown and Forsythe (1974) found that one-way ANOVA F statistic yields a test that is sensitive to a lack of homogeneity of within group variances. That is, the actual size of a test may differ greatly from the selected size when the groups have different underlying population variances. Second, we find that when homogeneity is assumed, ANOVA F test tends to ignore information provided by data. Given two group mean responses: $g_1 = (0, 0.09, 0.18, 0.27, 0.36)$ and $g_2 = (0, 0, 0, 0, 0.36)$, to achieve 80% of power, we need 68 patients per arm for g_1 and 53 patients per arm for g_2. This result is counterintuitive since g_1 offers more information by data but results in a larger sample size. The mathematical reason behind this result is that g_1 gives a smaller "variation between sample means" and a larger "variation within the samples". A smaller F is derived then which requires more sample size to achieve the same power.

6 Discussion

In this article, we compared the performance of MCP-Mod, ordinal linear contrast test (OLCT), ANOVA F test and Max T test, and showed that under monotonic assumption, MCP-Mod and OLCT yield similar performance with different dose response curves, and are in general more powerful than the other two methods. OLCT also performs reasonably well with mild violation of monotonic dose-response relationships. When there is a possibility for serious non-monotonic dose response (e.g., inversed U shape), OLCT may not be appropriate and MCP-Mod could be a preferred choice.

As mentioned in Sect. 5, OLCT method depends on two assumptions: correct MTD and monotonicity. Over the years, our experiences indicate that these two critical assumptions as stated above are often necessary for most of phase II study designs. Correct MTD is an important foundation irrespective of design methods stated in this article. On the other hand, monotonic assumption is relevant in the comparison. In general, it is believed that monotonic dose response is reasonable for more than 90% of programs. Potential exceptions include CNS trials or biological therapies.

Thomas and Ting (2007) summarized the findings based on a meta-analysis of clinical dose response in a large drug development portfolio. Their report covered a wide range of studies across different therapeutic areas in non-oncology small molecule compounds, and concluded that almost all compounds in the portfolio showed monotonic response. It should be noted that, in practice, when dose response reach its plateau at median dose, there is about 50% probability that median dose appears to be more efficacious than a higher dose. There are plenty of cases where a non-monotonic dose response curve in one study was subsequently confirmed to be a false signal by a second study. Thus when a non-monotonic shape is observed, it is worthwhile to pause and think twice before jumping into the conclusion.

Our results indicate that performance of OLCT is comparable with that of MCP-Mod. However, OLCT is simpler, more efficient, and more robust. Simplicity of this method makes it very useful—it is easy to communicate with non-statisticians, easy to implement and interpret. When there is not much prior knowledge about the underlying efficacy dose-response relationship, and that the project team is willing to assume MTD is correct and the efficacy dose-response relationship is monotonic, then OLCT can be an ideal choice. When implementing MCP-Mod with the existing software, there could be difficulties when models do not converge, and lack of transparency of the calculations behind the scene. These experiences could result in frustrations for users. Debugging MCP-Mod code can also be challenging. On the other hand, OLCT is simple and clear. Whenever the performance is not good, users can easily use these findings to debug the computer code and the OLCT method can be adjusted. The R code for MCP-Mod is confusing in many cases. For practitioners who have limited understanding of MCP-Mod, or who are not comfortable with the complexity of MCP-Mod software, OLCT is a useful alternative.

R and SAS codes that we used to produce Table 4 are available upon request. It should be clear to readers that the complexity and difficulty in coding when implementing these methods. These codes only reflect the difference in complexity at the design stage. When performing data analysis, MCP-Mod will go through the model selection process and the estimation process. The analysis code could be more complicated.

References

Bretz, F., Pinheiro, J. C., & Branson, M. (2005). Combining multiple comparisons and modeling techniques in dose-response studies. *Biometrics, 61*(3), 738–748.

Brown, M. B., & Forsythe, A. B. (1974). Robust tests for the equality of variances. *Journal of the American Statistical Association, 69*(346), 364–367.

Dunnett, C. W. (1955). A multiple comparison procedure for comparing several treatments with a control. *Journal of the American Statistical Association, 50*(272), 1096–1121.

Hamlett, A., Ting, N., Hanumara, R. C., & Finman, J. S. (2002). Dose spacing in early dose response clinical trial designs. *Drug Information Journal, 36*(4), 855–864.

Hochberg, Y., & Tamhane, A. C. (2009). *Multiple comparison procedures*. New York: Wiley.

ICH Harmonised Tripartite Guideline (2017). Dose-response information to support drug registration E4. In *International Conference on Harmonisation of Technical Requirements for Registration of Pharmaceuticals for Human Use. March 1994*. Available at http://www.ich.org/fileadmin/Public_Web_Site/ICH_Products/Guidelines/Efficacy/E4/Step4/E4_Guideline.pdf. Accessed 16 Oct 2017.

Mullard, A. (2015). Regulators and industry tackle dose-finding issues. *Nature Reviews. Drug Discovery, 14*(6), 371.

Penel, N., & Kramar, A. (2012). What does a modified-fibonacci dose-escalation actually correspond to? *BMC Medical Research Methodology, 12*(1), 103.

Pinheiro, J., Bornkamp, B., Glimm, E., & Bretz, F. (2014). Model-based dose finding under model uncertainty using general parametric models. *Statistics in Medicine, 33*(10), 1646–1661.

Quinlan, J. A., & Krams, M. (2006). Implementing adaptive designs: Logistical and operational considerations. *Therapeutic Innovation & Regulatory Science, 40*(4), 437.

Ruberg, S. J. (1989). Contrasts for identifying the minimum effective dose. *Journal of the American Statistical Association, 84*(407), 816–822.

Thomas, N., & Ting, N. (2007). Minimum effective dose (mined). In *Wiley encyclopedia of clinical trials*. Hoboken, NJ: Wiley.

Ting, N. (2009). Practical and statistical considerations in designing an early phase II osteoarthritis clinical trial: A case study. *Communications in Statistics Theory and Methods, 38*(18), 3282–3296.

Wang, X., & Ting, N. (2012). A proof-of-concept clinical trial design combined with dose-ranging exploration. *Pharmaceutical Statistics, 11*(5), 403–409.

Williams, D. (1971). A test for differences between treatment means when several dose levels are compared with a zero dose control. *Biometrics, 27*, 103–117.

Williams, D. (1972). The comparison of several dose levels with a zero dose control. *Biometrics, 28*, 519–531.

Landmark-Constrained Statistical Shape Analysis of Elastic Curves and Surfaces

Justin Strait and Sebastian Kurtek

1   Introduction

Shape is a fundamental property of objects observed in images, and is often defined as the appearance of their outlines. In the case of two dimensional images, the outlines of objects form planar open and closed curves. In the case of three dimensional images, such as medical ones including magnetic resonance images (MRIs), the outlines of structures form surfaces. Due to improvements in imaging technology, shape datasets have become ubiquitous in many different applications including biology, medicine, biometrics, graphics, bioinformatics, and many others. As a result, statistical shape analysis is an emerging discipline within statistics that seeks to make inferences about a population of objects, represented by their corresponding shapes. To develop statistical procedures applicable to shapes, one must first represent them mathematically; this is not a simple task. Consider a lightbulb, for example. The shape of a lightbulb is easily recognizable. However, it is important to note that if the lightbulb is moved to a different location in the image, rotated, or re-scaled, its shape does not change. Thus, mathematically, shape is a property of an object, which is invariant when the object is translated in space, rotated, or re-scaled. Because of these required invariances, new tools for analyzing shapes are required. That is, standard univariate or multivariate statistical methods are often not directly applicable in this context, because shape spaces are nonlinear and follow a quotient structure. Additionally, shape analysis often requires tools from functional data analysis (Ramsay and Silverman 2005) due to the infinite dimensionality of shape representation spaces. The goal of statistical shape analysis is to reproduce basic statistical techniques while taking into account these extra

J. Strait (✉) • S. Kurtek
Department of Statistics, The Ohio State University, Columbus, OH, USA
e-mail: strait.50@osu.edu; kurtek.1@stat.osu.edu

© Springer International Publishing AG 2017
D.-G. Chen et al. (eds.), *New Advances in Statistics and Data Science*,
ICSA Book Series in Statistics, https://doi.org/10.1007/978-3-319-69416-0_12

197

challenges. The developed techniques can then be used in real-life applications, most notably in medical imaging, where the shapes of anatomical structures can potentially be used to diagnose and monitor various types of diseases.

Many methods have been developed to analyze the shapes of objects observed in images. In the case of surfaces, one of the most popular approaches in medical imaging studies shapes of objects by embedding them in volumes and deforming the volumes (Beg et al. 2005; Grenander and Miller 1998; Joshi et al. 1997) (termed deformable templates and Large Deformation Diffeomorphic Metric Mapping or LDDMM). Others have studied 3D shape variability using level sets (Malladi et al. 1996), medial axes (Bouix et al. 2001; Gorczowski et al. 2010), or point clouds via the iterative closest point algorithm (Almhdie et al. 2007). The case of curves has also been considered under many different representations. In statistics, the most widely-used method was developed by Kendall (1984), where shapes were represented using a finite set of "important" points known as landmarks. The landmarks can be selected manually or automatically. Most often, they are provided by an application domain expert and correspond to similar salient features across a population of shapes; such landmarks are referred to as anatomical. On the other hand, mathematical landmarks correspond to points which in some sense capture the most important properties of the shapes (e.g., peaks and valleys). By reducing the representation of an object to a set of landmarks, one can alter multivariate statistical techniques to account for desired shape invariances, and use them for shape analysis. Developments of these techniques are described in many places (Bookstein 1986; Dryden and Mardia 1992, 1998; Small 1996).

The ability to apply classical multivariate analyses to landmark shapes is intriguing, but not without drawbacks. Landmark-based methods require the user to summarize the full outline of an object into a finite set of points. This leads to a loss of information, which may affect statistical conclusions. In addition, selecting landmarks is not a simple task; it is not clear how many points should be selected, or if there is an "optimal" configuration of points which best represents the objects' outlines. One could select a large number of landmarks to better approximate the shape; however, this leads to a very high-dimensional problem, which can be quite challenging computationally. To overcome these challenges, several groups proposed methods that retain all information provided about the object's outline. In this setting, one defines infinite-dimensional representations, which additionally requires invariance to re-parameterizations of the functions representing the curve or surface (in addition to the similarity group, which includes translation, rotation and scale). In the case of curves, parameterization determines how fast it is traversed. In the case of surfaces, parameterization defines its grid or mesh. Thus, changing the parameterization of curves or surfaces is a shape preserving transformation. In a statistical shape analysis context, re-parameterizing an object can be used to determine which geometric features of objects are in correspondence with each other.

Several authors have studied this new set of shape frameworks in-depth. Zahn and Roskies (1972) and Klassen et al. (2004) in the case of curves, and Brechbühler et al. (1995) and Styner et al. (2006) in the case of surfaces, achieve parameterization invariance through normalization (to arc-length for curves and equal area for surfaces). Unfortunately, these methods do not match geometric features of objects across a population of shapes, and thus result in suboptimal correspondences and subsequent statistical results (Kurtek et al. 2011b, 2012a,b; Srivastava et al. 2011). On the other hand, there is a set of methods in the statistics literature that seek "optimal" correspondences across a population of shapes; these methods are based on elastic metrics and are thus referred to as elastic in short. Instead of normalizing parameterizations, they seek a "best" re-parameterization to match one object to another. This process is often also referred to as registration. Such methods have been developed for statistical shape analysis of curves in Younes (1998), Younes et al. (2008), Joshi et al. (2007), Srivastava et al. (2011) and Kurtek et al. (2012b), and surfaces in Kurtek et al. (2010, 2011a,b, 2012a), Jermyn et al. (2012) and Samir et al. (2014). One of the main benefits of using elastic methods for shape analysis is that the metric used to calculate distances between shapes measures the amount of bending and stretching required to deform one object into another, thus providing a natural interpretation. However, elastic metrics in general are very difficult to work with due to their complex structure (Mio et al. 2007). Recent approaches developed elastic representations of curves and surfaces that greatly simplify the problem at hand (Jermyn et al. 2012; Kurtek et al. 2010; Srivastava et al. 2011).

In this manuscript, we describe an approach to statistical shape analysis that unifies the recent elastic method with previous landmark-based approaches. As mentioned earlier, relying on landmarks reduces the amount of information used in statistical analyses. However, while elastic shape analysis overcomes this problem, these methods treat all points as equally important. Thus, if special landmark locations (e.g., anatomical features) are known, standard elastic shape analysis methods are not able to emphasize these points. Thus, the ability to combine elastic shape analysis with landmark information allows us to overcome both drawbacks. As a motivating example, in medical imaging, an anatomical structure of interest is often represented as a surface. Additionally, the doctor marks special points on the structure, which can be used to detect abnormalities. These points (landmarks) are certainly valuable for statistical inferences, and thus including them in the analysis is necessary.

As another motivating example, consider the dog shapes shown in Fig. 1. In the left panel is a representation of the dog via a curve while in the right panel we show the outline of a dog as a surface. In both cases, it appears natural to place anatomical landmarks at the dogs' legs, tail and snout. In the surface case, one can also clearly see the dog's ears where additional landmarks can be marked. All of these points are important to representing the structure of the full dog outline, and should thus be incorporated into the shape analysis framework. Additionally, good landmark correspondences across shapes provide improved registration over unconstrained elastic methods as shown by Strait et al. (2017) and Kurtek et al. (2013a).

The idea of incorporating landmark constraints into elastic representations of shape had not been explored much in the past. Liu et al. (2010) imposed soft landmark constraints on the analysis by augmenting the elastic shapes with an auxiliary function constructed using the landmark locations. Two recent papers

Fig. 1 Landmark-
constrained curve and surface
representations of a dog.
Landmarks segment the full
curve outline of the dog into
six pieces. Landmarks are
shown as black points on the
curve or surface

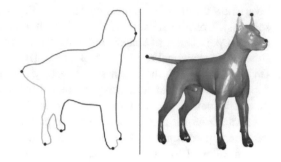

provide statistical shape analysis tools for both (curves and surfaces) that are able
to incorporate hard landmark constraints into elastic representations (Kurtek et al.
2013a; Strait et al. 2017). The methods presented in this manuscript are largely
based on those works. The rest of this paper is organized as follows. In Sect. 2, we
present tools for landmark-constrained registration and elastic comparison of shapes
of curves and surfaces. Sect. 3 provides methods for averaging and summarization
of variability of a sample of shapes. Throughout these two sections we illustrate the
approach using multiple examples. Finally, we give a brief summary in Sect. 4.

2 Landmark-Constrained Shape Analysis

In this section, we describe a landmark-constrained elastic shape analysis framework for curves and surfaces. We begin by briefly discussing a technical issue that
arises when using standard $\mathbb{L}^2$-based methods in this setting. We describe this issue
for curves only, but note that it also arises in the same way for surfaces.

Let $\mathscr{F}$ represent an appropriate representation space of curves made precise
later. Also, let Γ be the set of all diffeomorphisms of the curve domain. The set
Γ contains all possible re-parameterizations of curves, and for an object $f \in \mathscr{F}$ and
an element $\gamma \in \Gamma$, $f \circ \gamma$ represents its re-parameterization. Given this setup, many
works in literature adopt the standard approach of measuring distances between
elements of $\mathscr{F}$ using the $\mathbb{L}^2$ norm. Unfortunately, this framework is inappropriate
for statistical shape analysis of parameterized curves as was previously shown in
multiple places (Kurtek et al. 2010; Srivastava et al. 2011; Younes 1998). We
elaborate next. Let $f_1, f_2 \in \mathscr{F}$ be two parameterized curves, and $\gamma \in \Gamma$ a re-
parameterization function. Then, it is easy to show that the $\mathbb{L}^2$ norm is not preserved
under the action of Γ, i.e., $\|f_1 - f_2\| \neq \|f_1 \circ \gamma - f_2 \circ \gamma\|$. Thus, in this setup, a common
re-parameterization of two curves changes the distance between them (this is also
termed "lack of isometry"). This theoretical problem prevents one from defining
a parameterization-invariant statistical framework for shape analysis. Thus, in the
following sections, we describe an approach which uses new representations of
curves and surfaces that satisfy this property under the $\mathbb{L}^2$ metric. Furthermore, we

show that one can seamlessly incorporate hard landmark constraints into these representations. For more detailed descriptions of these methods please refer to Srivastava et al. (2011), Strait et al. (2017), Jermyn et al. (2012) and Kurtek et al. (2013a).

2.1 Unconstrained Representation Spaces of Curves and Surfaces

Curves Let $\mathscr{F}$ denote the space of two-dimensional, absolutely continuous curves with domain $D = [0, 1]$ (planar open curves). The framework is also applicable to closed curves with domain $D = \mathbb{S}^1$ with minimal changes. Let $\Gamma = \{\gamma : [0, 1] \to [0, 1] | \gamma(0) = 0, \ \gamma(1) = 1, \ 0 < \dot{\gamma} < \infty\}$ denote the unconstrained re-parameterization group, where $\dot{\gamma}$ is the derivative of γ. As stated earlier, this group does not act on $\mathscr{F}$ by isometries under the $\mathbb{L}^2$ metric. To circumvent this issue, for a curve $f \in \mathscr{F}$, we define the square-root velocity function (SRVF) representation of curves (Srivastava et al. 2011) as $q^{SRVF}(t) = \frac{\dot{f}(t)}{\sqrt{|\dot{f}(t)|}}$, where $|\cdot|$ is the Euclidean norm in $\mathbb{R}^2$. The inverse mapping is defined as $f(t) = f(0) + \int_0^t q^{SRVF}(r)|q^{SRVF}(r)|dr$; thus, the mapping from curve to SRVF is a bijection up to a translation. An important fact about the SRVF is that the action of Γ becomes $(q^{SRVF}, \gamma) = (q^{SRVF} \circ \gamma)\sqrt{\dot{\gamma}}$. Note that the SRVF representation can be used for curves of any dimension, though the focus here is on two-dimensional curves.

Surfaces In similar fashion, one can define a new representation of surfaces. In this case, let $\mathscr{F}$ represent the space of all smooth embeddings of $\mathbb{S}^2$ in $\mathbb{R}^3$ and let Γ be the set of all diffeomorphisms from $\mathbb{S}^2$ to itself. Again, Γ serves as the re-parameterization group for spherical surfaces. In this work, we only consider closed or spherical surfaces, but this framework is readily applicable to other types of surfaces including quadrilateral, hemispherical, cylindrical, etc. For a closed surface $f \in \mathscr{F}$, $f \circ \gamma$ represents its re-parameterization (i.e., the action of the re-parameterization group is the same as in the case of curves). To define a new representation of surfaces that allows parameterization-invariant shape analysis, let $n(s) = \frac{\partial f}{\partial u}(s) \times \frac{\partial f}{\partial v}(s) \in \mathbb{R}^3$ denote the normal vector to the surface at the point $s = (u, v) \in \mathbb{S}^2$. Jermyn et al. (2012) defined the square-root normal field (SRNF) as $q^{SRNF}(s) = \frac{n(s)}{\sqrt{|n(s)|}}$, where $|\cdot|$ denotes the Euclidean norm in $\mathbb{R}^3$. If a surface f is re-parameterized to $f \circ \gamma$, then its SRNF is given by $(q^{SRNF}, \gamma) = (q^{SRNF} \circ \gamma)\sqrt{J_\gamma}$, where J_γ is the determinant of the Jacobian of γ. Note that unlike in the case of curves, inversion of SRNFs cannot be performed analytically. The numerical inversion of SRNFs has been considered by Xie et al. (2014) and Laga et al. (2017), and is a difficult computational problem. As defined here, SRNFs are only applicable to shape analysis of two-dimensional surfaces embedded in $\mathbb{R}^3$.

Advantages of SRVFs and SRNFs There are two main benefits of these new mathematical representations of curves and surfaces: (1) the group Γ acts on the space of SRVFs or SRNFs by isometries under the $\mathbb{L}^2$ metric, and (2) the $\mathbb{L}^2$ metric on the space of SRVFs (SRNFs) corresponds to an elastic metric (partial elastic metric) on the original space of absolutely continuous curves (smooth surfaces). In both cases, the resulting representation space after transformation is $\mathbb{L}^2$, henceforth denoted by $\mathscr{Q}$. The relationship of these two representations to elastic metrics is an important property as they provide a measure of the amount of bending and stretching to deform one curve/surface into another. This allows natural interpretation of the shape distance between objects as well as natural shape deformation paths as will be seen in later sections. Further details on the elastic metric can be found in Srivastava et al. (2011), Mio et al. (2007) and Kurtek et al. (2012b). Note that whenever our discussion applies to either the SRVF or SRNF, we use q without the superscript to denote the representation.

Definition of the Pre-shape Space Recall that shape is defined as a property of an object that is invariant to translation, scale, rotation and re-parameterization. The SRVF and SRNF representations, and associated elastic metrics, are automatically invariant to translation due to their definition through first derivatives only. For curves, scale invariance in this framework is achieved by re-scaling to unit length via $\int_0^1 |\dot{f}(t)|dt = \int_0^1 |q^{SRVF}(t)|^2dt = \|q^{SRVF}\|^2 = 1$. For surfaces, we re-scale them to have unit area: $\int_{\mathbb{S}^2} |n(s)|ds = \int_{\mathbb{S}^2} |q^{SRNF}(s)|^2ds = \|q^{SRNF}\|^2 = 1$. Thus, the resulting SRVFs or SRNFs lie on the unit Hilbert sphere, which forms the pre-shape space: $\mathscr{C} = \{q \in \mathscr{Q}|\|q\| = 1\}$ (in the case of closed curves there is an additional closure condition). We refer to $\mathscr{C}$ as the pre-shape space because up to this point, we have only accounted for translation and scaling variabilities. Invariance to rotation and re-parameterization is obtained differently, using equivalence classes.

2.2 Landmark-Constrained Shape Space for Curves

We begin by introducing landmark constraints into the SRVF representation as they play an important role in the rotation and re-parameterization steps. Suppose that in addition to the curve f, we are given k discrete landmarks marked on f, $\{f(t_1), \ldots, f(t_k)\} \in \mathbb{R}^2$. Also, let $SO(2)$ denote the group of all rotations in 2D (also called the special orthogonal group). To take into consideration the landmark constraints that were marked on the curve f, we must redefine the set of allowed re-parameterizations as a subgroup of the unconstrained re-parameterization group Γ whose elements respect landmark matching. For this purpose, we define $\Gamma_0 = \{\gamma : [0, 1] \rightarrow [0, 1]|\gamma(0) = 0, \gamma(1) = 1, 0 < \dot{\gamma} < \infty, \gamma(t_i) = t_i, i = 1, \ldots, k\} \subset \Gamma$ as the landmark-constrained re-parameterization group. Applying two elements, $O \in SO(2)$ and $\gamma \in \Gamma_0$, to a curve f yields the transformed curve $O(f \circ \gamma)$, where the landmark points remain unmoved; the SRVF of this transformed curve is given by $O(q^{SRVF} \circ \gamma)\sqrt{\dot{\gamma}}$. Then, the landmark-constrained shape space, denoted by $\mathscr{S}$, is defined by the set of equivalence classes $[q^{SRVF}] = \{O(q^{SRVF} \circ \gamma)\sqrt{\dot{\gamma}}|O \in SO(2), \gamma \in \Gamma_0\}$ (note that these SRVF equivalence classes correspond to equivalence classes on the space of the original curves given by $[f] = \{O(f \circ \gamma) | O \in SO(2), \gamma \in \Gamma_0\}$. Thus, the landmark-constrained shape space is a quotient space: $\mathscr{S} = \mathscr{C}/(SO(2) \times \Gamma_0)$. The equivalence classes $[q^{SRVF}]$ represent the landmark-constrained shapes uniquely, and the shape space $\mathscr{S}$ provides the desired invariances to translation, scaling, rotation, and landmark-constrained re-parameterization.

Next, we define a suitable metric on $\mathscr{S}$. As mentioned earlier, an important property of the elastic metric on the space of absolutely continuous curves is that, under the SRVF representation, it is equivalent to the standard $\mathbb{L}^2$ metric (Srivastava et al. 2011). We begin by defining the elastic distance between two curves using their SRVF representation on $\mathscr{C}$. Since the pre-shape space $\mathscr{C}$ is a Hilbert sphere, the geodesic distance between two curves represented via their SRVFs $q_1, q_2 \in \mathscr{C}$ is given by $d_{\mathscr{C}}(q_1^{SRVF}, q_2^{SRVF}) = \theta = \cos^{-1}(\langle q_1^{SRVF}, q_2^{SRVF} \rangle)$, where $\langle \cdot, \cdot \rangle$ is the $\mathbb{L}^2$ inner product; the corresponding geodesic path (optimal deformation path) is given analytically by $\alpha(q_1^{SRVF}, q_2^{SRVF})(\tau) = \frac{1}{\sin(\theta)}(\sin((1-\tau)\theta)q_1^{SRVF} + \sin(\tau\theta)q_2^{SRVF})$, $\tau \in [0, 1]$. The rotation and landmark-constrained re-parameterization groups act on $\mathscr{C}$ by isometries, which allows the $\mathbb{L}^2$ metric to descend from the pre-shape space to the quotient shape space. Then, the landmark-constrained geodesic distance in the shape space $\mathscr{S}$ is given by:

$$d([f_1], [f_2]) \equiv d_{\mathscr{S}}([q_1^{SRVF}], [q_2^{SRVF}]) = \min_{O \in SO(2), \gamma \in \Gamma_0} d_{\mathscr{C}}(q_1^{SRVF}, O(q_2^{SRVF} \circ \gamma)\sqrt{\dot{\gamma}}).$$

(1)

The optimization over $SO(2)$ and Γ_0 is often referred to as the registration process, which aligns geometric features across shapes. The optimal rotation is found using Procrustes analysis, which involves singular value decomposition (SVD). To optimize over Γ_0, one can take a product space approach where the complete optimization problem is separated into an optimization over the unconstrained re-parameterization group Γ for each segment formed using the landmark constraints (see left panel of Fig. 1). See Strait et al. (2017) and Robinson (2012) for the implementation details. Once the optimal pair (O^*, γ^*) is found, one can compute the geodesic path in the SRVF shape space using $\alpha(q_1^{SRVF}, O^*(q_2^{SRVF} \circ \gamma^*)\sqrt{\dot{\gamma}^*})$, and map it back to the space of absolutely continuous curves for visualization purposes. This procedure provides the landmark-constrained elastic geodesic path and distance between shapes of two curves.

2.3 Landmark-Constrained Shape Space for Surfaces

In contrast to the elastic curve framework, it is not a simple task to invert an arbitrary SRNF to obtain its original surface (Laga et al. 2017; Xie et al. 2014). Thus, in this case, we work directly in the space of smooth surfaces under the pullback of the $\mathbb{L}^2$ metric from the SRNF space; this is the previously mentioned partial elastic metric (Jermyn et al. 2012). We provide some details next.

Throughout this section, with a slight abuse of notation, we use $\mathscr{C}$ as the pre-shape space of smooth surfaces rather than their SRNF representations. Let each surface $f \in \mathscr{C}$ be annotated by k landmark points. Let $s_1, \ldots, s_k$ be the locations of these landmarks on $\mathbb{S}^2$ such that $f(s_i) \in \mathbb{R}^3$, $i = 1, \ldots, k$ are the given landmarks on the parameterized surface f. To form the landmark constrained shape space we define $\Gamma_0 = \{\gamma : \mathbb{S}^2 \to \mathbb{S}^2 | \gamma$ is a diffeomorphism, $\gamma(s_i) = s_i, i = 1, \ldots, k\} \subset \Gamma$ as the landmark-constrained re-parameterization group for spherical surfaces. The rotation group $SO(3)$ acts on the pre-shape space as $(O, f) = Of$; the constrained re-parameterization group Γ_0 acts on $\mathscr{C}$ as before by composition $(f, \gamma) = (f \circ \gamma)$. Then, an equivalence class of a surface f is given by $[f] = \{O(f \circ \gamma) | O \in SO(3), \gamma \in \Gamma_0\}$, and represents a landmark-constrained shape of a spherical surface uniquely. The set of all such equivalence classes is defined to be the landmark-constrained elastic shape space denoted by $\mathscr{S}$. As in the case of curves, because $SO(3)$ and Γ_0 act on $\mathscr{C}$ by isometries, the partial elastic metric descends from the pre-shape space to the quotient space $\mathscr{S}$.

The shape geodesic between two landmark-constrained surfaces f_1 and f_2, such that $f_j(s_i), i = 1, \ldots, k$, and $j = 1, 2$, denote the landmarks on them, is defined as:

$$d_{\mathscr{S}}([f_1], [f_2]) = \min_{O \in SO(3), \gamma \in \Gamma_0} \left(\min_{\substack{F : [0,1] \to \mathscr{C} \\ F(0) = f_1, \ F(1) = O(f_2 \circ \gamma)}} \left(\int_0^1 \langle\langle \frac{dF}{dt}(t), \frac{dF}{dt}(t) \rangle\rangle^{(1/2)} dt \right) \right),$$

(2)

where $F(t)$ is a path in $\mathscr{C}$ and $\langle\langle \cdot, \cdot \rangle\rangle$ is the partial elastic metric. The quantity $L[F] = \int_0^1 \langle\langle \frac{dF}{dt}(t), \frac{dF}{dt}(t) \rangle\rangle^{(1/2)} dt$ denotes the length of the path F. The inside minimization problem seeks the shortest path (geodesic) between f_1 and $O(f_2 \circ \gamma)$ in $\mathscr{C}$; the solution can be found using a path-straightening algorithm (Klassen and Srivastava 2006; Kurtek et al. 2012a; Samir et al. 2014). In the presented results, we approximate the geodesic using a straight line path. The outside minimization problem seeks an optimal landmark-constrained registration between f_1 and f_2, which is a search for an optimal rotation $O^* \in SO(3)$ and an optimal landmark-constrained re-parameterization $\gamma^* \in \Gamma_0$. The search for O^* is again performed using Procrustes analysis. To find γ^*, we require two steps: (1) an initialization that matches given landmark points on f_1 and f_2, and (2) a gradient descent search over Γ_0 that finds the optimal landmark-constrained re-parameterization. We begin with a description of the first step.

Initial Landmark Matching First, we must find two initial diffeomorphisms $\gamma_1, \gamma_2 : \mathbb{S}^2 \to \mathbb{S}^2$ that map the selected landmarks on surfaces f_1 and f_2 with locations $\{\tilde{s}_1, \ldots \tilde{s}_k\} \in \mathbb{S}^2$ and $\{\bar{s}_1, \ldots \bar{s}_k\} \in \mathbb{S}^2$, respectively, to a standard set of landmarks $(s_1, \ldots, s_k \in \mathbb{S}^2)$. We briefly describe this procedure for γ_1. In general, the deformations between the landmarks can be very large. Thus, we divide the original problem into l smaller deformation steps. We first connect each pair of matched landmarks on $\mathbb{S}^2$ with a geodesic (great circle) and sample it uniformly using l steps. Then, we begin by solving for the first small deformation that matches the first point to the second point on this geodesic path for all landmarks. Let η_j be the tangent vector to $\mathbb{S}^2$ at $\tilde{s}_j$ such that $\exp_{\tilde{s}_j}(\eta_j) = s_j$; exp denotes the exponential map on the unit two-sphere. For brevity, we do not provide the full expression for the exponential map, but note that it is available analytically. Then, using a Gaussian kernel, we define a vector field over $\mathbb{S}^2$ according to $V(s) = \sum_{j=1}^{k} K(s, s_j)\eta_j$ in such a way that $V(s_j) = \eta_j$. This is a simple interpolation step that uses the landmark vector fields to define a full vector field over $\mathbb{S}^2$. The desired small deformation at each point s is obtained by computing $\exp_s(V_s)$. This is repeated for each of the l small steps. The desired large deformation γ_1, which guarantees that the landmarks on f_1 are matched exactly to the standard landmarks, is obtained through composition of the l small deformations. The procedure can be repeated for the second surface f_2 in the same manner. This general procedure is also described in Kurtek et al. (2013a).

Gradient Descent Optimization Over Γ_0   One can perform the optimization over Γ_0 directly as suggested by Eq. (2). However, the correspondence between the partial elastic metric on the space of smooth closed surfaces and the $\mathbb{L}^2$ metric on the space of SRNFs allows us to greatly simplify the problem. Given two surfaces f_1 and f_2 with matched landmarks, the optimization over Γ_0 is solved using the energy $E_{\gamma_{id}}(\gamma) = \|q_1^{SRNF} - \phi_{q_2^{SRNF}}(\gamma)\|^2$, where q_1^{SRNF}, q_2^{SRNF} are the SRNFs of f_1 and f_2 and $\phi_{q_2^{SRNF}}(\gamma) = (q_2^{SRNF} \circ \gamma)\sqrt{J_\gamma}$. An algorithm for finding optimal landmark-constrained re-parameterizations of surfaces via this energy is given in Kurtek et al. (2013a, 2010, 2011b) and is omitted here for brevity. We refer the interested reader to those papers for the details.

2.4   Motivating Examples

Landmark-Constrained Curves   The utility of landmark-constrained shape analysis for curves is presented in Fig. 2 for two complicated outlines of elephants. These elephants are fairly similar with two noticeable differences. First, the trunk of the first elephant is oriented downwards, but upwards for the second one. Also, the first elephant has four distinct legs (with very wide gaps in-between), while the second elephant has no gap between the second and third legs; visually, this feature looks like one large leg, although it is obvious that it should represent two legs. By identifying these special, salient features (i.e., the feet and trunk) as landmarks, we force them to be in correspondence. In some cases, this is a necessary constraint to enforce, as a standard unconstrained elastic shape analysis framework may not know how to handle the lack of a gap between the two legs on the second elephant or the very different orientations of the trunks.

The landmark-constrained geodesic distance between this pair of shapes is 0.7803, which provides an accurate measure of their shape differences; this claim is supported by the image displayed in the bottom panel of Fig. 2, which shows seven equally-spaced points along the shape space geodesic path where the initial

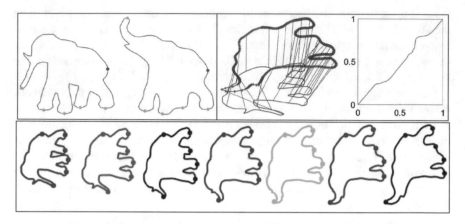

Fig. 2 Top left: Outlines of two elephants used for shape comparison. The starting point
(a landmark) is shown in red, while additional landmarks are in green. Top right: Correspondence
of features between the two elephants and the optimal landmark-constrained re-parameterization
function. Bottom: Landmark-constrained geodesic path between the two elephants, with landmarks
marked along the path

shape is the first elephant and the final shape is the second elephant. This path shows
how one can optimally deform the first elephant into the second, while preserving
the landmarks (marked by points in the figure); it represents a natural deformation
between the two given elephant shapes. The landmarks remain in correspondence
throughout, and one can clearly see the expected shift in the orientation of the
trunk as well as the reasonable transformation from being able to see all four legs
distinctly to the gap disappearing between the middle two legs.

The top-right panel of Fig. 2 shows two additional plots associated with the
landmark-constrained elastic matching obtained for the two elephants. The left plot
shows the correspondence of points on the first elephant (red) to the points on the
second elephant (blue); the landmark-constrained analysis ensured that geometric
features around the trunks and legs match each other well. The right plot shows
the optimal matching function (landmark-constrained diffeomorphism). Deviations
from a straight, 45° line indicate the elastic nature of the matching problem.

Landmark-Constrained Surfaces Figure 3 displays a motivating example for the
surface case. In the top left panel, we show two highly articulated surfaces of
a standing cat and a standing horse. On top of each surface, we marked seven
landmark points corresponding to natural features of the two animals (ears, legs
and tail; the landmark on the tail of the horse is occluded). In the bottom panel,
we show the initial landmark matching procedure. The leftmost spherical domain
contains the two sets of landmarks as given on the surfaces (red for cat and black
for horse). First, we compute an optimal rotation of the domain to match the two
landmark sets as well as possible (this is an area-preserving element of Γ). The
result is given on the middle sphere. Note that the landmarks are now closer than

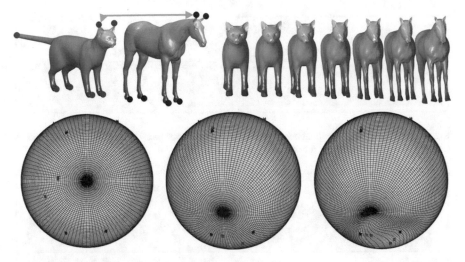

Fig. 3 Motivating example for landmark-constrained elastic shape analysis of spherical surfaces

previously. Finally, we compute the nonlinear, large deformation that matches the two sets of landmarks exactly. For reference, we still show the original landmark locations. We also display an intermediate matching result in magenta. After initial landmark matching, we compute the landmark-constrained registration and geodesic between the two surfaces. The geodesic path is displayed in the top right panel of the figure. The path preserves important features of the two animal models; the two surfaces naturally deform into each other.

2.5   Additional Examples

Figure 4 provides four additional examples of geodesic paths on the landmark-constrained shape space of curves. All examples in this manuscript were generated using the MPEG-7 dataset.[1] All of these examples were selected because of the potential for ambiguities in the matching of features using unconstrained elastic shape analysis (i.e., without landmarks). The first example compares two octopi, where the arms are in drastically different locations. Without the ability to constrain the comparison at the arm locations, the result may not display a natural path between the two shapes. However, placing eight meaningful landmarks allows for the geodesic path to show a natural movement of the octopus arms. Next to the octopus example is a comparison of two crowns, the first of which has five distinct tips, while the second one appears to have more than five tips. The landmark

---

[1]http://www.dabi.temple.edu/~shape/MPEG7/dataset.html.

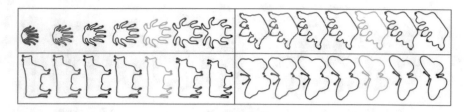

Fig. 4 Landmark-constrained geodesic paths for several examples from the MPEG-7 dataset. Corresponding landmarks are marked along each path

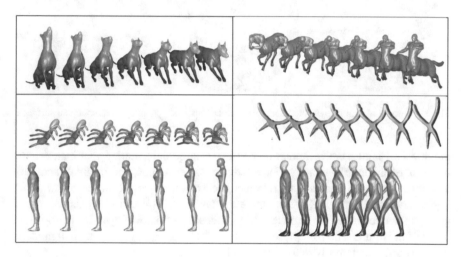

Fig. 5 Landmark-constrained geodesic paths for several examples from the TOSCA and SHREC 2007 datasets

constraints in this case allow the extra tips to grow out of the gaps between tips in the first crown. The last two comparisons consider cows and butterflies, respectively. As in the previous examples, the addition of landmarks to the elastic representation provides valid deformations between shapes.

Next, we provide several examples of landmark-constrained geodesic paths (approximated using linear paths) between shapes of very complex spherical surfaces including dogs, cats, horses and human bodies. The models used in all of the examples in this manuscript were obtained from the TOSCA (Bronstein et al. 2008) and SHREC 2007 (Girogi et al. 2007) databases. The results are presented in Fig. 5. We do not show the marked landmarks in these cases, which were chosen as extreme points on the surfaces, i.e., legs, ears, tails, etc. In all examples, geometric features are nicely preserved along the geodesic paths. Furthermore, all of the deformations are natural: movement of arms and legs reflects our intuition. For example, the first path deforms a sitting dog into a laying dog. Note that at each point along the path the head of the dog is slightly lowered while the front limbs simply extend out. Figure 6 presents two examples where we compare landmark-

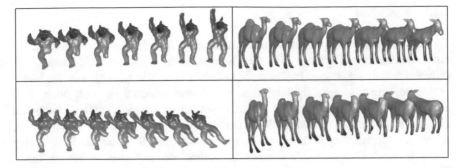

Fig. 6 Comparison of two landmark-constrained elastic geodesic paths (top) to their unconstrained elastic counterparts (bottom)

constrained geodesics (top) to unconstrained ones (bottom). It is clear that, in both examples, landmarks add valuable information, which improves the comparison of the given shapes.

3 Statistical Analysis of Landmark-Constrained Shapes

In this section, we provide two useful tools for statistical shape analysis of landmark-constrained curves and surfaces: computing the sample mean and summarizing variability using tangent principal component analysis (tPCA).

3.1 Sample Averaging

We begin by defining an intrinsic mean called the Karcher mean. Let $\{f_1, f_2, \ldots, f_n\}$ denote a sample of curves or surfaces. Then, the sample Karcher mean is given by $[\bar{f}] = \arg\min_{[f] \in \mathscr{S}} \sum_{i=1}^{n} d([f], [f_i])^2$. A gradient-based approach for finding the Karcher mean is given in Dryden and Mardia (1998) and Le (2001), and is omitted here for brevity; a specific implementation of this algorithm for SRVFs and SRNFs can be found in Kurtek et al. (2013b) and Kurtek et al. (2016), respectively. Further theoretical results and properties of Karcher means are given in Bhattacharya (2008), Bhattacharya and Bhattacharya (2012) and Bhattacharya and Lin (2017). Note that the resulting Karcher mean is defined as an entire equivalence class, which is how we defined shapes. For visualization purposes and subsequent covariance computation, we select one representative element $\bar{f} \in [\bar{f}]$. Next, we present several averaging results for landmark-constrained shapes of curves and closed surfaces.

3.1.1 Examples

We present two examples of Karcher averaging for a collection of landmark-constrained curves. Figure 7 shows the first example: a sample of 20 bones with different features. Some of the bones are slightly bent, and the edges of the bones vary from sharp to smooth. Four landmarks were selected on each bone. Two elastic averages are displayed; the middle average was computed without landmark constraints, while the right one includes landmarks. In this case, the two averages are somewhat similar; they both indeed look like bones, and it appears as if averaging over a somewhat large sample size has "smoothed" out any unusual features that a few of the bones may have. The difference in the two averages being fairly small suggests that landmark information may not be as crucial in this example.

The second example features a sample of 12 camels displayed in Fig. 8; these camels vary in the number of clearly visible legs as well as the number of humps the animal has. Unconstrained Karcher averaging (without landmarks) does not preserve the legs well, as shown in the middle panel of Fig. 8. Thus, landmark-

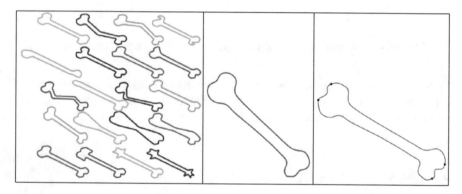

Fig. 7 Left: Sample of 20 bone curves. Middle: Average of bones without landmark constraints. Right: Average of landmark-constrained bones (with landmarks annotated in black)

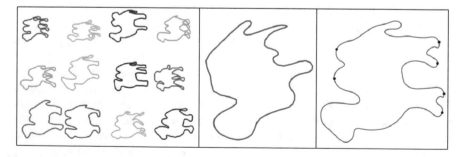

Fig. 8 Left: Sample of 12 camel outlines. Middle: Average of camels without landmark constraints. Right: Average of landmark-constrained camels (with landmarks annotated in black)

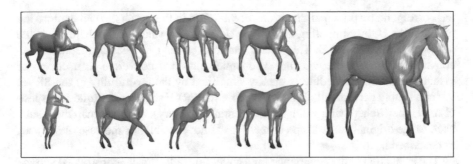

Fig. 9 Left: Sample of eight horse surfaces. Right: Landmark-constrained average of the eight horse shapes

constrained Karcher averaging appears to be a better option to preserve as many features in the camels as possible. Six landmarks were selected on each camel (one for each of the four legs and one for each of the two possible humps). The landmark-constrained average camel shape is shown in the right panel of Fig. 8. Since all but two of the camels have two humps, the average also has two distinct humps. However, the Karcher mean's legs show some signs of occlusion as the gap (particularly in the front pair of legs) is fairly small. This is inherited from the camels in the sample which share that property. For both examples, the gradient descent algorithm converged after approximately 500 iterations.

Finally, we close this section with one example of averaging shapes of landmark-constrained surfaces. The example is presented in Fig. 9 and considers a sample of eight horse shapes. The horses mostly differ in their pose. We selected eight landmarks on each horse corresponding to the two ears, the snout, the four legs and the tail. The resulting average is presented in the right panel. It is a nice representative of the given data where all features have been preserved. The pose of the average horse is approximately neutral.

3.2 Summarization of Variability

Tangent principal component analysis (tPCA) is a useful way to visualize principal directions of variability in shape datasets. We first describe this procedure for landmark-constrained curves. Given the Karcher mean shape, we compute the shooting vectors v_i, $i = 1, \ldots, n$ by projecting all of the SRVFs into the linear tangent space at $\bar{q}$, the SRVF of $\bar{f}$, using the inverse exponential map. At the implementation stage, the shooting vectors are sampled using N points allowing us to use multivariate tools on this tangent space to perform tPCA. We first compute the sample covariance matrix given by $K = \frac{1}{n-1} \sum_{i=1}^{n} v_i v_i^T$ (assuming that the v_is are stacked into long vectors). The SVD of K is given by $K = U\Sigma U^T$, where Σ is a diagonal matrix of principal component variances and the columns of U are

the corresponding principal directions of variation in the data. One can explore the
ith direction U_i by computing $v = t\sqrt{\Sigma_{ii}}U_i$ (for some value of t), where Σ_{ii} is the
ith diagonal element of Σ. This vector can then be mapped back to the landmark-
constrained shape space via the exponential map and converted to a curve for
visualization. This procedure is greatly simplified by the invertibility of the SRVF.
We can simply perform all of the analysis on the SRVF shape space (quotient space
of the Hilbert sphere with a simple differential geometry), and then map the results
back to the original curve shape space. This is not possible for the case of surfaces
as described next.

The evaluation of the covariance for a collection of landmark-constrained surface
shapes is performed as follows. First, we find the shooting vectors from the
estimated Karcher mean $\bar{f}$ to each of the surfaces in the sample, $v_i = \frac{dF_i^*}{dt}|_{t=0}$,
where $i = 1, \ldots, n$ and F^* denotes a geodesic path in the landmark-constrained
shape space $\mathscr{S}$ (computed using path-straightening as before). To generate a much
lower dimensional, orthonormal basis denoted by $\{B_j | j = 1, \ldots, m\}$, $m \leq n$, we
apply the Gram-Schmidt procedure under the partial elastic metric $\langle\langle \cdot, \cdot \rangle\rangle$ to the
observed shooting vectors $\{v_i, i = 1, \ldots, n\}$. We approximately represent each
original shape using a low dimensional coefficient vector $c_i = \{c_{i,j}, j = 1, \ldots, m\}$,
where $c_{i,j} = \langle\langle v_i, B_j \rangle\rangle$. The sample covariance matrix can be computed in the
coefficient space as $K = \frac{1}{n-1}\sum_{i=1}^{n} c_i c_i^T \in \mathbb{R}^{m \times m}$ and tPCA can be performed
using K as before. This results in the principal directions of variation in the given
data U and the diagonal matrix of principal component variances Σ. To explore the
principal direction $U_i \in \mathbb{R}^m$, we can compute the corresponding shooting vector as
$v = t\sqrt{\Sigma_{ii}}\sum_{j=1}^{m} U_{i,j}B_j$ ($\sqrt{\Sigma_{ii}}$ denotes the ith diagonal element of Σ). One can then
map this vector to a surface f using the exponential map. The exponential map in
this case must be computed under the non-standard partial elastic metric introduced
earlier, which is not a simple task. This can be accomplished using a tool called
parallel transport, which was derived for this representation of surfaces by Xie et al.
(2013). For brevity, we do not provide details here but rather refer the interested
reader to that paper. In the current results, we approximate the exponential map
using a straight line.

3.2.1 Examples

Like in many standard statistical analyses, one may want to understand the
variability in a population given a collection of shapes. This can be done by looking
at principal directions of variation obtained through tPCA. The top panel of Fig. 10
shows the top two principal directions of variation in the bone data. The primary
direction includes a slight bending of the bone, as well as different patterns at
the ends of the bone (especially at the top end). The second direction controls
the thickness of the middle portion of the bone. Similarly, the middle panel of
Fig. 10 displays the two principal directions of variation for the collection of camel
shapes. The primary direction captures the variability in the presence of a gap

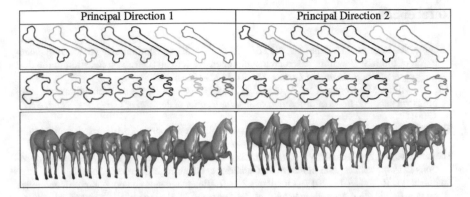

Fig. 10 Visualization of the two principal directions of variation for the bone, camel and horse examples. From left to right for each direction: $-1.5, -1, -0.5, 0$ (mean), $+0.5, +1, +1.5$ standard deviations from the mean

between the front legs or the rear legs (or both) among the sample of shapes. The second one appears to capture some more differences in the leg structure as well as the variability in the humps. Finally, the bottom panel of Fig. 10 displays the same results for the sample of horse surfaces. The principal direction mainly reflects the up-down movement of the horse's head and the pose of the front two legs. The second direction captures changes in the pose of the back legs and the overall body.

4 Summary

We present a framework for landmark-constrained shape analysis of curves and surfaces. The framework is based on elastic metrics and corresponding, simplifying representations termed the square-root velocity function and the square-root normal field. The elastic metrics combined with anatomical landmarks provide intuitive correspondences between shapes and result in natural geodesic deformations. We also provide tools for statistical analysis including averaging and summarization of variability using tangent principal component analysis. The resulting sample shape averages and principal directions of variability provide natural summaries of complex datasets.

Acknowledgements We would like to thank Dr. Hamid Laga (Murdoch University) for providing the spherically parameterized meshes for the TOSCA and SHREC 2007 datasets. This research was partially supported by NSF DMS 1613054 (SK).

References

Almhdie, A., Léger, C., Deriche, M., & Lédée, R. (2007). 3D registration using a new implementation of the ICP algorithm based on a comprehensive lookup matrix: Application to medical imaging. *Pattern Recognition Letters, 28*(12), 1523–1533.

Beg, M., Miller, M., Trouvé A., & Younes, L. (2005). Computing large deformation metric mappings via geodesic flows of diffeomorphisms. *International Journal of Computer Vision, 61*(2), 139–157.

Bhattacharya, A. (2008). Statistical analysis on manifolds: A nonparametric approach for inference on shape spaces. *Sankhya: The Indian Journal of Statistics, 70-A*(Part 2), 223–266.

Bhattacharya, A., & Bhattacharya, R. (2012). *Nonparametric inference on manifolds with applications to shape spaces. IMS monograph*. Cambridge: Cambridge University Press.

Bhattacharya, R., & Lin, L. (2017). Omnibus CLTs for Frechet means and nonparametric inference on non-Euclidean spaces. *Proceedings of the American Mathematical Society, 145*, 413–428.

Bookstein, F. L. (1986). Size and shape spaces for landmark data in two dimensions. *Statistical Science, 1*(2), 181–222.

Bouix, S., Pruessner, J., Collins, D., & Siddiqi, K. (2001). Hippocampal shape analysis using medial surfaces. *NEUROIMAGE, 25*, 1077–1089.

Brechbühler, C., Gerig, G., & Kübler, O. (1995). Parameterization of closed surfaces for 3D shape description. *Computer Vision and Image Understanding, 61*(2), 154–170.

Bronstein, A. M., Bronstein, M. M., & Kimmel, R. (2008). *Numerical geometry of non-rigid shapes*. New York: Springer.

Dryden, I. L., & Mardia, K. V. (1992). Size and shape analysis of landmark data. *Biometrika, 79*(1), 57–68.

Dryden, I. L., & Mardia, K. V. (1998). *Statistical shape analysis*. New York: Wiley.

Girogi, D., Biasotti, S., & Oaraboschi, L. (2007). Shape retrieval contest 2007: Watertight models track. In *Proceedings of Computer Graphics Forum*.

Gorczowski, K., Styner, M., Jeong, J., Marron, J., Piven, J., Hazlett, H., et al. (2010). Multi-object analysis of volume, pose, and shape using statistical discrimination. *IEEE Transactions on Pattern Analysis and Machine Intelligence, 32*(4), 652–666.

Grenander, U., & Miller, M. (1998). Computational anatomy: An emerging discipline. *Quarterly of Applied Mathematics, LVI*(4), 617–694.

Jermyn, I. H., Kurtek, S., Klassen, E., & Srivastava, A. (2012). Elastic shape matching of parameterized surfaces using square root normal fields. In *Proceedings of European Conference on Computer Vision* (pp. 804–817).

Joshi, S., Miller, M., & Grenander, U. (1997). On the geometry and shape of brain sub-manifolds. *Pattern Recognition and Artificial Intelligence, 11*, 1317–1343.

Joshi, S. H., Klassen, E., Srivastava, A., & Jermyn, I. H. (2007). A novel representation for Riemannian analysis of elastic curves in $\mathbb{R}^n$. In *Proceedings of the IEEE Conference on Computer Vision and Pattern Recognition* (pp. 1–7).

Kendall, D. G. (1984). Shape manifolds, Procrustean metrics, and complex projective shapes. *Bulletin of London Mathematical Society, 16*, 81–121.

Klassen, E., & Srivastava, A. (2006). Geodesics between 3D closed curves using path-straightening. In *Proceedings of ECCV. Lecture Notes in Computer Science* (pp. I:95–106). Berlin/Heidelberg: Springer.

Klassen, E., Srivastava, A., Mio, W., & Joshi, S. H. (2004). Analysis of planar shapes using geodesic paths on shape spaces. *IEEE Transactions on Pattern Analysis and Machine Intelligence, 26*(3), 372–383.

Kurtek, S., Klassen, E., Ding, Z., Avison, M. J., & Srivastava, A. (2011a). Parameterization-invariant shape statistics and probabilistic classification of anatomical surfaces. In *Proceedings of Information Processing in Medical Imaging*.

Kurtek, S., Klassen, E., Ding, Z., Jacobson, S. W., Jacobson, J. L., Avison, M. J., et al. (2011b). Parameterization-invariant shape comparisons of anatomical surfaces. *IEEE Transactions on Medical Imaging*, *30*(3), 849–858.

Kurtek, S., Klassen, E., Ding, Z., & Srivastava, A. (2010). A novel Riemannian framework for shape analysis of 3D objects. In *Proceedings of IEEE Conference on Computer Vision and Pattern Recognition* (pp. 1625–1632).

Kurtek, S., Klassen, E., Gore, J. C., Ding, Z., Srivastava, A. (2012a). Elastic geodesic paths in shape space of parameterized surfaces. *IEEE Transactions on Pattern Analysis and Machine Intelligence*, *34*(9), 1717–1730.

Kurtek, S., Srivastava, A., Klassen, E., & Ding, Z. (2012b). Statistical modeling of curves using shapes and related features. *Journal of the American Statistical Association*, *107*(499), 1152–1165.

Kurtek, S., Srivastava, A., Klassen, E., & Laga, H. (2013a). Landmark-guided elastic shape analysis of spherically-parameterized surfaces. *Computer Graphics Forum (Proceedings of Eurographics)*, *32*(2), 429–438.

Kurtek, S., Su, J., Grimm, C., Vaughan, M., Sowell, R. T., & Srivastava, A. (2013b). Statistical analysis of manual segmentations of structures in medical images. *Computer Vision and Image Understanding*, *117*(9), 1036–1050.

Kurtek, S., Xie, Q., Samir, C., & Canis, M. (2016). Statistical model for simulation of deformable elastic endometrial tissue shapes. *Neurocomputing*, *173*(P1), 36–41.

Laga, H., Xie, Q., Jermyn, I. H., & Srivastava, A. (2017, in press). Numerical inversion of SRNF maps for elastic shape analysis of genus-zero surfaces. *IEEE Transactions on Pattern Analysis and Machine Intelligence*. arXiv:1610.04531v1.

Le, H. (2001). Locating Frechet means with application to shape spaces. *Advances in Applied Probability*, *33*(2), 324–338.

Liu, W., Srivastava, A., & Zhang, J. (2010). Protein structure alignment using elastic shape analysis. In *Proceedings of the First ACM International Conference on Bioinformatics and Computational Biology* (pp. 62–70).

Malladi, R., Sethian, J. A., & Vemuri, B. C. (1996). A fast level set based algorithm for topology-independent shape modeling. *Journal of Mathematical Imaging and Vision*, *6*, 269–290.

Mio, W., Srivastava, A., & Joshi, S. H. (2007). On shape of plane elastic curves. *International Journal of Computer Vision*, *73*(3), 307–324.

Ramsay, J. O., & Silverman, B. W. (2005). *Functional data analysis* (2nd ed.). *Springer series in statistics*. New York: Springer.

Robinson, D. T. (2012). *Functional data analysis and partial shape matching in the square root velocity framework*. Ph.D. thesis, Florida State University.

Samir, C., Kurtek, S., Srivastava, A., & Canis, M. (2014). Elastic shape analysis of cylindrical surfaces for 3D/2D registration in endometrial tissue characterization. *IEEE Transactions on Medical Imaging*, *33*(5), 1035–1043.

Small, C. G. (1996). *The statistical theory of shape*. New York: Springer.

Srivastava, A., Klassen, E., Joshi, S. H., & Jermyn, I. H. (2011). Shape analysis of elastic curves in Euclidean spaces. *IEEE Transactions on Pattern Analysis and Machine Intelligence*, *33*, 1415–1428.

Strait, J., Kurtek, S., Bartha, E., & MacEachern, S. N. (2017). Landmark-constrained elastic shape analysis of planar curves. *Journal of the American Statistical Association*, *112*(518), 521–533.

Styner, M., Oguz, I., Xu, S., Brechbuhler, C., Pantazis, D., Levitt, J., et al. (2006). Framework for the statistical shape analysis of brain structures using SPHARM-PDM. In *Proceedings of MICCAI Open Science Workshop*.

Xie, Q., Jermyn, I. H., Kurtek, S., & Srivastava, A. (2014). Numerical inversion of SRNFs for efficient elastic shape analysis of star-shaped objects. In *European Conference on Computer Vision* (pp. 485–499).

Xie, Q., Kurtek, S., Le, H., & Srivastava, A. (2013). Transport of deformations along paths in shape space of elastic surfaces. In *Proceedings of International Conference on Computer Vision*.

Younes, L. (1998). Computable elastic distance between shapes. *SIAM Journal of Applied Mathematics*, *58*(2), 565–586.

Younes, L., Michor, P. W., Shah, J., Mumford, D., & Lincei, R. (2008). A metric on shape space with explicit geodesics. *Matematica E Applicazioni*, *19*(1), 25–57.

Zahn, C. T., & Roskies, R. Z. (1972). Fourier descriptors for plane closed curves. *IEEE Transactions on Computers*, *21*(3), 269–281.

Phylogeny-Based Kernels with Application to Microbiome Association Studies

Jian Xiao and Jun Chen

1 Introduction

The human microbiome is the collection of microorganisms (mostly bacteria) and their genomes associated with an individual body location. It plays an important role in promoting human health. For example, the human gut microbiome can harvest otherwise inaccessible nutrients, synthesize certain vitamins, promote the proper development of the immune system and protect us from pathogens (Turnbaugh et al. 2007). Increasingly more human microbiome studies have implicated the human microbiome in the pathogenesis of many human diseases such as obesity, diabetes, inflammatory bowel disease (IBD), irritable bowel syndrome (IBS), vaginosis and cancers (Cho 2012; Holmes et al. 2011; Honda and Littman 2012; Kinross et al. 2011; Plottel and Blaser 2011; Pughoeft and Versalovic 2011). Higher Firmicutes to Bacteroidetes ratios and reduced species diversity have been observed in obese humans (Ley et al. 2005, 2006). Two recent studies found that the abundance of phylum Fusobacteria increased significantly in the gut microbiome of colorectal cancer patients (Castellarin et al. 2012; Kostic et al. 2012). These findings have profound implications. If the microbiome effect is causal, new therapeutic strategies can be designed to treat diseases by modulating the microbiome composition (Collison et al. 2012; Virgin and Todd 2011). Even if the microbiome alteration is a result of disease process, the affected taxa in the microbiome can still serve as biomarkers for disease prevention and early diagnosis (Knights et al. 2011; Segata et al. 2011).

J. Xiao
Division of Biomedical Statistics and Informatics, Center for Individualized Medicine,
Mayo Clinic, Rochester, MN 55905, USA

J. Chen (✉)
Division of Biomedical Statistics and Informatics, Department of Health Science Research and
Center for Individualized Medicine, Mayo Clinic, Rochester, MN 55905, USA
e-mail: chen.jun2@mayo.edu

© Springer International Publishing AG 2017
D.-G. Chen et al. (eds.), *New Advances in Statistics and Data Science*,
ICSA Book Series in Statistics, https://doi.org/10.1007/978-3-319-69416-0_13

The development of next generation sequencing methods such as 454 pyrosequencing and Illumina Solexa sequencing enables researchers to study the microbiome composition by directly sequencing the environmental DNAs. One commonly used sequencing strategy involves sequencing a variable region of the 16S ribosomal RNA (rRNA) gene in the bacterial genome, and this variable region serves as 'fingerprint' for species identification. A basic bioinformatics workflow first clusters these 16S sequence reads into small sequence units based on sequence similarities, either by comparing to a curated reference set of 16S rRNA gene sequences or by de novo clustering method (Chen et al. 2013b). These small sequence units are termed as operational taxonomic units (OTUs) and, at 97% similarity level, they are thought to approximate the bacterial species. Each OTU has a representative DNA sequence, and a taxonomic lineage can be assigned to each OTU by comparing their sequence to existing 16S rRNA gene databases. Finally, a phylogenetic tree can be inferred based on the aligned OTU sequences, characterizing their evolutionary relationships. Therefore, a typical 16S data set is usually summarized as a table of counts of the detected OTUs, together with a phylogenetic tree among these OTUs. Sparsity (excessive zeros or zero-inflation) and phylogenetic tree structure are two key features of 16S-based microbiome data.

One challenge of statistical analysis of microbiome data involves appropriately modeling the microbiome data in relation to disease phenotypes or environmental covariates. Due to the complex interaction between bacterial species and the environment/disease and non-normality of the count data, traditional linear models are not appropriate for microbiome data. Kernel-machine (KM) methods, which allow modeling complex nonlinear relationships and potential interactive effects, are particularly appealing for microbiome data. Moreover, KM methods allow easy incorporation of prior structure information by defining a problem-specific kernel function. KM methods have been proven to be an effective approach for the analysis of complex genomic and genetic data, especially for testing the association between a group of genetic/genomic features and an outcome. The popularity of KM methods for genomic/genetic data is mainly due to the work of Liu et al. (2007, 2008), who connected the KM-based semi-parametric regression models with generalized mixed effects models and derived a score test for testing the significance of the expression of a gene pathway on a normal or binary outcome. Later, many variants of KM-based association tests have been proposed, ranging from the sequence kernel association test (SKAT) for human genetic data, to the microbiome regression-based kernel association test (MiRKAT) for human microbiome data (Kwee et al. 2008; Lee et al. 2012; Wu et al. 2010, 2011b, 2013; Zhao et al. 2015).

KM methods require a kernel function $K(\cdot, \cdot)$, which can be regarded as a similarity measure between observations. Though any generic kernels can be used, a well-defined kernel, which incorporates the field knowledge, is usually more powerful. For microbiome data, the phylogenetic tree provides important prior knowledge as how these bacterial species are related, and hence incorporating the phylogenetic tree into analysis can potentially improve the efficiency and power of statistical analysis of microbiome data. This was clearly demonstrated in the context of lower-dimensional embedding, canonical correlation analysis, regression analysis and multiple testing of microbiome data (Chen and Li 2013; Chen et al. 2013a, 2015; Purdom 2011; Zhao et al. 2015; Xiao et al. 2017). KM methods have also been applied to microbiome data (Chen and Li 2013; Zhao et al. 2015). Among these, MiRKAT is the most successful KM method designed for testing the association between the microbiome and an outcome variable (Zhao et al. 2015). Instead of inventing new microbiome-based kernels, MiRKAT converts distance measures into kernels, given the availability of various ecological distances for microbiome data. Since each distance measure represents an individual view of the microbiome, it is only powerful when the distance captures the relationship between the microbiome and the outcome and becomes powerless if the distance does not reflect the underlying biological relationship. Thus it is beneficial to consider multiple distance measures to have a comprehensive view of the microbiome in order not to miss important biologically relevant associations. Therefore, MiRKAT proposed an omnibus test, which combines multiple distance measures to improve the robustness and power of the test. By default, it uses three phylogeny-based distances: unweighted, generalized and weighted UniFrac distances, and one phylogeny-independent distance: Bray-Curtis distance (Chen et al. 2012; Lozupone and Knight 2005, 2008). The unweighted UniFrac distance (Lozupone and Knight 2005), which is defined as the fraction of the branch length of the tree that leads to descendants from either sample, but not both, is a qualitative measure that uses only the presence and absence information. It is efficient in detecting the community membership change or the abundance change in rare lineages, given that more prevalent species are likely to be present in all samples (Chen et al. 2012). In contrast, the weighted UniFrac distance (Lozupone and Knight 2008), which weighs the branches of the phylogenetic tree based on the abundance difference, is more sensitive to changes in abundant lineages. The generalized UniFrac distance (Chen et al. 2012) fills the gaps that the weighted and unweighted UniFrac distance do not over, and has been shown to be more powerful to detect changes in moderately abundant lineages. Bray-Curtis distance (Beals 1984), on the other hand, does not take into account the phylogenetic relationship among OTUs, and quantifies the dissimilarity between two samples on the basis of the OTU counts only. It is powerful to detect phylogenetically non-related changes.

One inherent problem with the 'distance-to-kernel' approach is the choice of distance measures. Though the above choice of distance measures seems reasonable in practice, it is not clear whether it constitutes the optimal combination to include in the omnibus test. Including too many biologically irrelevant distance measures will reduce the statistical power due to multiple testing while too few distance measures may miss relevant microbiome associations. Moreover, the 'flexibility' of choosing distance measures opens up the possibility of p-value hacking, where the 'best' p-value is reported after trying out different combinations of distance measures.

Here we circumvent the difficulty of choosing an optimal combination of distance measures by inventing a new phylogeny-based and fully parameterized kernel function. The kernel function is defined based on the OTU abundances and the phylogenetic tree, and are capable of detecting a broad range of microbiome changes. Microbiome change can occur in many forms. The change could be in the abundant, moderately abundant or rare lineages at different phylogenetic depth. For example, obesity has been associated with the change in the bacterial phyla, which are high up on the phylogenetic tree, while other diseases or traits may affect a much deeper level such as the genus level (Martiny et al. 2015). Moreover, the change can be highly nonlinear. Through the use of three parameters, the new kernel can capture microbiome effects in bacterial lineages of different abundance levels and different phylogenetic depths, and allows modeling a wide range of nonlinear relationships. Each parameter has a nice biological interpretation and, by tuning the parameter, we can gain insights about how the microbiome interacts with the environment.

We demonstrated the performance of the phylogeny-based kernel using KM-based association test. We show that the omnibus test based on our new kernel outperforms MiRKAT based on traditional distance-converted kernels. We finally applied the phylogeny-based kernel to a real gut microbiome data from a diet-microbiome association study. We identified more nutrients associated with the gut microbiome using the phylogeny-based kernels.

2 Methods

In this paper, we directly define a three-parameter kernel function based on the OTU abundance data and the phylogenetic tree among OTUs. Before introducing the new kernel, we firstly define a phylogeny-induced correlation structure among OTUs, which is based on the observation that closely related OTUs usually have similar biological characteristics, and their traits tend to be correlated with the correlation depending on the divergence time between the OTUs.

2.1 Phylogeny-Induced Correlation Structure Among OTUs

Assume we have p OTUs on a phylogenetic tree, we define the trait correlation between OTU i and j using the following model, which is a direct extension of the trait evolution model by Martin and Hansen (1997):

$$C_{ij}(\rho, \theta) = e^{-\rho M_{ij}^{\theta}}, \ i, j = 1, \ldots, p,$$

where $\mathrm{M} = (M_{ij})$ is the $p \times p$ matrix of patristic distances between OTUs, i.e., the length of the shortest path linking the OTUs on the tree. The parameter $\rho \in [0, \infty)$ characterizes the evolutionary rate. If $\rho = 0$, there is no evolution at all since $C_{ij} = 1, \forall i, j$ and all traits are identical. While $\rho \to \infty$, the traits evolve so fast that there is no correlation between traits. From a statistical perspective, ρ controls the depth of phylogenetic grouping with a large ρ value grouping OTUs at

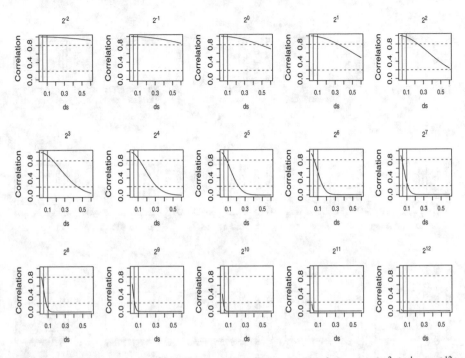

Fig. 1 The relationship between M (X axis) and C(ρ,θ) (Y axis) with $\theta=2$ and $\rho=2^{-2}, 2^{-1}, \ldots, 2^{12}$ (numbers on top). Blue and red lines represent species level (3%) and family level (10%) divergence respectively

a lower phylogenetic depth. The phylogenetic grouping is very similar in concept to taxonomic grouping, where OTUs from various taxonomic ranks (e.g. phylum, family, genus) are grouped. Thus by varying ρ, we can achieve various phylogenetic resolutions by grouping OTUs at different phylogenetic depths. When $\rho \to \infty$, we have the finest OTU-level resolution. Compared to the trait evolution model by Martin and Hansen (1997), we have an extra parameter θ, which controls the decay rate of the correlation with respect to the patristic distance. The effect can be best seen from Figs. 1 and 2, where we set $\theta = 2$ and 16 respectively and plot the correlation coefficients C_{ij} as a function of the patristic distances M_{ij}. When $\theta=2$, the correlation decays slowly with the patristic distances, and the grouping is 'soft' meaning no clear boundary as for where the grouping takes place. When $\theta=16$, the correlation drops abruptly from (nearly) 1 to (nearly) 0 at a certain distance threshold depending on ρ, and the grouping is 'hard', where OTUs with patristic distances less than a threshold are grouped together. Therefore, by varying θ, we can achieve soft and hard grouping of the OTUs, making the model more flexible.

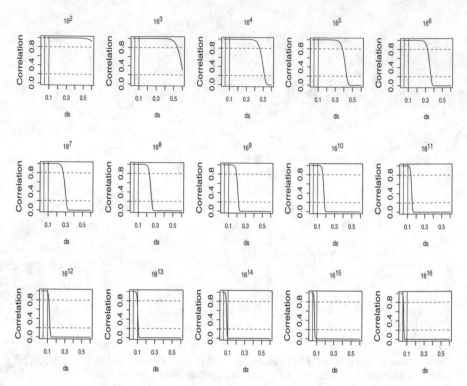

Fig. 2 The relationship between M (X axis) and C(ρ,θ) (Y axis) with $\theta=16$ and $\rho=16^2, 16^2,\ldots, 16^{16}$ (numbers on top). Blue and red lines represent species level (3%) and family level (10%) divergence respectively

2.2 A Phylogeny-Based Kernel for Microbiome Data

With the phylogeny-induced correlation structure, we next define the phylogeny-based kernel function. Let $z = (z_1,\ldots,z_n)^T$, where $z_i = (z_{i1},\ldots,z_{ip})^T$ denotes observed (normalized) abundance vector for the p OTUs from ith sample. Then we define the three-parameter phylogeny-based kernel function as

$$K_{\text{phy}}(z_i, z_j; \gamma, \rho, \theta) = \mathbf{f}(z_i, \gamma)^T \mathbf{C}(\rho, \theta)\mathbf{f}(z_j, \gamma),$$

where $\mathbf{f}(z_i, \gamma) = (f(z_{i1}, \gamma),\ldots,f(z_{ip}, \gamma))^T, f$ denotes a transformation function with parameter γ. With some abuse of notation, we also denote $K_{\text{phy}}(\gamma, \rho, \theta)$ as the kernel matrix evaluated at the data points z.

Remark 1 The OTU abundance data has a very skewed distribution, i.e., a few highly abundant OTUs with a large number of low-abundance and rare OTUs. The OTU data also contain excessive zeros, which makes the modeling very difficult. To improve the modeling capability of the kernel, we propose a power transform on z_i:

$$f(z_{ij}, \gamma) = \begin{cases} z_{ij}^{\gamma} & z_{ij} \neq 0 \\ 0 & z_{ij} = 0, \end{cases}$$

$j = 1, \ldots, p$ and γ is a constant ($0 \leq \gamma \leq 2$). The above transformation is similar to the Box-Cox transformation and can approximate a wide range of nonlinear functions including the *log* function by the parameter γ. The parameter γ also controls the weights on OTUs of different abundance levels. When γ is large, the effects of abundant OTUs will dominate. As γ becomes smaller, these less abundant OTUs will contribute more weights. When $\gamma = 0$, the abundance data is reduced to presence/absence data. Since the majority of the OTUs are low-abundance/rare, small γ favors these OTUs. Thus γ is designed to improve the efficiency of the proposed kernel in capturing microbiome effects from OTU lineages of different abundance levels. Note that the effect of γ is very similar to the α parameter in generalized UniFrac distance (Chen et al. 2012) and it also has some feature weighting/selection function (Wu et al. 2016).

Remark 2 The derivation of the phylogeny-based kernel function can be best understood based on a generalized mixed effects model

$$g(E(y_i)) = \beta_0 + \mathbf{f}(z_i, \gamma)^T \beta,$$

where $g(.)$ is a known link function, β_0 is the intercept and $\beta = (\beta_1, \cdots, \beta_p)^T$ are random effects for the p OTUs following a multivariate normal distribution

$$\beta \sim MVN(0, \tau^2 C(\rho, \theta)),$$

where τ^2 is variance component, and $C(\rho, \theta))$ is the phylogeny-induced correlation matrix. Thus we incorporate the phylogenetic tree information through a prior MVN distribution on the OTU effects. The model above is equivalent to

$$g(E(y_i)) = \beta_0 + h_i, \quad \mathbf{h} = (h_1, \cdots, h_p)^T \sim MVN(0, \tau^2 K_{\text{phy}}(\gamma, \rho, \theta)),$$

where $\mathbf{h}$ are aggregated OTU effects and K_{phy} is the phylogeny-based kernel matrix evaluated on the data points.

Remark 3 There exists some connection between the proposed kernel and existing kernels. For example, when $\rho \to \infty$ and $\gamma = 1$, it is easily seen that the phylogeny-based kernel becomes regular kernel $K_{\text{regular}} = zz^T$.

2.3   Kernel-Machine (KM) Association Test

To demonstrate the performance of the proposed kernel, we apply our kernel to KM-based association test, which was implemented in MiRKAT (Zhao et al. 2015).

KM-based association tests share a common framework, and are based on a score test, which compares similarity in the features to similarity in the outcome.

We first review KM-based linear and logistic regression framework briefly (Liu et al. 2007, 2008). Specifically, for subject i ($i = 1, \ldots, n$), we denote x_i a $q \times 1$ vector of covariates and z_i a $p \times 1$ vector of OTU abundances. We assume an intercept is included in x_i. Then for a normally distributed continuous outcome variable y_i, the outcome y_i depends on x_i and z_i through the following linear model

$$y_i = x_i^T \beta + h(z_i) + \varepsilon_i, \tag{1}$$

and, for a dichotomous outcome variable (e.g., $y = 1$ or 0), we use the logistic model

$$\text{logit}(P(y_i = 1)) = x_i^T \beta + h(z_i), \tag{2}$$

where β is a $q \times 1$ vector of regression coefficients, $h(z_i)$ is a smooth function from a functional space and the errors ε_i are assumed to be independent and follow $N(0, \sigma^2)$. Model (1) and (2) models covariate effects parametrically and the OTU effects non-parametrically. One popular choice of the functional space is the RKHS (Reproducible Kernel Hilbert Space), which is specified using a known kernel function $K(\cdot, \cdot)$ (Cristianini and Shawe-Taylor 2000). From Mercer's theorem, under some regularity conditions, a kernel function $K(\cdot, \cdot)$ implicitly specifies a unique function space spanned by a particular set of orthogonal basis functions (features) $\{\phi_j(z)\}_{j=1}^J$. In other words, any $h(z) \in \mathcal{H}_K$ can be represented using a set of bases as $h(z) = \sum_{j=1}^J \omega_j \phi_j(z) = \phi(z)^T \omega$ (the primal representation), where ω is a vector of coefficients. Equivalently, $h(z)$ can also be represented using the kernel function $K(\cdot, \cdot)$ as $h(z) = \sum_{l=1}^L \alpha_l K(z_l^*, z)$ (the dual representation), for some integer L, some constants α_i and some $\{z_1^*, \ldots, z_L^*\} \in R^p$.

2.3.1 Single Kernel-Based KM Association Test

Given γ, ρ and θ, under model (1) and (2) for microbiome data, when only a single kernel is considered, we estimate the coefficients β and $h(z)$ by maximizing the following penalized log-likelihood:

$$pl(h, \beta) = \sum_{i=1}^n \log L(h, \beta; y_i, x_i, z_i) - \frac{1}{2} \lambda ||h||^2_{\mathcal{H}_{K_{phy}(\gamma, \rho, \theta)}}$$

$$= \sum_{i=1}^n \log L(h, \beta; y_i, x_i, z_i) - \frac{1}{2} \lambda \alpha^T K_{phy}(\gamma, \rho, \theta) \alpha.$$

Through an important relationship between KM regression and mixed models (Liu et al. 2007, 2008; Gianola and Van Kaam 2008), $h(z)$ can be viewed as a subject-specific random effect that follows a MVN distribution with mean 0 and variance $\tau^2 K_{\text{phy}}(\gamma, \rho, \theta)$ (See Remark 2). Then, testing for an association between the microbiome composition and the outcome is equivalent to testing the null hypothesis that $H_0 : \tau^2 = 0$. Under the mixed-model framework, this can be done with a standard variance-component score test (Lin 1997). In particular, the score statistic is computed as

$$Q = \frac{1}{2\phi}(y - \hat{y}_0)^T K_{\text{phy}}(\gamma, \rho, \theta)(y - \hat{y}_0), \tag{3}$$

where $\hat{y}_0$ is the fitted mean of y under H_0 and ϕ is the dispersion parameter. For linear KM regression, $\phi = \hat{\sigma}^2$, the estimated error variance under the null model. For logistic KM regression, $\phi = 1$.

Under the null hypothesis, Q asymptotically follows a weighted mixture of χ^2 distribution. This can be best seen for the continuous-outcome case, where

$$y = X\beta + \varepsilon, \quad \varepsilon \sim MVN(0, \phi I).$$

Denote $P_0 = I - X(X^T X)^{-1} X^T$ the projection matrix into the residual space, we have

$$Q = \frac{1}{2\phi}\varepsilon^T P_0 K_{\text{phy}}(\gamma, \rho, \theta) P_0 \varepsilon.$$

Suppose λ_i is the ith eigenvalue of $P_0 K_{\text{phy}}(\gamma, \rho, \theta) P_0$, then asymptotically

$$Q \sim \sum_{i=1}^{n} \lambda_i \chi_i^2,$$

given a consistent estimator of ϕ. Similar results have also been derived for the binary-outcome case (Liu et al. 2008). P value can thus be analytically obtained through higher-order moment matching (Liu et al. 2009) or by the exact methods (Davies 1980) with possible small-sample adjustments via resampling (Lee et al. 2012). However, the comparatively small sample sizes for many microbiome studies and the complexity of the phylogeny-based kernels considered here lead to very conservative tests. Thus, MiRKAT (Zhao et al. 2015) further considers the use of new, alternative small-sample adjustments for both continuous and dichotomous traits (Chen et al. 2016).

2.3.2 Multiple Kernel-Based Optimal KM Association Test

As noted, although KM association test is valid even if a poor kernel is chosen, better kernel choices can lead to improved power. The optimal MiRKAT method (Zhao et al. 2015) extends the single kernel-based MiRKAT to simultaneously consider multiple kernels. The basic idea is to combine the strength of different kernels to detect a wide range of microbiome changes since each kernel is only powered to detect a specific type of microbiome change. The optimal MiRKAT performs testing with each individual kernel, obtains the p value for each of the tests, selects the minimum p value as the test statistic, and then evaluates the significance via a residual permutation approach. The purpose of the residual permutation is to derive the empirical null distribution of the test statistic. Specifically, we first obtain the residuals under the null model by fitting a linear and a logistic regression model for continuous and binary outcomes, respectively. Then outcomes under the null are generated by either permuting the residuals for continuous outcomes or using Fisher's non-central hypergeometric distribution to generate 1/0 values for binary outcomes. We refer the readers to Zhao et al. (2015) for more technical details. In this paper, we use the similar strategy to simultaneously consider multiple phylogeny-based kernels (different values of γ, ρ and θ). We label our method as optimal phylogenetic tree-kernel association test (PTKAT). We search the best combination of (γ, ρ, θ) over a pre-defined grid. The grid was chosen to strike a balance between power and computational efficiency.

3 Simulation Studies

In this section, we carry out various simulations to evaluate the performance of our proposed phylogeny-based kernel in the context of testing the association between the microbiome composition and an outcome. We compare our method (PTKAT) to the optimal MiRKAT method, where four distance-converted kernels, the weighted and unweighted UniFrac kernels, the Bray-Curtis kernel and the generalized UniFrac kernel with α value 0.5, are selected as the candidate kernels for the optimal MiRKAT method. For PTKAT, we use a grid of values from $\{16^{4k-2}|k = -7, -6, \cdots, 0\} \bigcup \{16^{2k-2}|k = 1, 2, \cdots, 12\}$ for parameter ρ, $\{0.001, 0.1, 0.5, 1, 2\}$ for parameter γ, and $\{2, 16\}$ for parameter θ. We let the outcome (binary or continuous) depend on the abundance of a cluster of OTUs with different abundance levels to reflect the clustered signals usually observed in microbiome data. Both linear and nonlinear OTU effects are considered in the simulations. Performance is evaluated with the type I error and the statistical power of detecting significant associations at an α level of 0.05.

3.1 Simulation Details

For all simulation settings, we simulate $n = 100$ samples for continuous outcomes and 50 cases and 50 controls for binary outcomes. We base our simulations on a real microbiome data set from a study of the human upper respiratory tract (Chen and Li 2013), which consists of an abundance table of 778 OTUs, together with a phylogenetic tree. We fit a Dirichlet-multinomial model (DMM) to the OTU counts and estimate the mean proportion vector and the dispersion parameter. We then simulate the counts using DMM with the estimated parameter values and a total read count drawn from a negative binomial distribution (depth = 5000 and size = 25). We next normalize the OTU counts into proportion data z, which has a unit sum for each sample.

We partition the 778 OTUs into 10 clusters using the partitioning-around-medoids (PAM) algorithm based on the patristic distances between OTUs. We pick three representative clusters with minimum, medium and maximum abundance (denoted as level 1 to level 3) and generate the outcomes based on the OTU abundances within the cluster. Given an OTU cluster (let $\mathcal{J}$ contain the OTU indices for the cluster), we consider the following specific models:

Gaussian outcome case
Linear OTU effects:

$$y_i = scale(\sum_{k \in \mathcal{J}} z_{ik})b_{causal} + \varepsilon_i, \ i = 1, \ldots, n,$$

Non-linear OTU effects:

$$y_i = scale(\sum_{k \in \mathcal{J}} z_{ik}^{\gamma})b_{causal} + \varepsilon_i, \ i = 1, \ldots, n,$$

where $scale(.)$ is the scaling function to standardize the data into mean 0 and variance 1 and $\gamma = 0.001$. The coefficients for OTU effects b_{causal} are drawn from $N(0, \sigma_b^2)$ and the random errors ε_i are drawn from $N(0, 1)$. The variance parameter σ_b^2 characterizes the effect size and we let σ_b^2 vary from 0 to 1 with a step size 1/6 to create a power curve.

Binary outcome case
Linear OTU effects:

$$\log(\frac{\pi_i}{1 - \pi_i}) = scale(\sum_{k \in \mathcal{J}} z_{ik})b_{causal}, \ i = 1, \ldots, n,$$

Non-linear OTU effects:

$$\log(\frac{\pi_i}{1 - \pi_i}) = scale(\sum_{k \in \mathcal{J}} z_{ik}^{\gamma})b_{causal}, \ i = 1, \ldots, n,$$

where $\pi_i = P(y_i = 1 | z_i, b_{causal})$ and $\gamma = 0.001$. The coefficients for OTU effects b_{causal} are drawn from $N(0, \sigma_b^2)$ as in the Gaussian outcome. We vary σ_b^2 from 0 to 2 with a step size 1/3 to create the power curve. All the simulation settings are replicated 1000 times.

Remark 4 For the nonlinear case, the small γ value converts the abundance data into nearly binary data (presence/absence). It represents an extreme case of nonlinearity, where the abundance does not matter. The nonlinear case corresponds to the biological scenario where the species richness (the number of OTUs) within a high-level taxonomic group such as the phylum Firmicutes is associated with the outcome.

3.2 Results on Simulated Data

As expected, from Table 1, both PTKAT and MiRKAT control the type I error at the nominal level of $0.01, 0.05$ and 0.10 under the null ($\sigma_b^2 = 0$) and the power increases with the effect size. The results for Gaussian and binary outcomes are very similar (Figs. 3 and 4 vs. Figs. 5 and 6). For linear OTU effects (Figs. 3 and 5), PTKAT and MiRKAT do not dominate each other. PTKAT has a better performance when the associated cluster has low abundance while MiRKAT performs better when the associated cluster is more abundant. Overall, the power difference is very moderate. For nonlinear effects (Fig. 4 and 6), the trend is opposite. MiRKAT is slightly more powerful than PTKAT when the associated cluster is less abundant. However, PTKAT becomes much more powerful than MiRKAT when the cluster becomes more abundant, and the power difference could be up to 50%. The suboptimal performance of MiRKAT under such scenarios is due to the insufficient coverage of the four distance-converted kernels used in the omnibus test. In contrast, PTKAT is more robust than MiRKAT, and the three-parameter kernel covers a wider range of microbiome changes, explaining the huge power gain in the nonlinear scenarios.

4 Application to a Real Data Set

Finally, we demonstrate the performance of phylogeny-based kernel by the analysis of a real microbiome data set from a study of long-term dietary effects on the human gut microbiome (Wu et al. 2011a). Diet strongly affects human health, partly by modulating gut microbiome composition. In this cross-sectional study, 98 healthy volunteers were enrolled, and habitual long-term diet information was collected using a food frequency questionnaire. The intake amounts of 214 nutrients were calculated based on questionnaires and further standardized by total caloric intake. Stool samples were collected, from which DNA was extracted, and the V1–V3 region of the 16S rRNA gene was sequenced using 454 pyrosequencing.

Table 1 Simulation results for empirical type-I error

Response type	Model	Abundance level	Methods	Level 0.01	Level 0.05	Level 0.10
Gaussian	Linear	Low	PTKAT	0.002	0.047	0.108
			MiRKAT	0.010	0.049	0.110
		Medium	PTKAT	0.001	0.049	0.101
			MiRKAT	0.009	0.054	0.100
		High	PTKAT	0	0.045	0.092
			MiRKAT	0.009	0.043	0.101
Gaussian	Nonlinear	Low	PTKAT	0	0.044	0.083
			MiRKAT	0.009	0.057	0.110
		Medium	PTKAT	0	0.051	0.102
			MiRKAT	0.002	0.041	0.090
		High	PTKAT	0.002	0.055	0.105
			MiRKAT	0.005	0.042	0.099
Binomial	Linear	Low	PTKAT	0	0.037	0.086
			MiRKAT	0.011	0.042	0.098
		Medium	PTKAT	0	0.046	0.109
			MiRKAT	0.010	0.045	0.103
		High	PTKAT	0	0.058	0.108
			MiRKAT	0.005	0.047	0.105
Binomial	Nonlinear	Low	PTKAT	0	0.038	0.080
			MiRKAT	0.006	0.042	0.081
		Medium	PTKAT	0	0.041	0.104
			MiRKAT	0.013	0.051	0.086
		High	PTKAT	0.001	0.036	0.090
			MiRKAT	0.015	0.053	0.104

16S sequence tags were denoised before being analyzed by the QIIME pipeline (Caporaso et al. 2010) with the default parameter settings, yielding 3071 OTUs after discarding the singleton OTUs. A phylogenetic tree among these OTUs was constructed using the FastTree algorithm.

We test for the association of these 214 nutrients with the gut microbiome composition to demonstrate the performance of PTKAT. We exclude very rare OTUs, which occur in less than 10% of the samples. We normalize the OTUs count data into proportions before running the analysis. The same parameter setting is used for PTKAT and MiRKAT as in the simulation study. Figure 7 plots the number of significant nutrients at different p-value cutoffs (raw p-value) for PTKAT and MiRKAT. Overall, PTKAT identifies more nutrients than MiRKAT at various significance levels. We finally apply Benjamini-Hochberg (BH) based false discovery rate (FDR) control to correct for multiple testing (Benjamini and Hochberg 1995). At an FDR of 15%, our procedure identifies 15 nutrients while MiRKAT does not identify any nutrient at this cutoff. Most of the identified nutrients are from the category 'fat' and the effect of dietary fat on the gut microbiome has

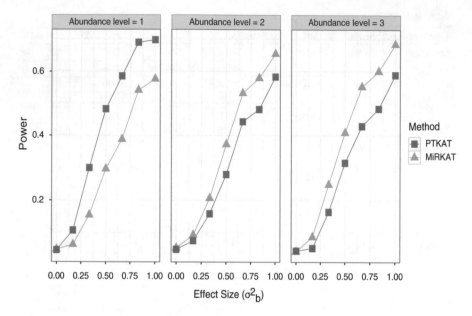

Fig. 3 Power curves for Gaussian outcome case with linear OTU effects. The cluster becomes more abundant from level 1 to level 3

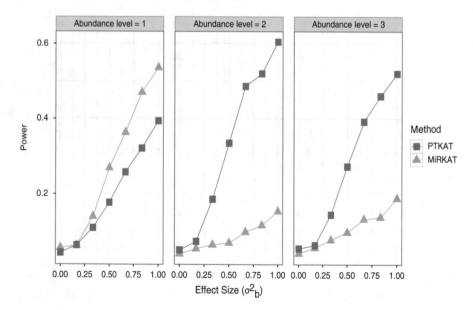

Fig. 4 Power curves for Gaussian outcome case with nonlinear OTU effects. The cluster becomes more abundant from level 1 to level 3

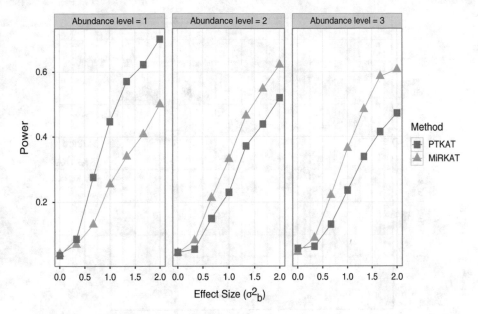

Fig. 5 Power curves for binary outcome case with linear OTU effects. The cluster becomes more abundant from level 1 to level 3

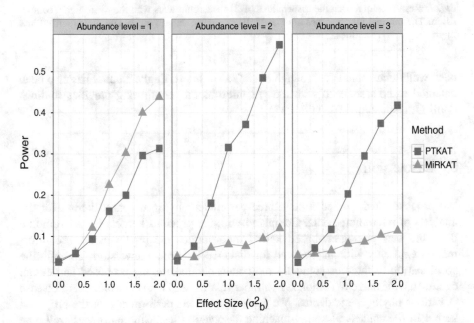

Fig. 6 Power curves for binary outcome case with nonlinear OTU effects. The cluster becomes more abundant from level 1 to level 3

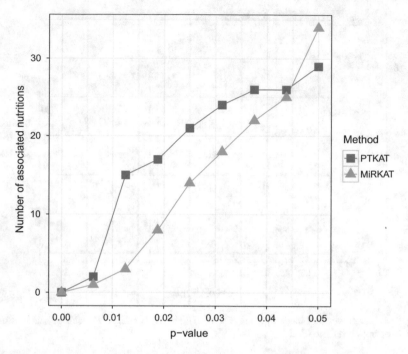

Fig. 7 Results from testing the associations of 214 micronutrients with the microbiome composition. The nutrient intake values are standardized against caloric intake and dichotomized into 'high' and 'low' categories

been well documented (Turnbaugh et al. 2006). Interestingly, alcohol has also been detected to be associated with the gut microbiome, confirming previous findings (Bull-Otterson et al. 2013) (Table 2).

5   Discussion

We proposed and studied a new three-parameter phylogeny-based kernel for the analysis of microbiome data. Compared with the previous kernels for microbiome data, the new phylogeny-based kernel incorporates the phylogenetic tree information explicitly without the need for distance-to-kernel conversion. Through the specification of three ecologically motivated parameters, the proposed kernel can capture a wide range of complex, nonlinear relationship with environment or disease at various phylogenetic depths. We demonstrated the performance of the proposed kernel in the context of kernel-machine association test. Simulations as well as a real data application revealed the robustness of the proposed kernel.

Table 2 Nutrients identified by PTKAT and MiRKAT with an FDR of 15%

Nutrient ID	Nutrient name	PTKAT	MiRKAT
tfat	Total fat	0.150	0.546
poly	Polyunsaturated fat	0.150	0.307
chol	Cholesterol	0.150	0.307
alco	Alcohol	0.150	0.307
f225	Docosapentaenoic fatty acid (DPA)	0.150	0.686
trn02	Total trans fat	0.150	0.307
cys	Cystine	0.150	0.307
germa	Added germ from wheats	0.150	0.392
pfn602	Omega 6	0.150	0.392
n602	Omega 6, no gamma	0.150	0.392
pfa183n3c02	Alpha linolenic fatty acid	0.150	0.307
ag18302	Alpha + Gamma linolenic acid	0.150	0.307
pfn602_wo	Omega 6 w/o suppl.	0.150	0.307
n602_wo	Omega 6, no gamma 18:3	0.150	0.307
aspart	Aspartame	0.150	0.307

The 'PTKAT' and 'MiRKAT' columns show the BH procedure (Benjamini and Hochberg 1995) adjusted p-values for PTKAT and MiRKAT, respectively

There is concern that the phylogenetic tree may not be useful or the phylogenetically clustered signal is a very strong assumption. This can happen when the tree constructed based on 16S sequences does not reflect the truly evolutionary relationship between species or the tree is contaminated with heavy noises. Moreover, it is also likely that disease/environment may only affect phylogenetically non-related species. Therefore, the tree information should be taken cautiously. Interestingly, the proposed kernel can be reduced to a regular tree-independent kernel if the tuning parameter $\rho \to \infty$, which adds to the robustness of the proposed kernel.

The proposed kernel only depends on a pairwise distance matrix between OTUs. Thus the tree construction step is not necessary and the distance can be defined directly based on the divergence of OTU sequences. The proposed kernel can also be used in other kernel methods for microbiome data such as kernel-based prediction, dimension reduction, clustering, and canonical correlation analysis (Akaho 2001; Hoffmann 2007; Ober et al. 2011; Scholkopf et al. 1999).

There is still room for improvement for the proposed kernel. The current implementation focuses on the overall similarity as captured by the kernel, and it is expected to perform optimally when the signal is dense. However, when the signal is sparse, the described kernel approach may not work well due to the signal dilution of irrelevant OTUs when constructing the kernels. In such case, it may be more powerful by performing variable selection in the kernel framework or performing association tests for all the nodes on the tree, coupled by multiple testing correction. KerNel Iterative Feature Extraction (KNIFE) provides a general framework for incorporating variable selection into kernel machine methods (He et al. 2016). Allowing multiple phylogenetic depths in the kernel is also

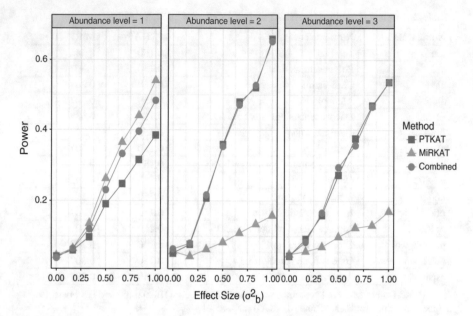

Fig. 8 Power curves for Gaussian outcome case with nonlinear OTU effects. The cluster becomes more abundant from level 1 to level 3. The combined test uses the kernels from PTKAT and MiRKAT

an interesting topic. The parameter ρ in the proposed kernel governs a global phylogenetic depth. However, the environment and disease may affect different bacterial lineages at different phylogenetic depths. Thus it may be beneficial to allow different ρ's for different bacterial lineages. Finally, it is possible to combine the proposed phylogeny kernels and the traditional kernels used by MiRKAT to further increase the robustness of the test since PTKAT does not dominate MiRKAT in the simulations. We have conducted additional simulations by combining both kernels. Figure 8 shows an example of the combined test with Gaussian outcome and nonlinear OTU effects. This strategy does make the test more robust.

Acknowledgements The work is supported by Mayo Clinic Gerstner Family Career Award and Center for Individualized Medicine.

References

Akaho, S. (2001). A kernel method for canonical correlation analysis. In *Proceedings of the International Meeting of the Psychometric Society*. Tokyo: Springer.

Beals, E. W. (1984). Bray-Curtis ordination: An effective strategy for analysis of multivariate ecological data. *Advances in Ecological Research, 14*, 55.

Benjamini, Y., & Hochberg, Y. (1995). Controlling the false discovery rate: A practical and powerful approach to multiple testing. *Journal of the Royal Statistical Society. Series B, 57*, 289–300.

Bull-Otterson, L., Feng, W., Kirpich, I., Wang, Y., Qin, X., Liu, Y., et al. (2013). Metagenomic analyses of alcohol induced pathogenic alterations in the intestinal microbiome and the effect of Lactobacillus rhamnosus GG treatment. *PloS One, 8*, e53028.

Caporaso, J. G., Kuczynski, J., Stombaugh, J., Bittinger, K., Bushman, F.D., Costello, E.K., et al. (2010). QIIME allows analysis of high-throughput community sequencing data. *Nature Methods, 7*, 335–336.

Castellarin, M., Warren, R., Freeman, J., Dreolini, L., Krzywinski, M., Strauss, J., et al. (2012). Fusobacterium nucleatum infection is prevalent in human colorectal carcinoma. *Genome Research, 22*, 299–306.

Chen, J., Bittinger, K., Charlson, E. S., Hoffmann, C., Lewis, J., Wu, G.D., et al. (2012). Associating microbiome composition with environmental covariates using generalized UniFrac distances. *Bioinformatics, 28*, 2106–2113.

Chen, J., Bushman, F., Lewis, J., Wu, G.D., & Li, H. (2013a). Structure-constrained sparse canonical correlation analysis with an application to microbiome data analysis. *Biostatistics, 14*, 244–258.

Chen, J., Chen, W., Zhao, N., Wu, M.C., & Schaid, D.J. (2016). Small sample kernel association test for human genetic and microbiome association studies. *Genetic Epidemiology, 40*, 5–9.

Chen, J., & Li, H. (2013). Kernel methods for regression analysis of microbiome compositional data. In M. Hu, Y. Liu, & J. Lin (Eds.), *Topics in Applied Statistics: 2012 Symposium of the International Chinese Statistical Association* (pp. 191–201). Boston: Springer.

Chen, L., Han, L., Kocher, J. P., Li, H., & Chen, J. (2015). glmgraph: An R package for variable selection and predictive modeling of structured genomic data. *Bioinformatics, 31*, 3991–3993.

Chen, W., Zhang, C. K., Cheng, Y., et al. (2013b). A comparison of methods for clustering 16S rRNA sequences into OTUs. *PloS One, 8*, e70837.

Cho, I., & Blaser, M. (2012). The human microbiome: At the interface of health and disease. *Nature Reviews Genetics, 13*, 260–270.

Collison, M., Hirt, R. P., Wipat, A., Nakjang, S., Sanseau, P., & Brown, J.R. (2012). Data mining the human gut microbiota for therapeutic targets. *Briefings in Bioinformatics, 13*, 751–768.

Cristianini, N., & Shawe-Taylor, J.: *An introduction to support vector machines*. Cambridge: Cambridge University Press (2000)

Davies, R. (1980). The distribution of a linear combination of chi-2 random variables. *Journal of the Royal Statistical Society: Series C: Applied Statistics, 29*, 323–333.

Gianola, D., & Van Kaam, J. B. (2008). Reproducing kernel Hilbert spaces regression methods for genomic assisted prediction of quantitative traits. *Genetics, 178*, 2289–2303.

He, Q., Cai, T., Liu, Y., Zhao, N., Harmon, Q.E., Almli, L.M., et al. (2016). Prioritizing individual genetic variants after kernel machine testing using variable selection. *Genetic Epidemiology, 40*, 722–731.

Hoffmann, H. (2007). Kernel PCA for novelty detection. *Pattern Recognition, 40*(3), 863–874.

Holmes, E., Li, J. V., Athanasiou, T., Ashrafian, H., & Nicholson, J.K. (2011). Understanding the role of gut microbiome-host metabolic signal disruption in health and disease. *Trends in Microbiology, 19*, 349–359.

Honda, K., & Littman, D. (2012). The microbiome in infectious disease and inflammation. *Immunology, 30*, 759–795.

ICH Harmonised Tripartite Guideline: Dose-Response Information to Support Drug Registration E4. (1994, March). *International conference on harmonisation of technical requirements for registration of pharmaceuticals for human use.* Availableathttp://www.ich.org/fileadmin/Public_Web_Site/ICH_Products/Guidelines/Efficacy/E4/Step4/E4_Guideline.pdf. Accessed 16 Oct 2017.

Kinross, J., Darzi, A., & Nicholson, J. (2011). Gut microbiome-host interactions in health and disease. *Genome Medicine, 3*, 14.

Knights, D., Parfrey, L. W., Zaneveld, J., Lozupone, C., & Knight, R. (2011). Human-associated microbial signatures: Examining their predictive value. *Cell Host Microbe, 10*, 292–296.

Kostic, A., Gevers, D., Pedamallu, C. S., Michaud, M., Duke, F., Earl, A.M., et al. (2012). Genomic analysis identifies association of Fusobacterium with colorectal carcinoma. *Genome Research, 22*, 292–298.

Kwee, L. C., Liu, D., Lin, X., Ghosh, D., & Epstein, M.P. (2008). A powerful and flexible multilocus association test for quantitative traits. *American Journal of Human Genetics, 82*, 386–397.

Lee, S., Emond, M. J., Bamshad, M. J., Barnes, K.C., Rieder, M.J., Nickerson, D.A., et al. (2012). Optimal unified approach for rare-variant association testing with application to small-sample case-control whole exome sequencing studies. *American Journal of Human Genetics, 91*, 224–237.

Ley, R., Bäckhed, F., Turnbaugh, P. J., Lozupone, C.A., Knight, R.D., & Gordon, J.I. (2005). Obesity alters gut microbial ecology. *Proceedings of the National Academy of Sciences of the United States of America, 102*, 11070.

Ley, R., Turnbaugh, P. J., Klein, S., & Gordon, J.I. (2006). Microbial ecology: Human gut microbes associated with obesity. *Nature, 444*, 1022–1023.

Lin, X. (1997). Variance component testing in generalised linear models with random effects. *Biometrika, 84*, 309–326.

Liu, D., Ghosh, D., & Lin, X. (2008). Estimation and testing for the effect of a genetic pathway on a disease outcome using logistic kernel machine regression via logistic mixed models. *BMC Bioinformatics, 9*, 292.

Liu, D., Lin, X., & Ghosh, D. (2007). Semiparametric regression of multidimensional genetic pathway data: Least-squares kernel machines and linear mixed models. *Biometrics, 63*, 1079–1088.

Liu, H., Tang, Y., & Zhang, H. H. (2009). A new chi-square approximation to the distribution of non-negative definite quadratic forms in non-central normal variables. *Computational Statistics and Data Analysis, 53*, 853–856.

Lozupone, C. A., & Knight, R. (2005). UniFrac: A new phylogenetic method for comparing microbial communities. *Applied and Environmental Microbiology, 71*, 8228–8235.

Lozupone, C. A., & Knight, R. (2008). Species divergence and the measurement of microbial diversity. *FEMS Microbiology Review, 32*, 557–578.

Martin, E. P., & Hansen, T. F. (1997). Phylogenies and the comparative method: A general approach to incorporating phylogenetic information into the analysis of interspecific data. *The American Naturalist, 149*, 646–667.

Martiny, B. H., Jones, S. E., Lennon, J. T., & Martiny, A.C. (2015). Microbiomes in light of traits: A phylogenetic perspective. *Science, 350*, aac9323.

Ober, U., Erbe, M., Long, N., Porcu, E., Schlather, M., & Simianer, H. (2011). Predicting genetic values: A kernel-based best linear unbiased prediction with genomic data. *Genetics, 188*, 695–708.

Plottel, C. S., & Blaser, M. J. (2011). Microbiome and malignancy. *Cell Host Microbe, 10*, 324–335.

Pughoeft, K., & Versalovic, J. (2011). Human microbiome in health and disease. *Annual Review of Pathology, 7*, 99–122.

Purdom, E. (2011). Analysis of a data matrix and a graph: Metagenomic data and the phylogenetic tree. *Annals of Applied Statistics, 5*, 2326–2358.

Scholkopf, B., Smola, A., & Muller, K. R. (1999). Kernel principal component analysis. In B. Scholkopf, C. J. C. Burges, & A. J. Smola (Eds.), *Advances in kernel methods SV learning* (pp. 327–352). Cambridge, MA: MIT.

Segata, N., Izard, J., Waldron, L., Gevers, D., Miropolsky, L., Garrett, W.S., et al. (2011). Metagenomic biomarker discovery and explanation. *Genome Biology, 12*, 60.

Turnbaugh, P., Ley, R., Hamady, M., Fraser-Liggett, C., Knight, R., & Gordon, J.I. (2007). The human microbiome project. *Nature, 449*, 804–810.

Turnbaugh, P., Ley, R., Mahowald, M., Magrini, V., Mardis, E.R., & Gordon, J.I. (2006). An obesity-associated gut microbiome with increased capacity for energy harvest. *Nature, 444*, 1027–1031.

Virgin, H., & Todd, J. (2011). Metagenomics and personalized medicine. *Cell, 147*, 44–56.

Wu, C., Chen, J., Kim, J., & Pan, W. (2016). An adaptive association test for microbiome data. *Genome Medicine, 8*, 56.

Wu, G. D., Chen, J., Hoffmann, C., Bittinger, K., Chen, Y.Y., Keilbaugh, S.A., et al. (2011). Linking long-term dietary patterns with gut microbial enterotypes. *Science, 334*, 105–108.

Wu, M. C., Kraft, P., Epstein, M. P., Taylor, D.M., Chanock, S.J., Hunter, D.J., et al. (2010). Powerful SNP-set analysis for case-control genome-wide association studies. *American Journal of Human Genetics, 86*, 929–942.

Wu, M. C., Lee, S., Cai, T., Li, Y., Boehnke, M., & Lin, X. (2011). Rare-variant association testing for sequencing data with the sequence kernel association test. *American Journal of Human Genetics, 89*, 82–93.

Wu, M. C., Maity, A., Lee, S., Simmons, E.M., Harmon, Q.E., Lin, X., et al. (2013). Kernel machine SNP-set testing under multiple candidate kernels. *Genetic Epidemiology, 37*, 267–275.

Xiao, J., Cao, H., & Chen, J. (2017). False discovery rate control incorporating phylogenetic tree increases detection power in microbiome-wide multiple testing. *Bioinformatics, 33*, 2873–2881.

Zhao, N., Chen, J., Carroll, I. M., Ringel-Kulka, T., Epstein, M.P., Zhou, H., et al. (2015). Testing in microbiome-profiling studies with MiRKAT, the microbiome regression-based kernel association test. *American Journal of Human Genetics, 96*, 797–807.

Accounting for Differential Error in Time-to-Event Analyses Using Imperfect Electronic Health Record-Derived Endpoints

Rebecca A. Hubbard, Joanna Harton, Weiwei Zhu, Le Wang, and Jessica Chubak

1 Introduction

Electronic health records (EHR) have great potential as a data source for investigating questions about use and outcomes of clinical interventions in a real-world setting. However, poor data quality, including missing and erroneous data elements, constitutes a major challenge to valid inference based on this data source. Because EHR data are collected for clinical and administrative rather than research purposes, data elements that are considered low priority from a clinical perspective may be recorded inconsistently. For instance, information on behavioral risk factors such as smoking or alcohol consumption may be inconsistently assessed and recorded by medical providers. This inconsistency can lead to substantial under estimation of the prevalence of these risk factors and differential misclassification if risk factors are more likely to be assessed for some patients than for others. Addressing the limitations of erroneous and inconsistent data is a necessary first step to realizing the promise of EHR data for research.

EHR provide a uniquely valuable data source for studying cancer survivors because they provide information on cancer recurrence, an important outcome that is notably not available in population-based cancer registry data or in diagnosis codes. Aging of the population coupled with improvements in early detection and cancer treatment have led to a steady increase in the population of patients with a personal history of cancer. As a result, the population of cancer survivors included

R.A. Hubbard (✉) • J. Harton • L. Wang
Department of Biostatistics, Epidemiology & Informatics, University of Pennsylvania, Philadelphia, PA, USA
e-mail: rhubb@upenn.edu; jograce@upenn.edu; wangle@upenn.edu

W. Zhu • J. Chubak
Kaiser Permanente Washington Health Research Institute, Seattle, WA, USA
e-mail: zhu.w@ghc.org; chubak.j@ghc.org

© Springer International Publishing AG 2017
D.-G. Chen et al. (eds.), *New Advances in Statistics and Data Science*,
ICSA Book Series in Statistics, https://doi.org/10.1007/978-3-319-69416-0_14

over 15.5 million individuals as of 2016 and is anticipated to grow to over 26 million individuals by 2040 (Bluethmann et al. 2016). Understanding risk factors for cancer recurrence and mortality in this population is therefore of increasing importance. However, data sources are lacking to support such studies. Population-based cancer registries do not collect data on cancer recurrence. As a result, a number of attempts have been made to use medical claims to identify recurrences (Earle et al. 2002; Lamont et al. 2006; Chubak et al. 2012; Hassett et al. 2014). However, validation studies have demonstrated that in many cases classification accuracy of these approaches is fair or poor (Hassett et al. 2014; Warren et al. 2016). More detailed information about utilization and results of diagnostic tests as well as treatments for cancer available in the EHR have the potential to improve classification accuracy of algorithms for identifying cancer recurrence, but are unlikely to completely eliminate error and misclassification.

The ability to extract dates of event occurrence from EHR would increase the clinical relevance of research studies conducted in this context. For instance, in the case of cancer recurrence, knowledge of the timing of recurrence is important for planning appropriate surveillance schedules and providing patients with accurate information on prognosis. Indeed, as survival rates have improved, the expected length of disease-free survival has emerged as a key measure to support informed decision-making (Warren and Yabroff 2015). Despite this, the majority of studies that have investigated cancer recurrence using EHR data have focused on defining a binary recurrence outcome, with little attention paid to the precise timing of recurrence. Motivated by an EHR-based algorithm for second breast cancers, we previously investigated the accuracy of a cancer recurrence date derived from an EHR-based measure (Chubak et al. 2015). In this prior study, we found that the EHR-based algorithm could identify the date of breast cancer recurrence within 60 days of the true date in 82% of cases. However, for a small subset of patients, the EHR-derived date differed from the true date by a year or more.

Estimates of survival functions and hazard ratios are biased in the presence of imperfect ascertainment of a time-to-event outcome (Snapinn 1998; Meier et al. 2003; Zee and Xie 2015). In the case of non-differential outcome misclassification, association estimates tend to be biased towards the null (Magder and Hughes 1997; Neuhaus 1999). When information on the sensitivity and specificity of the imperfect time-to-event outcomes is available, this can be incorporated into the model to obtain unbiased estimates (Richardson and Hughes 2000; Meier et al. 2003). Alternatively, a validation subsample can be included in the analysis along with a larger sample for whom only the imperfect outcome is available in order to obtain bias-corrected estimates (Zee and Xie 2015). In the context of EHR-based studies, obtaining gold standard outcome data through manual review of medical records can be extremely costly and time consuming. It is therefore desirable to conduct analyses using results of existing validation studies.

In this context of event times assigned on the basis of EHR, error in the outcome measure takes two forms. First, an error may be made in classifying an individual as to whether an event has occurred during follow-up. Second, among those classified as having experienced an event, error may exist in the precise timing of the event. In our previous analysis, we conducted simulation studies to quantify the magnitude of bias arising in a Cox proportional hazards regression model using such an imperfect time-to-event measure as the outcome and found that bias in hazard ratios was minimal unless misclassification of event status was differential with respect to exposure status (Chubak et al. 2015). Unfortunately, in the context of EHR-based studies, differential error is not uncommon because patients may differ in their interactions with the healthcare system, leading to more accurate or precise outcome ascertainment according to patient characteristics.

As illustrated by the case of error in ascertainment of time to cancer recurrence, error in time-to-event outcomes derived from the EHR differs from cases previously investigated in the biostatistical literature in several important respects. First, the structure of the error consists of not only misclassification as to whether an event occurred but also error in the precise timing of the event. Second, information on the operating characteristics of an EHR-based algorithm for identifying the outcome of interest is typically only available at the person-level. That is, the standard approach to validation of EHR-based algorithms computes sensitivity and specificity or positive and negative predictive values for the algorithm applied to all EHR for a given individual relative to their true status as ever having experienced an event. This person-level validation does not provide information at the level of an individual follow-up visit or suspected event which is required by previously proposed approaches (Snapinn 1998; Meier et al. 2003). Finally, while past work has noted that the direction of bias is not uniformly toward or away from the null in the case of differential measurement error, the case of differential error has generally received less attention than that of non-differential error. However, in the case of EHR-derived outcomes, where the health status and healthcare seeking behavior of the individual will strongly influence the type and timing of information populated in their EHR, differential error may be the norm. This particularly challenging case thus warrants further investigation.

The current study was motivated by the need to identify statistical methods that can correct for bias in hazard ratio estimates induced by misclassification and measurement error in EHR-derived time-to-event outcomes, with a special focus on the challenge posed by differential measurement error. Motivated by the study of second breast cancer events described above, we investigated alternative approaches to account for this error. We first discuss naive and adjusted approaches to estimating associations for a mismeasured time-to-event outcome derived from the EHR and then describe a simulation study designed to investigate the ability of existing approaches to correct bias arising in the case of differential error (Sect. 2). In Sect. 3, we present the results of our simulation studies. Finally, in Sect. 4, we conclude with general considerations for analyses of EHR-derived time-to-event endpoints and discuss areas for future research.

2 Methods

We conceive of EHR data as a set of records documenting encounters between a patient and a given healthcare system. Each record consists of a date, procedure and diagnosis codes, free text notes describing the encounter, and, when relevant, additional information describing the encounter such as test results or other findings. Because the timing of these encounters varies in response to a patient's healthcare needs and healthcare seeking behavior and is not fixed according to a study protocol, it is tempting to conceive of EHR data as representing a continuous time representation of a patient's health. However, despite the unscheduled nature of encounters, each represents a discrete encounter, with information about patient health unavailable in the elapsed periods between encounters. Data of this structure more closely reflect a discretely sampled process than one that is continuously observed and can be described using a survival model in discrete time, which accounts for the inherent interval censoring of the observation process (Kalbfleisch and Prentice 1980).

EHR-derived outcomes must be based on the presence or absence of a combination of codes or other pieces of information in the medical record. For instance, Chubak et al. (2012) proposed algorithms for breast cancer recurrence that made use of combinations of codes denoting mastectomy, radiation therapy, and diagnosis of a secondary malignant neoplasm. Each of these events will occur at a different time and all will lag behind the biological time of cancer recurrence making it impossible to precisely pinpoint the date of cancer recurrence. It may be preferable to aggregate data across a fixed time period, such as a week or month, resulting in a discrete time process where time is measured in units corresponding to the level of aggregation. Within each interval the event of interest is defined based on the presence or absence of the corresponding codes or other EHR data. For instance, in the case of breast cancer recurrence we could define the date of recurrence as the first month in which the necessary combination of codes is observed. An advantage of this discrete time approach is that it provides a concrete unit of time for validation studies to target. Rather than providing information on concordance between EHR-derived and true event status at the person-level, this information could be reported based on discrete windows of time. Similarly, if the operating characteristics of an EHR algorithm are known at the person level, performance within windows of fixed length can be calculated, subject to certain assumptions about variation in operating characteristics over time (see Sect. 2.4). Below we describe the discrete proportional hazards approach corresponding to this discrete-time formulation and extensions to accommodate error in time-to-event outcomes.

2.1 Definitions and Notation

Our data take the form $\{t_i, d_i\}$, for $i = 1, \ldots N$, where t_i is the earlier of the time of the event of interest or a censoring time if the study ends or the participant moves out of catchment of the EHR and d_i is a binary indicator taking the value 1 if the participant experienced an event while under observation and 0 otherwise. For instance, in our breast cancer recurrence example t_i represents the number of months after a primary breast cancer diagnosis at which diagnosis or treatment codes indicative of a second breast cancer event appear in the EHR. Censoring may have a number of causes, but an important cause to consider in EHR-based studies is disenrollment from the healthcare system or health insurance plan or moving outside the catchment area of the healthcare system. It is important that information on patient enrollment in the healthcare system is available and incorporated into time-to-event studies in order to ensure that the apparent lack of occurrence of the event of interest is not simply due to the fact that the patient is no longer seeking care within the healthcare system.

We assume that t_i is unobserved but that we have an imperfect proxy, t_i^o. We further assume that once a subject is observed to have experienced an event, follow-up ends. True events occurring after t_i^o are thus censored at t_i^o. The true event status, d_i, is also unobserved. Instead d_i^o, an imperfect event status indicator, is available and takes the value 1 if the imperfect outcome occurs before censoring and 0 otherwise. We further assume that each subject has available a vector of covariates X_i and that scientific interest lies in estimating the association between these covariates and the event time. Like information on outcome status, time-varying covariate status can be updated within each discrete time interval based on presence or absence of records indicative of a particular condition or exposure.

2.2 Discrete Proportional Hazards Model

The discrete proportional hazards model (Kalbfleisch and Prentice 1980) is appropriate for outcomes that are assessed at discrete, equally spaced time points such as those resulting from discretization of follow-up time as described above. Let $\lambda_0 = \{\lambda_{01}, \lambda_{02}, \ldots, \lambda_{0T}\}$ represent the baseline hazard at time 1 to T. The baseline hazard is allowed to vary flexibly over time, with no constraints placed on λ_{0k}. For subject i with covariates X_i, the discrete hazard at time j is given by $1 - (1 - \lambda_{0j})^{\exp(X_i'\beta)}$. We write the likelihood as

$$f(t_i, d_i; X_i, \beta, \lambda_0) = \prod_{j=1}^{t_i-1} \left\{ (1 - \lambda_{0j})^{\exp(X_i'\beta)} \right\} \times \left\{ 1 - (1 - \lambda_{0t_i})^{\exp(X_i'\beta)} \right\}^{d_i}$$

$$\times \left\{ (1 - \lambda_{0t_i})^{\exp(X_i'\beta)} \right\}^{(1-d_i)}.$$

This represents the product of $t_i - 1$ contributions to the likelihood at time points at which no event occurred followed by a term representing the final likelihood contribution for subjects who experience the event and a term representing the final likelihood contribution for censored subjects. Analogous to Cox proportional hazards regression, in many cases λ_0 can be considered a nuisance parameter and the primary target of inference will be β which represents the association between covariates and the hazard of the event of interest. This model corresponds to a generalized linear model for Bernoulli distributed data with complementary log-log link function. Estimates can be obtained using standard software for generalized linear models.

2.3 Adjustment for Error in Event Times

In the context of EHR data, the true event times are unobserved and we instead attempt to make inference about the relationship between covariates and the outcome of interest by applying an algorithm to available EHR data. t_i^o can be obtained by applying the algorithm within each discrete time period and represents the first time period in which the algorithm returns a positive result. For instance, using an algorithm for colorectal cancer recurrence described by Warren et al. (2016), we might divide time after treatment for a primary colorectal cancer diagnosis into months and within each month look for codes for chemotherapy, radiation therapy, or colorectal cancer-directed surgery. In this example, t_i^o represents the first month in which such codes appear in a patient's EHR, and d_i^o represents a binary indicator of whether such codes were ever observed over the course of available follow-up data for a patient or were never observed.

One approach to the analysis of such data is to reformulate the discrete proportional hazards likelihood to account for the possibility that, within each discrete time period, the outcome of interest may have been misclassified. We briefly describe such an adjusted discrete proportional hazards model, originally proposed by Meier et al. (2003). Let θ represent the probability that the algorithm correctly classifies an interval where an event truly has occurred (i.e., sensitivity) and ϕ represent the probability that the algorithm correctly classifies an interval where there truly has been no event (i.e., specificity). It is important to note that θ and ϕ correspond to the operating characteristics of the EHR-based approach within each discrete interval and not with respect to correct classification of an individual over the complete follow-up period, as is typically reported in EHR-based validation studies.

Below we illustrate a sample observation pattern for a participant in a study of breast cancer recurrence who experienced a recurrence t_i months after her primary cancer diagnosis and whose EHR data reflected a recurrence based on a pre-existing algorithm t_i^o months after the primary diagnosis.

$$\underbrace{1, 2, \cdots, t_i - 1,}_{t_i - 1 \text{ true negatives}} \overbrace{t_i}^{\substack{\text{True} \\ \text{recurrence}}} \underbrace{, \cdots, t_i^o - 1,}_{t_i^o - t_i \text{ false negatives}} \overbrace{t_i^o}^{\substack{\text{EHR} - \text{based} \\ \text{recurrence}}}$$

Note that this observation pattern corresponds to $t_i - 1$ true negative observations followed by $t_i^o - t_i$ false negatives and a single true positive observation at time t_i^o. In terms of θ and ϕ, the probability of this pattern of observations can be expressed as $\phi^{t_i-1}(1-\theta)^{t_i^o - t_i}\theta$.

More generally, we can express the probability of observed event times and statuses as functions of θ and ϕ as

$$f(t_i^o, d_i^o | t_i = t_i^o, d_i = 0, \theta, \phi) = \phi^{t_i^o-1}\phi^{1-d_i^o}(1-\phi)^{d_i^o} \doteq \Gamma_i \tag{1}$$

$$f(t_i^o, d_i^o | t_i \le t_i^o, d_i = 1, \theta, \phi) = \phi^{t_i-1}(1-\theta)^{t_i^o - t_i}(1-\theta)^{1-d_i^o}\theta^{d_i^o} \doteq \Delta_{it_i} \tag{2}$$

The observed data likelihood can then be obtained by marginalizing over all possible combinations of true event time and status,

$$f(t_i^o, d_i^o; \ X_i, \boldsymbol{\beta}, \lambda_0, \theta, \phi) = \left[\prod_{j=1}^{t_i^o}(1-\lambda_{0j})^{\exp(X_i'\beta)}\right]\Gamma_i + \left\{1 - (1-\lambda_{01})^{\exp(X_i'\beta)}\right\}\Delta_{i1}$$

$$+ \sum_{k=2}^{t_i^o}\left[\prod_{j=1}^{k-1}\left\{(1-\lambda_{0j})^{\exp(X_i'\beta)}\right\} \times \left\{1 - (1-\lambda_{0k})^{\exp(X_i'\beta)}\right\}\Delta_{ik}\right]. \tag{3}$$

By numerically maximizing this observed data likelihood function with respect to $\boldsymbol{\beta}$ and $\boldsymbol{\lambda_0}$ we can obtain maximum likelihood estimates that correctly account for the imperfect accuracy of θ and ϕ.

2.4   Incorporating Person-Level Validation Data

If a discrete time approach were considered prior to undertaking a validation study for a proposed EHR algorithm, it would be possible to directly obtain estimates of θ and ϕ by conducting chart review to obtain gold-standard outcome information and comparing this against algorithm classification within each discrete time-period. However, given the high cost and labor intensity of manual chart review, it is often the case that EHR-based studies rely on prior validation of a given algorithm in which case it is likely that sensitivity and specificity will only be available across a longer period of time than we would prefer to use in our discrete-time model. For instance, the motivating study by Chubak et al. (2012) validated an algorithm for second breast cancer events comparing the algorithm applied to the complete set of

EHR available for a given woman over her period of follow-up to her true event status at the end of follow-up. Sensitivity and specificity over this entire follow-up period are expected to be substantially different from sensitivity and specificity computed within a single, relatively brief time period such as a week or month.

Information from a prior validation study available at the person-level can be used to compute θ and ϕ under a set of fairly strong assumptions about temporal variation in classification accuracy. Specifically, if we are willing to assume that θ and ϕ are constant over the follow-up period we can relate these quantities to the observed person-level sensitivity and specificity. Let $\hat{P}(d^o = 1|d = 1)$ represent a person-level measure of sensitivity estimated in a prior validation study and $\hat{P}(d^o = 0|d = 0)$ represent the estimated person-level specificity. We assume information on the distribution of follow-up time for cases and controls is also available. We can obtain estimates $\hat{\theta}$ and $\hat{\phi}$ based on these validation results using the equations

$$\hat{P}(d^o = 1|d = 1) = \sum_{k=1}^{M} \left[1 - (1 - \hat{\theta})^k\right] P(t^o = k|d = 1) \tag{4}$$

$$\hat{P}(d^o = 0|d = 0) = \sum_{k=1}^{M} \hat{\phi}^k P(t^o = k|d = 0), \tag{5}$$

where M is the maximum follow-up length and $P(t^o = k|d = 1)$ and $P(t^o = k|d = 0)$ are the distribution of follow-up time in cases and controls, respectively. Although the complete specification of these follow-up distributions will not be reported by a validation study, simple approximations based on the reported means and standard deviations or medians and interquartile ranges can be used.

Note that in addition to assuming θ and ϕ constant over follow-up, this approach assumes that, in the validation sample, individuals with $d_i = 1$ had already experienced the event prior to the period included in the validation study. Both of these assumptions are potentially unrealistic and could be relaxed, although this results in more complex expressions. Specifically, if information about changes in coding or other practices within the healthcare system are known and suggest a particular functional form for θ and ϕ they could be replaced with time-dependent analogues θ_k and ϕ_k both here and in Eqs. (1) and (2). However, with only information on person-level sensitivity and specificity available, strong assumptions about the functional form of these relationships will still be required in order for θ_k and ϕ_k to be identifiable. We posit that in the absence of very strong prior information about how these parameters vary over time, assuming that they remain constant is a reasonable simplifying assumption.

2.5 Differential Error in Event Times

In the context of EHR-based studies, we are particularly interested in the setting where θ and ϕ may differ according to patient characteristics. Let θ_Z and ϕ_Z represent covariate-specific values of the discrete-time period sensitivity and specificity and Z_{ik} represent a vector of possibly time-varying characteristics associated with algorithm accuracy. If these quantities are known they can simply be incorporated into Eqs. (1) and (2), and the estimation procedure is otherwise unchanged. If data on a validation subsample is available they can be estimated using this data. For instance, given interval-level data on true and imperfect event status, d_{ik} and d_{ik}^o, respectively, we can use an appropriate regression framework such as

$$\theta_{Z_{ik}} \doteq E(d_{ik}^o | Z_{ik}, d_{ik} = 1) = g^{-1}(Z'_{ik}\alpha)$$
$$\phi_{Z_{ik}} \doteq 1 - E(d_{ik}^o | Z_{ik}, d_{ik} = 0) = 1 - g^{-1}(Z'_{ik}\gamma),$$

where $g(.)$ represents a suitable link function.

However, as discussed above, it is often the case that validation data are not available and that a study relies on operating characteristics reported by prior validation studies. In these cases it is unlikely that sensitivity and specificity will be reported in suitably stratified sub-groups to encompass variation in performance of the algorithm for outcome ascertainment across all of the many potentially relevant patient sub-groups. In this case, the investigator must rely on adjustment using the marginal values of θ and ϕ which will incompletely account for differential error in outcome ascertainment. We anticipate this will be a common challenge in EHR-based studies and therefore investigate this case in simulation studies described below.

2.6 Simulation Study Design

Motivated by the BRAVA study of second breast cancer events (Chubak et al. 2012) we conducted a series of simulation studies to compare the performance of alternative approaches to accounting for an imperfect time-to-event outcome, focusing on the case of cancer recurrence derived from EHR data. We previously developed an administrative data-derived measure for time to second breast cancer event and compared this measure to true time of second breast cancer event based on chart review (Chubak et al. 2015). We found that our administrative data algorithm identified the true date of second breast cancer event with a mean error of 0 days and interquartile range of about 15 days. We used these estimates of the magnitude of error in a time-to-event outcome in our simulation study, assuming that these are representative of what might be expected in a similar study based on EHR data. Parameters of the distributions of event times and censoring times in our simulation study were also selected to produce event and censoring rates approximately mirroring those observed in the BRAVA study.

In our simulation studies we first evenly divided the population into exposed and unexposed groups. We then simulated a true time-to-event (in months) for each individual by simulating an exponential random variable. The rate of events in the unexposed group was 0.004 (corresponding to a mean time to second breast cancer of 240 months). The event rate in the exposed group was set to $0.004 \times \exp(\beta)$ for values of the hazard ratio ranging from 1 to 5 (log hazard ratio, β, ranging from 0 to 1.6). Next we simulated a censoring time for each individual from a Weibull distribution with shape = 2.1 and scale = 84. This parametric distribution as well as the choice of shape and scale parameters were motivated by the distribution observed in data from the BRAVA study. Any simulated individual with more than 120 months of follow-up was administratively censored at 120 months. We next assigned a sensitivity and specificity for detecting an event prior to censoring conditional on exposure status for each individual. Conditional on true event status, i.e. event time prior to censoring time, we simulated observed event status, d_i^o from either a Bernoulli distribution with p equal to sensitivity (for individuals experiencing a true event) or with p equal to 1-specificity (for individuals not experiencing a true event). All individuals with simulated $d_i^o = 0$, censored individuals, were assigned t_i^o equal to their simulated censoring time. Individuals with $d_i^o = 1$ and $d_i = 1$, true positive events, were assigned t_i^o equal to their true event time plus a normally distributed error term with mean, μ, and variance, σ^2, varying across simulation scenarios. Finally, for individuals with $d_i^o = 1$ and $d_i = 0$, false positive events, we simulated t_i^o from a Weibull distribution with shape = 1.1 and scale = 37.2, corresponding to a mean observed event time of approximately 36 months, motivated by the distribution observed in the BRAVA study. All censoring and event time variables were rounded to the nearest month. We simulated a cohort of size 4000 for all scenarios and repeated each scenario 1000 times.

Our simulations focus on the setting of differential measurement error. Across all simulations, sensitivity in the exposed group was set to 0.91 and specificity was set to 0.982. Corresponding values for the unexposed group were 0.86 and 0.99. These values were selected to preserve marginal sensitivity and specificity of 0.89 and 0.99, respectively, similar to values observed in the BRAVA study. We hypothesized that higher sensitivity and lower specificity would be expected in exposed individuals compared to unexposed in settings where exposure results in more frequent contact with the healthcare system, such as greater burden of comorbid disease. We investigated two scenarios for differential misclassification of recurrence times. First, we simulated dates assuming that the person-level sensitivity and specificity of the algorithm varied according to exposure status but that, if correctly classified as an event, the distribution of error in the date assigned did not vary according to exposure. In these scenarios μ was fixed at 0 for the exposed and unexposed groups. We varied the strength of the log hazard ratio (β) relating exposure status to hazard of recurrence and the standard deviation of the error in dates (σ). Second, we investigated scenarios where there was both differential misclassification and differential error in dates assigned. In these scenarios we again varied β as well as the difference in the mean of the date error distribution between exposed and unexposed individuals.

In each simulated data set we estimated the association between exposure and outcome using the following approaches:

1. Unadjusted discrete proportional hazards model
2. Adjusted discrete proportional hazards model using exposure-specific θ and ϕ
3. Adjusted discrete proportional hazards model using marginal θ and ϕ

For the adjusted approaches, we assumed that person-level sensitivity and specificity were available such as would be the case if a prior validation study had been performed and used Eqs. (4) and (5) along with the empirical distribution of follow-up times in cases and controls to obtain estimates of θ and ϕ. Under approach 2, we estimated these quantities separately for the two exposure groups while for approach 3 we obtained estimates of accuracy parameters pooling all data. Note that both approaches represent a misspecified error correction because the model used to account for error in the dates differs from the model used to simulate the data.

For all simulation scenarios, bias was estimated by averaging the log hazard ratios across replications of the simulation and computing the difference relative to the true log hazard ratio used in the simulation of the data.

3   Results

3.1   Non-differential Error in Dates

We first present results for the case where the mean and standard deviation of the error in simulated dates were assumed independent of exposure status. Note that although error in dates is non-differential in this scenario, classification accuracy of event status was assumed to be exposure status dependent. Figure 1a, illustrates bias in the three discrete proportional hazards models as a function of σ, the standard deviation of the error in dates among true positive individuals, which was assumed to be the same for exposed and unexposed individuals. Across all values of σ investigated, bias was smallest when a separate bias correction was made for exposed and unexposed individuals (approach 2), intermediate for the naive approach (approach 1), and largest when a marginal bias correction was made (approach 3). This indicates that, in this setting, the imperfect marginal bias correction resulted in more bias than making no bias correction at all. Similar results were observed when σ was fixed at 1 and β was allowed to vary (Fig. 1b). For all three methods, bias decreased for increasing values of β but was smallest across all values of β investigated for the exposure-dependent adjusted discrete proportional hazards model (approach 2) and largest for the marginally adjusted discrete proportional hazards model (approach 3).

Fig. 1 Bias in log hazard ratio (β) as a function of σ (panel **a**) and β (panel **b**) under differential classification accuracy and non-differential date error. Dashed line with squares provides estimates for unadjusted method (approach 1), solid line with triangles provides estimates for exposure-group specific adjusted method (approach 2), and dashed-and-dotted line with circles provides estimates for marginal adjusted method (approach 3)

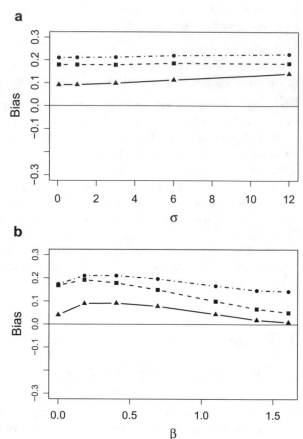

3.2 Differential Error in Dates

We next present results for the case where the mean of the error in simulated dates was allowed to differ between exposed and unexposed groups. In Fig. 2a, the mean of the error in the recurrence date in the exposed group was held constant at 3 months while mean error in the unexposed group was varied across the range from 3 to 24 months. When the difference in the mean date error was similar in exposed and unexposed groups, all three methods overestimated the log hazard ratio with the exposure group-specific adjustment (approach 2) having the smallest positive bias while the marginal bias correction (approach 3) had the largest bias, similar to what we observed in the case of non-differential error in dates. However, as mean date error in the unexposed group increased, bias of the exposure status-specific approach systematically decreased while bias in the other two approaches increased slightly. In these scenarios, recurrence in the unexposed group is detected systematically later than in the exposed group, resulting in overestimation of the positive exposure

Fig. 2 Bias in log hazard ratio (β) as a function of difference in mean date error (panel **a**) and β (panel **b**) under differential classification accuracy and differential mean error in dates. Dashed line with squares provides estimates for unadjusted method (approach 1), solid line with triangles provides estimates for exposure-group specific adjusted method (approach 2), and dashed-and-dotted line with circles provides estimates for marginal adjusted method (approach 3)

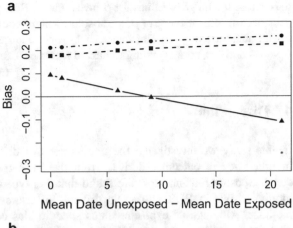

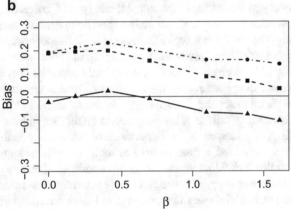

hazard ratio when using the uncorrected and marginally corrected approaches. The systematic decrease in the bias in the exposure group-specific adjustment approach suggests that this approach is overcorrecting, resulting in underestimation of β when the mean error in the date of the unexposed group was approximately 10 months greater than that in the exposed group or larger. Despite this overcorrection, the absolute magnitude of the bias of the exposure group-specific adjustment was smaller than the bias in the marginally adjusted or naive approaches for all values of differential date error investigated.

Finally, we fixed the mean date error at 9 months in the unexposed group and 3 months in the exposed group and investigated the effect of varying log hazard ratios, β, on the performance of the three methods (Fig. 2b). Similar to the pattern observed in the case of non-differential date error, bias in all three methods decreased as β increased. The exposure group-specific bias correction (approach 2) resulted in negative bias for values of β greater than 0.4 indicating over-correction for error in the ascertainment of recurrence times while the other two approaches had positive bias across the range of values for β investigated. Because bias in all three methods decreased across the range of β, the absolute magnitude of the bias in β was smallest for the unadjusted approach (approach 1) for the largest values of β investigated, $\beta = 1.4$ and 1.6, corresponding to hazard ratios of 4 and 5.

4 Discussion

In this study we investigated the implications of differential measurement error in time-to-event outcomes derived from the EHR for bias in estimates of outcome/exposure relationships. We found that this type of measurement error commonly arising in EHR studies is difficult to address using existing statistical methods. Although an exposure-status specific bias correction decreased bias in many of the settings investigated, this type of correction is difficult to implement in practice because exposure status-specific operating characteristics for EHR-derived algorithms are not typically reported. Unlike cohort studies with outcome assessment at defined study visits occurring at fixed intervals, operating characteristics for EHR-derived outcomes are typically reported only at the level of the individual rather than the level of the assessment or discrete time-point. In this setting, it is difficult to accurately derive operating characteristics at the discrete time-point level resulting in failure of bias-correction methods to adjust for measurement error. This finding underscores the importance of conducting validation studies and reporting their results at a finer timescale, with the goal of supporting future time-to-event studies. Providing validation results conditional on key patient characteristics would also better support future studies by providing the information necessary to correct for differential measurement error at least with respect to these characteristics.

Understanding and appropriately adjusting for error in EHR-derived variables is a critical first step in conducting valid research using this data source. Despite this, a comprehensive review of health outcomes research studies conducted using EHR data published between 2000 and 2007 found that only 24% included a validation component (Dean et al. 2009). As the frequency of use of EHR data for research increases, several studies have highlighted the variable data quality of EHR and have cautioned against using these data without investigating data quality or considering the clinical and administrative processes that generated it (Hripcsak and Albers 2013; Hersh et al. 2013; Weiskopf and Weng 2013; Overhage and Overhage 2013). In addition to data quality issues, all of the standard considerations that arise when using observational data such as the risk of confounding also pertain to EHR data. But if data quality issues are not addressed, no amount of confounding control will allow meaningful inference to be made on the basis of inaccurate data.

Many prior studies have investigated effects of measurement error in outcomes on exposure/outcome association parameter estimates. When parameters of the error distribution are unknown it is theoretically possible to obtain maximum likelihood estimates for the joint likelihood for both the association parameters and the error distribution parameters. However, in practice, the likelihood tends to be so flat that this task is impracticable (Carroll et al. 2006). The alternative approach investigated here is to assume parameters of the error distribution are known and estimate association parameters conditional on these known values. While promising if validation data are available, previous work has demonstrated that misspecification of sensitivity and specificity can result in substantial bias in association parameter estimates (Meier et al. 2003). In the current study we have expanded this finding to investigate the case where sensitivity and specificity are estimated based on available validation data but the parametric form of the error distribution has been misspecified. In this case as well, we found that misspecification of the error model results in an inability to effectively remove bias from association parameter estimates.

Our investigations were motivated by a real world study of second breast cancer events using EHR data from an integrated healthcare system. The distributions and parameter values used in our simulation studies were selected to approximate the features of this data set. While this provides insight into the implications of error in time-to-event outcomes in scenarios similar to this study, findings may differ in other settings. For instance, results may be more robust to misclassification and misspecification of the error distribution if a time-to-event outcome is classified with perfect specificity but imperfect sensitivity. Additionally, the bias correction approach we have investigated assumed that algorithm operating characteristics based on a prior study were available but that the validation data themselves were not. In the case where investigators have access to the raw validation data, operating characteristics at the individual study assessment level could be directly estimated conditional on relevant patient characteristics, facilitating more precise and accurate bias correction. We anticipate that bias correction would perform better in this setting, but note that in many studies validation data will not be available.

In the bias correction approach investigated in this paper, we assumed that information on sensitivity and specificity was only available at the person-level and made use of a simplifying assumption that sensitivity and specificity were constant with respect to time. In the context of cancer recurrence, if the main cause of misclassification for patients who have not yet experienced a recurrence is a cancer diagnosis code assigned to routine visits for cancer surveillance purposes and the frequency of surveillance visits does not vary over time then specificity would remain constant over time. In contrast, if the recommended frequency of surveillance visits decreases over time then this would tend to result in an increase in algorithm specificity. Over relatively short periods of time (e.g., several years) it may be reasonable to assume that no substantial changes in surveillance schedules or medical records coding that would lead to systematic variation in sensitivity and specificity have occurred. The appropriateness of this assumption depends on the outcome under study and the causes of outcome misclassification.

If productive use is to be made of EHR data, additional work must be conducted to mitigate, characterize, and account for data quality issues. Characterization includes understanding the processes and procedures within the healthcare system that lead to the generation of these data. Attempting to understand the error in EHR data without devoting attention to the means by which they are created is akin to analyzing data from an observational study without reading the study protocol. Such uninformed efforts are nearly certain to produce erroneous results.

Acknowledgements Research reported in this paper was supported by the National Cancer Institute of the National Institutes of Health under award number R01CA120562 and R21CA143242. The content is solely the responsibility of the authors and does not necessarily represent the official views of the National Institutes of Health.

References

Bluethmann, S. M., Mariotto, A. B., & Rowland, J. H. (2016). Anticipating the "silver tsunami": Prevalence trajectories and comorbidity burden among older cancer survivors in the united states. *Cancer Epidemiology, Biomarkers & Prevention, 25*(7), 1029–1036.

Carroll, R. J., Ruppert, D., Stefanski, L. A., & Crainiceanu, C. M. (2006). *Measurement error in nonlinear models: A modern perspective*. Boca Raton: CRC Press.

Chubak, J., Onega, T., Zhu, W., Buist, D. S., & Hubbard, R. A. (2015). An electronic health record-based algorithm to ascertain the date of second breast cancer events. *Medical Care.* https://doi.org/10.1097/MLR.0000000000000352. http://www.ncbi.nlm.nih.gov/pubmed/25856568.

Chubak, J., Yu, O., Pocobelli, G., Lamerato, L., Webster, J., Prout, M. N., et al. (2012). Administrative data algorithms to identify second breast cancer events following early-stage invasive breast cancer. *Journal of the National Cancer Institute, 104*(12), 931–940. https://doi.org/10.1093/jnci/djs233. http://www.ncbi.nlm.nih.gov/pubmed/22547340.

Dean, B. B., Lam, J., Natoli, J. L., Butler, Q., Aguilar, D., & Nordyke, R. J. (2009). Review: Use of electronic medical records for health outcomes research a literature review. *Medical Care Research and Review, 66*(6), 611–638.

Earle, C. C., Nattinger, A. B., Potosky, A. L., Lang, K., Mallick, R., Berger, M., et al. (2002). Identifying cancer relapse using seer-medicare data. *Medical Care, 40*(8), 75–81.

Hassett, M. J., Ritzwoller, D. P., Taback, N., Carroll, N., Cronin, A. M., Ting, G.V., et al. (2014). Validating billing/encounter codes as indicators of lung, colorectal, breast, and prostate cancer recurrence using 2 large contemporary cohorts. *Medical Care, 52*(10), E65–E73.

Hersh, W. R., Weiner, M. G., Embi, P. J., Logan, J. R., Payne, P. R., Bernstam, E. V., et al. (2013). Caveats for the use of operational electronic health record data in comparative effectiveness research. *Medical care, 51*(803), S30.

Hripcsak, G., & Albers, D. J. (2013). Next-generation phenotyping of electronic health records. *Journal of the American Medical Informatics Association, 20*(1), 117–121.

Kalbfleisch, J. D., & Prentice, R. L. (1980). *The statistical analysis of failure time data*. New York: Wiley.

Lamont, E. B., Herndon, J. E., Weeks, J. C., Henderson, I. C., Earle, C. C., Schilsky, R. L., et al. (2006). Measuring disease-free survival and cancer relapse using medicare claims from CALGB breast cancer trial participants (companion to 9344). *Journal of the National Cancer Institute, 98*(18), 1335–1338.

Magder, L. S., & Hughes, J. P. (1997). Logistic regression when the outcome is measured with uncertainty. *American Journal of Epidemiology, 146*(2), 195–203.

Meier, A. S., Richardson, B. A., & Hughes, J. P. (2003). Discrete proportional hazards models for mismeasured outcomes. *Biometrics 59*(4), 947–954.

Neuhaus, J. M. (1999). Bias and efficiency loss due to misclassified responses in binary regression. *Biometrika, 86*(4), 843–855.

Overhage, J. M., & Overhage, L. M. (2013). Sensible use of observational clinical data. *Statistical Methods in Medical Research, 22*(1), 7–13.

Richardson, B. A., & Hughes, J. P. (2000). Product limit estimation for infectious disease data when the diagnostic test for the outcome is measured with uncertainty. *Biostatistics, 1*(3), 341–354.

Snapinn, S. M. (1998). Survival analysis with uncertain endpoints. *Biometrics, 54*, 209–218.

Warren, J. L., & Yabroff, K. R. (2015). Challenges and opportunities in measuring cancer recurrence in the united states. *Journal of the National Cancer Institute, 107*(8), djv134.

Warren, J. L., Mariotto, A., Melbert, D., Schrag, D., Doria-Rose, P., Penson, D., et al. (2016). Sensitivity of medicare claims to identify cancer recurrence in elderly colorectal and breast cancer patients. *Medical Care, 54*(8), E47–E54.

Weiskopf, N. G., & Weng, C. (2013). Methods and dimensions of electronic health record data quality assessment: Enabling reuse for clinical research. *Journal of the American Medical Informatics Association, 20*(1), 144–151.

Zee, J., & Xie, S. X. (2015). Nonparametric discrete survival function estimation with uncertain endpoints using an internal validation subsample. *Biometrics, 71*(3), 772–781.

Part IV
Statistical Modeling and Data Analysis

Modeling Inter-Trade Durations in the Limit Order Market

Jianzhao Yang, Zhicheng Li, Xinyun Chen, and Haipeng Xing

1 Introduction

A limit order market is an order-driven market that automatically collects orders, and matches the buyers and sellers in a centralized *limit order book* (LOB) based on some priority rules. As frequencies of trading have become extremely high in recent years, a great number of order events can be generated for a single stock in a very short time period. For instance, the time interval between two order events has reached the level of a nanosecond (i.e., 10^{-9} s), and tends to be even finer with the rapid development of information technology. Such high frequency tradings bring unparalleled challenge to researchers on modeling and analyzing trading events. As an example, although the NASDAQ stock market was initially a quote-driven market in which only market makers facilitate transactions, nowadays it has become a hybrid market where customer limit orders are allowed in addition to on-exchange market making, by using the *electronic communication networks* (ECN). In terms of total market activities, the share of using ECN has increased dramatically in the past years, and recently trades through ECN account for more than 40% of the total trading volume in NASDAQ market (Fink et al. 2006; Hendershott 2003). Given

J. Yang • H. Xing (✉)
Department of Applied Mathematics and Statistics, University of New York, Stony Brook, NY 11794, USA
e-mail: Jianzhao.Yang@stonybrook.edu; xing@ams.sunysb.edu

Z. Li
Department of Economics, State University of New York, Stony Brook, NY 11794, USA
e-mail: Zhicheng.li@stonybrook.edu

X. Chen
Department of Finance, Economics and Management School, Wuhan University, Wuhan 430072, China
e-mail: xinyun.chen@whu.edu.cn

© Springer International Publishing AG 2017   259
D.-G. Chen et al. (eds.), *New Advances in Statistics and Data Science*,
ICSA Book Series in Statistics, https://doi.org/10.1007/978-3-319-69416-0_15

the high frequency feature of electronic limit orders in the market, providers of market liquidity have transferred from the orders given by traditional market makers to the LOB. In order to gain more insight into the market mechanism and merits of orders in different scenarios (Harris and Hasbrouck 1996) and optimize order execution strategies (Obizhaeva and Wang 2013), it becomes extremely important to understand the dynamics of the LOB for both market participants and academic researchers.

In this paper, we focus on empirical features of inter-trade durations in the LOB market. Inter-trade duration is not only an important variable in the LOB, but also highly related to the trading behaviors and price formation processes. Recent studies have demonstrated the following important properties about inter-trade duration. First, the transaction-time trade arrivals are intimately related to the calendar time volatility in price (Clark 1973; O'hara 1995; Engle and Russell 1998; Engle 2000; Bauwens and Veredas 2004). Specifically, the serial correlation in transaction-time trade arrival drives the serial correlation of calendar-time trade counts, which further drives the serial correlation in calendar-time volatility. This feature is crucially important in terms of risk management, portfolio allocation and asset pricing. Second, returns interact with inter-trade duration. For instance, short duration moves price more than long duration across stocks and across time (Manganelli 2005; Furfine 2007). Third, transaction-time trade arrival intensity is ultimately driven by serial correlation in the information flow that drives trading (Diamond and Verrecchia 1987; Dufour and Engle 2000a; Simonsen 2007). The time elapsed between transactions is believed to contain some messages on the information flow and these messages can be passed to market participants. Relevant information may be related to the valuation of the stock also.

Some stylized facts of inter-trade durations have been studied intensively over the past decades, such as, long-range dependence (i.e., trade duration tends to be persistent), heavy tailedness (i.e., extremely short or long trade duration can be often observed), and trading clustering (i.e., short duration follows short duration and long duration follows long duration); see discussions in Jasiak (1999), Bauwens and Giot (2000), Dufour and Engle (2000b), and Chen et al. (2013). Among these studies, one breakthrough in modeling financial market inter-trade duration is the *autoregressive conditional duration* (ACD) model of Engle and Russell (1998), which expresses the conditional expectation of duration as a linear function of past duration and past conditional expectation and is an analog of Engle (1982) autoregressive conditional heteroskedasticity model in duration analysis. Bauwens and Veredas (2004) extended the discussion and proposed a stochastic conditional duration (SCD) model, which is similar to the stochastic volatility model in Ghysels et al. (2004) and allows the conditional mean duration depending on some latent information.

These models have been generalized to discuss different features of the trade data in the past years. Bauwens and Giot (2000) extended the ACD model to the logarithmic ACD model. Zhang et al. (2001) embedded a regime switching structure into the ACD model so that the model has different persistence, conditional means, and error distributions in different regimes. Feng et al. (2004) proposed a linear non-Gaussian state-space version of the SCD model to capture the leverage effect of the expected durations. Simonsen (2007) extended the ACD model to examine the dependence between durations.

Besides the multiplicative framework discussed above, another way to analyze inter-trade durations is to use the assumption from the point process theory that durations between two events follow an exponential distribution conditional on the hazard rate (or trade arrival intensity) and hence directly model their hazard rates or intensities; see Russell (1999) and Bauwens and Hautsch (2009). Recently, inspired by the success of the *Markov-switching multifractal* (MSM) stochastic volatility model in forecasting persistent volatility of financial returns (Calvet and Fisher 2004). Chen et al. (2013) proposed a *Markov-switching multifractal inter-trade duration* (MSMD) model. This model uses an elegant structure and parsimonious parameters to generate rich dynamics of inter-trade durations, and the inter-trade durations are composed of multiple fractals, with each of them following a distinct hidden Markov process. Also because of this multifractal feature, the MSMD model can be used to analyze trading data of large sample sizes, and is computationally efficient. Chen et al. (2013) used the model to study trade durations of the 1993 NYSE stock data and showed that the model could capture the long memory property of the data.

The nice feature of the MSMD model indicates that it might be applied to analyze durations of today's LOB market. However, the frequency of the LOB data has a much larger range than that in the 1993 NYSE stock market. Specifically, the LOB data we collected from the NASDAQ market have a large dispersion in the inter-trade duration, as it ranges from 10^{-5} to 10^2 s, while the inter-trade duration in the 1993 NYSE stock data ranges from 1 s to several hundreds of seconds. Due to this limit, the MSMD model in Chen et al. (2013) could not fit the 2013 NASDAQ LOB data well. To overcome this problem, we extend the MSMD model by modifying their assumption on error distributions. In particular, we keep the multifractal feature of the MSMD model, but relax the assumption of a single exponential distribution for error distribution to mixtures of exponentials (i.e., Gamma or Weibull distributions). We show that the extended model fits the current LOB data better than the original one and demonstrate the empirical features of LOB data that can be captured by the modified model.

The rest of the paper is organized as follows. Section 2 demonstrates some stylized facts of inter-trade durations of the NASDAQ LOB data. Section 3 presents the details of our model and inference method, and compares our models with Chen's MSMD models. In Sect. 4, we apply the MSMD model and our extensions to analyze the inter-trade durations of the 2013 NASDAQ LOB stock data, and compare the pros and cons of these models. Section 5 provides conclusive remarks and our discussion for further research.

2 Empirical Facts

Our data are downloaded from LOBSTER (https://lobsterdata.com/), which provides high-quality LOB data of all NASDAQ stocks from June 2007. The LOB data reconstructed by LOBSTER are based on NASDAQ's Historical TotalView-ITCH data (i.e., the historic record of what NASDAQ calls), and contain event messages that record changes of the LOB.

Table 1 shows a sample of LOB event messages, which record LOB events of Microsoft Corporation (MSFT) on January 2, 2013. In the table, event type 1, 2, and 3 represents submission, cancellation and deletion of a limit order, respectively. Event type 4 represents execution of a visible limit order. Thus, from the event message file provided in the LOB, one can easily construct the inter-trade durations series for a particular stock during a specified time period.

To demonstrate some features of inter-trade durations in the LOB, we plot the time series of inter-trade durations for Microsoft Corporation on January 2, 2013 in Fig. 1. Note that some features of the data have been mentioned in the past literature, while some of them are only possessed by recent high frequency LOB data.

- Large variation: There are almost 9000 trades for Microsoft Corporation on 01/02/2013. In Fig. 1, we can see that some durations are extremely short (to the extent of 1×10^{-5} s), some are very long (to the extent of 100 s). In the histogram of logarithm of MSFT inter-durations, which is shown as Fig. 2, there is a bimodal distribution with two peaks at 1×10^{-3} s and 1×10^{1} s. The extremely large span of the durations is probably related to the high frequency trading and has never been discussed before.

- Huge dispersion: This refers to the standard deviation exceeding the mean to a huge extent. Standard homogeneous Poisson process suggests that the duration should follow an independent and identical exponential distribution. However, in the exponential $Q - Q$ plot for this duration series shown in Fig. 3, we find a non-exponential distribution with an extraordinarily heavy tail. We will show

Table 1 Message file of LOB events

Time (s)	Event type	Order ID	Size	Price	Direction
34200.678583052	1	8100758	200	272,700	1
34200.678585706	1	8100759	200	272,700	1
34200.678914184	1	8100869	12	272,600	1
34200.679079227	1	8100901	100	272,600	1
34200.680069341	4	8100320	99	272,700	1
34200.681045068	1	8101470	100	272,800	−1
34200.681700278	3	8100043	115	272,600	1
34200.681700278	4	8101470	100	272,800	−1

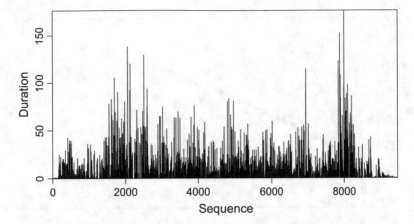

Fig. 1 MSFT inter-trade duration time series on January 2, 2013

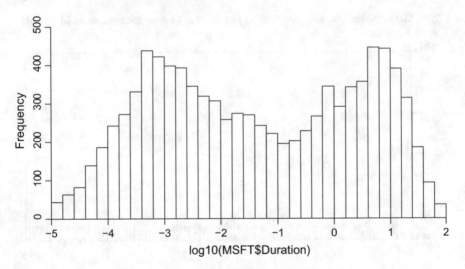

Fig. 2 Histogram of logarithm of MSFT inter-trade durations on 01/02/2013

in Sect. 4 that this dispersion is so large that even a combination of several exponential distributions (just like the MSMD) is still faint to model it.

- Persistence and long memory: It is not hard to see from Fig. 1 that the durations have a high persistence, i.e, short (or long) durations follow by short (or long) durations. Furthermore, the sample autocorrelation function decays very slowly and exhibits the so-called long memory property, which is shown in Fig. 4. This phenomenon is consistent with the discussion in many other studies (Deo et al. 2010; Pacurar 2008).

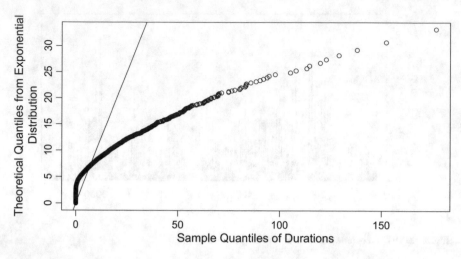

Fig. 3 Exponential and Inverse Gaussian QQ plot for MSFT inter-trade duration on 01/02/2013

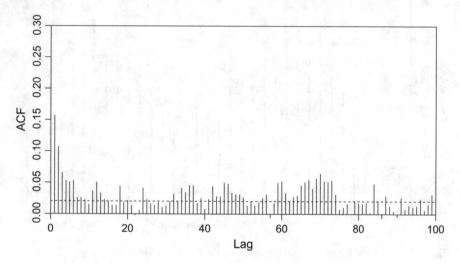

Fig. 4 Autocorrelations of MSFT inter-trade durations on 01/02/2013

3 Model and Estimation

3.1 Model Specification

We consider the following extension of the MSMD model (Chen et al. 2013). Denote $d_i = t_i - t_{i-1}$ the inter-trade durations, where t_i is the calendar time of ith trade and $i = 1, 2, \ldots N$. The durations d_i is assumed to have the form of

$$d_i = \psi_i \varepsilon_i, \tag{1}$$

where ε_i are *independent and identically distributed* (i.i.d.) random variables with mean 1 and variance σ^2. Same as that in the MSMD model, the conditional mean ψ_i is a latent variable that possess the following Markov-switching multifractal

$$\psi_i = \bar{\psi} \prod_{k=1}^{\bar{k}} M_{k,i}, \qquad (2)$$

in which the component $M_{k,i}$ ($1 \leq k \leq \bar{k}$) is an independent Markov renewal process specified below

$$M_{k,i} = \begin{cases} M & \text{drawn from distribution } G_M \text{ with probability } \gamma_k \\ M_{k,i-1} & \text{with probability} 1 - \gamma_k. \end{cases} \qquad (3)$$

The above specification suggests that, the kth component of the ith duration $M_{k,i}$ remains the same as that in the last duration with probability $1 - \gamma_k$, and takes a new value that is drawn from a fixed distribution G_M with probability γ_k. Furthermore, probabilities $(\gamma_1, \gamma_2, \cdots, \gamma_{\bar{k}})$ are parsimoniously parameterized by

$$\gamma_k = 1 - (1 - \gamma_{\bar{k}})^{b^{k-\bar{k}}}. \qquad (4)$$

Following Chen et al. (2013), we assume the distribution of the components G_M is binomial, which draws values m_0 and $2 - m_0$ with equal probabilities. Then the state vector and the corresponding transition matrix of $M_{k,i}$ are written as

$$M_{k,i} = \begin{cases} m_0 & \text{with probability } 1/2, \\ 2 - m_0 & \text{with probability } 1/2, \end{cases} \qquad (5)$$

$$P_k = \begin{bmatrix} 1 - \frac{1}{2}\gamma_k & \frac{1}{2}\gamma_k \\ \frac{1}{2}\gamma_k & 1 - \frac{1}{2}\gamma_k \end{bmatrix}. \qquad (6)$$

Since the components $M_{k,i}$ are independent, the transition matrix of M_i is given by

$$P = P_1 \otimes P_2 \otimes \cdots \otimes P_{\bar{k}}, \qquad (7)$$

where the $\otimes$ represents the Kronecker product.

We shall note that the model specification so far is essentially the same as the MSMD model, and such a specification has two prominent advantages. First, it has a "parameter-driven" structure since the conditional dynamics are driven by the history of the latent variable. The dynamics implied by the model allows more flexibility, compared to the traditionally ACD models that are "observation-driven" (i.e., conditional dynamics are driven by the history of observables). Such flexibility comes from the stochastic process of the latent variable, which follows a hidden Markov process. Although the number of controlling parameters is small (just $\bar{k}$, $\gamma_{\bar{k}}$, b, and m_0), each component of this Markov-switching multifractal has a distinct evolution path and the total number of states can reach $2^{\bar{k}}$. Second, such specification provides a natural long-memory duration generating mechanism by overlaying simple regime-switching processes with different degrees of persistence, which can be explained as reactions of different types of informed and uninformed traders.

In Chen et al. (2013)'s MSMD model, they assumed that ε_i in (1) are i.i.d. exponentials with mean 1. Although they argued that this assumption is general enough and only requires very weak regularity conditions, it actually imposes a strong constraint that limits its empirical applications, especially with application to the high frequency trading data. Therefore, we relax this assumption and allow the error term ε_i to follow a variety of distributions. Specifically, instead of using exponential distribution with mean 1, we consider the standard Weibull distribution and Gamma distribution with the unit mean for error ε_i. To distinguish from the original MSMD model with the unit-mean exponential distribution (denoted as the Exponential-MSMD), we denote the other two corresponding models as the Weibull-MSMD and the Gamma-MSMD models.

3.2 Maximum Likelihood

Denote the observed inter-trade durations as $d_{1:n} = \{d_1, d_2, \ldots d_n\}$. The log-likelihood function for $d_{1:n}$ can be expressed as

$$\ln \mathscr{L}(d_{1:n}|\theta) = \log f(d_1|\theta) + \sum_{i=2}^{n} \log f(d_i|d_{1:i-1}, \theta), \tag{8}$$

where θ includes the parameter in $f(\varepsilon)$ and $\{\bar{k}, m_0, b, \gamma_{\bar{k}}\}$. Since the mean levels ψ_i can not be observed, we need to use a weighted average of state-conditional likelihoods. Moreover, according to (2) and (5), the possible states of ψ_i can be as large as $2^{\bar{k}}$. This is due to the fact that each underlying Markov component $M_{k,i}$ has two independent states. Assume that the states of ψ_i are $\psi^{(j)}$, $j = 1 \ldots 2^{\bar{k}}$ and denote the probability of $\psi_i = \psi^{(j)}$ as $\mathbb{P}(\psi_i = \psi^{(j)})$. Then the log-likelihood (8) can be written as

$$\ln \mathscr{L}(d_{1:n}|\theta) = \sum_{j=1}^{2^{\bar{k}}} \mathbb{P}(\psi_1 = \psi^{(j)}|\theta) \cdot \log f(d_1|\psi^{(j)}, \theta)$$

$$+ \sum_{i=2}^{n} \sum_{j=1}^{2^{\bar{k}}} \mathbb{P}(\psi_i = \psi^{(j)}|d_{1:i-1}, \theta) \cdot \log f(d_i|\psi^{(j)}, \theta). \tag{9}$$

To compute the log-likelihood, we first initialize $t = 0$ by the long run equilibrium distribution associated with the Markov transition matrix $\boldsymbol{P}_{2^{\bar{k}} \times 2^{\bar{k}}}$ in (7). Then for $t = 1 \ldots n$, $\mathbb{P}(\psi_i = \psi^{(j)}|d_{1:i-1}, \theta)$ is computed by the previous probability distribution and the Markov transition matrix

$$\mathbb{P}(\psi_i = \psi^{(j)}|d_{1:i-1}, \theta) = \sum_{k=1}^{2^{\bar{k}}} \mathbb{P}(\psi_{i-1} = \psi^{(k)}|d_{1:i-1}, \theta) \cdot \boldsymbol{P}_{kj}, \qquad (10)$$

and the posterior distribution of the ψ_i is updated by the Bayes rule, i.e,

$$\mathbb{P}(\psi_i = \psi^{(j)}|d_{1:i}, \theta) \propto f(d_i|\psi^{(j)}, \theta)\mathbb{P}(\psi_i = \psi^{(j)}|d_{1:i-1}, \theta). \qquad (11)$$

We can iteratively compute (10) and (11), and obtain the log-likelihood function for all these observations from 1 to n for a given value of θ. Therefore we could use grid search to maximize the log-likelihood and obtain a maximum likelihood estimate for θ, i.e.,

$$\widehat{\theta} = \arg \max \ln \mathscr{L}(d_{1:n}|\theta). \qquad (12)$$

Note that in the calculation above, different distribution assumptions on ε_i lead to different functional forms of (12). In Chen et al.'s (2013) Exponential-MSMD model, $\varepsilon_i \sim$ Exponential(1), i.e.

$$f_E(\varepsilon) = \exp(-\varepsilon), \qquad (13)$$

then the density function of the duration d_i is

$$f_E(d_i; \psi_i) = \frac{\exp(-d_i/\psi_i)}{\psi_i}. \qquad (14)$$

In this case, $\theta = \{\bar{k}, m_0, b, \gamma_{\bar{k}}\}$.

In the Weibull-MSMD model with scale parameter $\Gamma\left(1 + \frac{1}{\kappa}\right)$, the unit mean assumption implies that the density of the error distribution is given by

$$f_W(\varepsilon; \kappa) = \kappa \left[\Gamma\left(1 + \frac{1}{\kappa}\right)\right]^{\kappa} \varepsilon^{\kappa-1} \exp\left\{-\Gamma\left(1 + \frac{1}{\kappa}\right)\varepsilon\right\}^{\kappa}. \qquad (15)$$

Hence the density function for the duration d_i is

$$f_W(d_i; \psi_i, \kappa) = \frac{\kappa}{d_i} \left[\Gamma\left(1 + \frac{1}{\kappa}\right)\right]^{\kappa} \left(\frac{d_i}{\psi_i}\right)^{\kappa} \exp\left\{-\Gamma\left(1 + \frac{1}{\kappa}\right)\left(\frac{d_i}{\psi_i}\right)\right\}^{\kappa} \qquad (16)$$

In this case, $\theta = \{\bar{k}, m_0, b, \gamma_{\bar{k}}, \kappa\}$.

In the Gamma-MSMD model with scale parameter $\frac{1}{\kappa}$, the unit mean assumption implies that the density of the error distribution is expressed as

$$f_G(\varepsilon; \kappa) = \frac{\varepsilon^{\kappa-1}}{\kappa^{-\kappa}\Gamma(\kappa)} \exp(-\varepsilon\kappa). \tag{17}$$

Thus the density function of the duration d_i is

$$f_G(d_i; \psi_i, \kappa) = \frac{\kappa^\kappa}{d_i \Gamma(\kappa)} \left(\frac{d_i}{\psi_i}\right)^\kappa \exp(-\kappa\frac{d_i}{\psi_i}). \tag{18}$$

In such a case, $\theta = \{\bar{k}, m_0, b, \gamma_{\bar{k}}, \kappa\}$.

4 Empirical Analysis

We use the original Exponential-MSMD model and the extended Weibull- and Gamma-MSMD models to analyze the LOB data of Google from January 8, 2014 to January 10, 2014, which contains 10,000 inter-trade durations in total. Figure 5 shows the time series plot of the data. One thing need to be mentioned is that we have used a procedure which is similar to that in Chen et al. (2013) to remove the calendar effect. The only difference is that the time interval we use is 5 min instead of 30-min intervals used in Chen et al. (2013). This is because that, for the current high frequency data, the information is updated much quicker than 20 years ago. Figure 6 shows the sample autocorrelation of the data. We can see that the inter-trade durations have significant correlation even until lag 100, exhibiting a strong long memory effect.

We fitted these three MSMD models to the sample data, and assumed the number of Markov components to be 3, 4 and 5 in each model. We coded the estimation procedure in MATLAB and implemented it on a desktop (3.4 GHz Intel Core i5). It took about 3 min to obtain the estimation results for exponential error distribution and about 5 min for Weibull or Gamma error distribution. The running time varies with different initial parameter values, $\bar{k}$ and optimization methods. Table 2 presents the estimation results. (We tried a larger range of $\bar{k}$ and various initial parameters, but

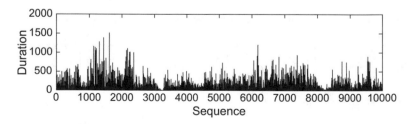

Fig. 5 Time series plot of Google inter-trade durations from 2014/01/08 10:30:03 to 2014/01/10 10:46:46, with number of observations 10,000 and calendar effect removed

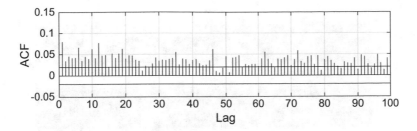

Fig. 6 Autocorrelation of the sample of Google inter-trade duration

Table 2 Estimation results of the sample durations of Google

	Exponential-MSMD			Weibull-MSMD			Gamma-MSMD		
	$\bar{k}=3$	$\bar{k}=4$	$\bar{k}=5$	$\bar{k}=3$	$\bar{k}=4$	$\bar{k}=5$	$\bar{k}=3$	$\bar{k}=4$	$\bar{k}=5$
m_0	1.99	1.96	1.92	1.98	1.96	1.922	1.35	1.31	1.33
	(0.00027)	(0.00069)	(0.0011)	(0.0006)	(0.0008)	(0.0011)	(0.022)	(0.024)	(0.025)
ψ	1486.72	288.62	153.17	400	301.62	175.50	76.12	31.35	86.69
	(51.15)	(9.91)	(6.21)	(18.45)	(11.32)	(8.73)	(4.32)	(2.10)	(5.92)
$\gamma_{\bar{k}}$	0.79	0.86	0.86	0.84	0.84	0.86	0.0055	0.0049	0.0056
	(0.04)	(0.037)	(0.041)	(0.033)	(0.040)	(0.046)	(0.0018)	(0.0017)	(0.0020)
b	1.001	1.001	1.001	1.001	1.001	1.002	6.10	1.89	2.63
	(0.12)	(0.085)	(0.075)	(0.11)	(0.09)	(0.081)	(3.71)	(0.63)	(0.97)
κ	N/A	N/A	N/A	0.79	0.88	0.90	0.196	0.198	0.197
				(0.0051)	(0.0064)	(0.0074)	(0.0021)	(0.0022)	(0.0021)
$\ln \mathscr{L}$	-30962	-30500	-30694	-30779	-30338	-30610	-29368	-29357	-29360

the best results we have gotten are shown here. Based on our experiments, a larger $\bar{k}$ will lead to a rapid increase in the computational cost but not necessarily improved the results.) We can see that the Exponential-MSMD and Weibull-MSMD models have a very small value of b (lower boundary is 1) and a large value of γ_k. This indicates that, in order to capture the dynamics of these high frequency data, both the Exponential-MSMD and Weibull-MSMD models require shifts among different states to be very frequent. One possible reason for this is that the single standard exponential or Weibull distribution can not capture large variations in a short time period. On the other hand, the result from fitting a Gamma-MSMD model indicates a stable Markov transition matrix, which demonstrates its high flexibility.

To further see if these results are reasonable, we simulate the inter-trade durations using parameters estimated in Table 2 and demonstrate them in Figs. 7, 8, and 9, respectively (here we use $\bar{k} = 4$). In these figures, the first four panels show the time series plots of simulated latent components $M_{t,i}$. It is clear that the latent processes in the Exponential- and Weibull-MSMD models switch regimes so quickly that even the slowest component M_1 is hard to be recognized. This is probably due to large variations of inter-trade durations in the LOB data. The fifth panels in Figs. 7, 8, and 9 show the evolution of ψ_i. We find from them that, for Exponential- and Weibull-MSMD models, ψ_i need frequently jump from its upper bounds to the lower bounds

270   J. Yang et al.

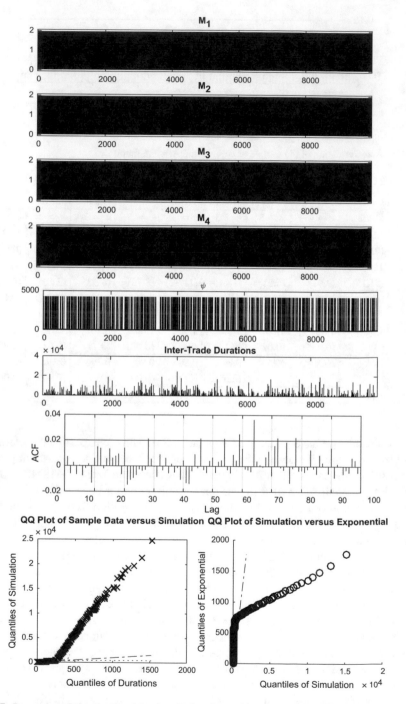

Fig. 7 Properties of the simulated inter-trade durations of Exponential-MSMD, with parameters calibrated from the sample of Google inter-trade duration from 2014/01/08 10:30:03 to 2014/01/10 10:46:46

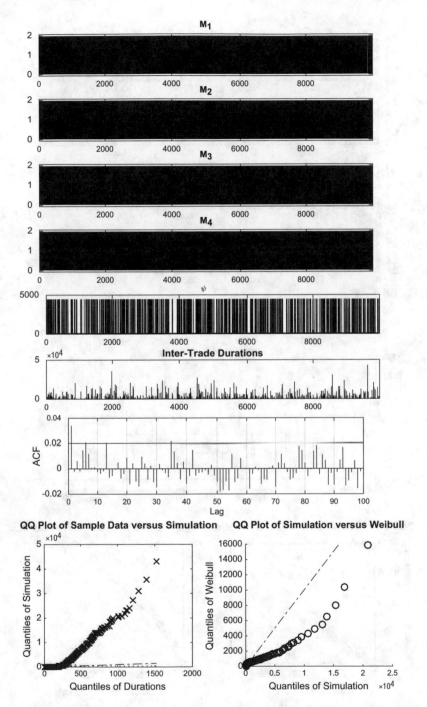

Fig. 8 Properties of the simulated inter-trade durations of Weibull-MSMD, with parameters calibrated from the sample of Google inter-trade duration from 2014/01/08 10:30:03 to 2014/01/10 10:46:46

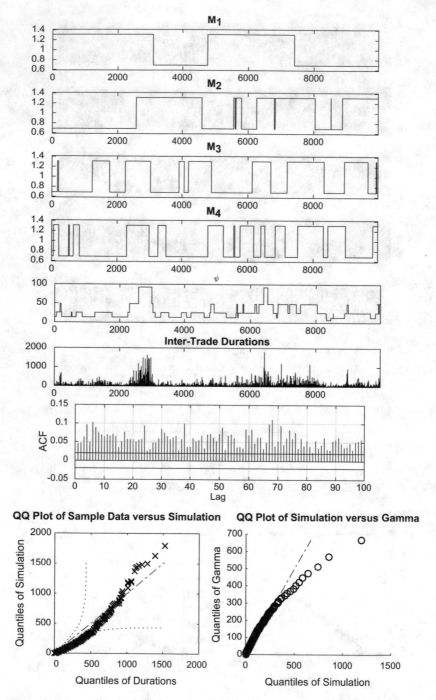

Fig. 9 Properties of the simulated inter-trade durations of Gamma-MSMD, with parameters calibrated from the sample of Google inter-trade durations from 2014/01/08 10:30:03 to 2014/01/10 10:46:46

to adapt to large variations of inter-trade durations in the high frequency LOB data. On the other hand, the latent process of the Gamma-MSMD model evolves steadily and we can clearly observe the difference from M_1 to M_4. The overall dynamic of ψ in the Gamma-MSMD model is clear and stable, suggesting the MSMD model with Gamma distribution fits the high frequency data better than the other two. Then we show the autocorrelation of simulated data from three MSMD models. Note that only the Gamma-MSMD model generates long memory phenomena. This indicates that, although the MSMD structure provides a natural long-memory by overlaying regime-switching components with different degrees of persistence, if latent components switch their regimes too fast, the benefit of multifractal feature in the MSMD models can be offset. We further compare these simulation with the real data using Q-Q plots. Both the Exponential- and Weibull-MSMD models exhibit a very long tail in durations, while the Gamma-MSMD model does not.

In the end, we compare the out-of-sample forecasting performance of the three models. We use the first 5000 data points as the training data, and the rest 5000 data points for out-of-sample prediction. To compare the forecasting performance, we consider the Mincer-Zarnowitz ordinary least squares (OLS) regressions for durations on a one-step forecasts,

$$X_{t+1} = \beta_0 + \beta_1 E_t(X_{t+1}) + \mu_t \qquad (19)$$

The results of out of sample prediction are presented in Figs. 10, 11, and 12 and summarized in Table 3. Both the figures and the table suggest that the Gamma-MSMD model performs better than the other two models.

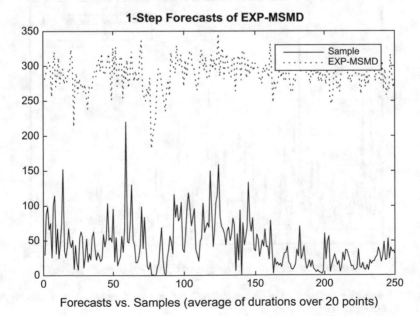

Fig. 10 Forecasting performance of Exponential-MSMD and its out-of-sample comparison with the real data of Google inter-trade durations

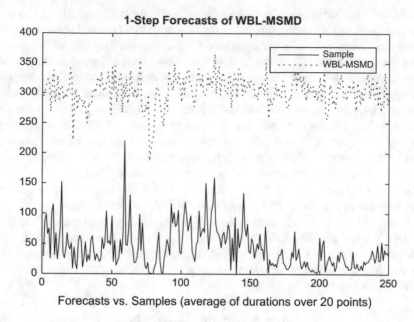

Fig. 11 Forecasting performance of Weibull-MSMD and its out-of-sample comparison with the real data of Google inter-trade durations

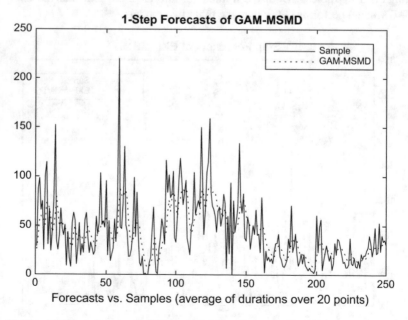

Fig. 12 Forecasting performance of Gamma-MSMD and its out-of-sample comparison with the real data of Google inter-trade durations

Table 3 Mincer-Zarnowitz OLS summary for three MSMD model to compare the forecasting performance

		Exponential-MSMD	Weibull-MSMD	Gamma-MSMD
R-square		0.218	0.224	0.493
β_0	Estimate	−132.23	−127.91	0.75
	S.E	21.25	20.34	2.85
	t-statistics	(−6.22)	−6.29	0.26
	p-value	2.07E−09	1.44E−09	0.79
β_1	Estimate	0.60	0.55	0.92
	S.E	0.07	0.067	0.06
	t-statistics	8.11	8.23	15.37
	p-value	2.25E−14	8.31E−15	6.7E−38

5 Conclusion

The ultra high frequency LOB data have brought much challenge to statistical analysis. To model the dynamics of inter-trade durations in the LOB data, we extend the Exponential-MSMD model that was originally proposed for the 1993 NYSE trade data and discuss two extensions, Weibull and Gamma distributions for error distributions. We compare the in-sample and out-of-sample performance of the original and extended models using the 2014 NASDAQ LOB data. We find that the Gamma-MSMD model performs better than the other two, due to the fact that inter-trade durations in the LOB data has a huge dispersion.

On the other hand, we note that the success of using the MSMD model to analyze inter-trade durations lies in the fact that the MSMD has an intrinsic Markov switching feature in its model structure. This motivates us to investigate what is the driving force for these regime switchings. Specifically, it is worthwhile in the future to look into which market factors play an important role in regime switchings and how these factors affect patterns of regime switchings in inter-trade durations.

References

Bauwens, L., & Giot, P. (2000). The logarithmic ACD model: An application to the bid-ask quote process of three NYSE stocks. *Annales d'Economie et de Statistique, 60*, 117–149.

Bauwens, L., & Hautsch, N. (2009). Modelling financial high frequency data using point processes. In T. Mikosch, J. Kreib, R. Davis, & T. G. Andersen (Eds.), *Handbook of financial time series* (pp. 953–979). New York: Springer-Verlag.

Bauwens, L., & Veredas, D. (2004). The stochastic conditional duration model: A latent variable model for the analysis of financial durations. *Journal of Econometrics, 119*(2), 381–412.

Calvet, L. E., & Fisher, A. J. (2004). How to forecast long-run volatility: Regime switching and the estimation of multifractal processes. *Journal of Financial Econometrics, 2(1)*, 49–83.

Chen, F., Diebold, F. X., & Schorfheide, F. (2013). A Markov-switching multifractal inter-trade duration model, with application to US equities. *Journal of Econometrics, 177*(2), 320–342.

Clark, P. K. (1973). A subordinated stochastic process model with finite variance for speculative prices. *Econometrica: Journal of the Econometric Society, 41*, 135–155.

Deo, R., Hsieh, M., & Hurvich, C. M. (2010). Long memory in intertrade durations, counts and realized volatility of NYSE stocks. *Journal of Statistical Planning and Inference, 140*(12), 3715–3733.

Diamond, D. W., & Verrecchia, R. E. (1987). Constraints on short-selling and asset price adjustment to private information. *Journal of Financial Economics, 18*(2), 277–311.

Dufour, A., & Engle, R. F. (2000a). Time and the price impact of a trade. *The Journal of Finance, 55*(6), 2467–2498.

Dufour, A., & Engle, R. F. (2000b). The ACD model: predictability of the time between consecutive trades. *University of Reading and University of California at San Diego, 35*(3), 463–497.

Engle, R.F. (1982). Autoregressive conditional heteroskedasticity with estimates of the variance of United Kingdom inflation. *Econometrica, 50*(4), 987–1007.

Engle, R. F. (2000). The econometrics of ultra-high-frequency data. *Econometrica, 68*(1), 1–22.

Engle, R. F., & Russell, J. R. (1998). Autoregressive conditional duration: A new model for irregularly spaced transaction data. *Econometrica, 65*, 1127–1162.

Feng, D., Jiang, G. J., & Song, P. X. K. (2004). Stochastic conditional duration models with leverage effect for financial transaction data. *Journal of Financial Econometrics, 2*(3), 390–421.

Fink, J., Fink, K. E., & Weston, J. P. (2006). Competition on the Nasdaq and the growth of electronic communication networks. *Journal of Banking & Finance, 30*(9), 2537–2559.

Furfine, C. (2007). When is inter-transaction time informative? *Journal of Empirical Finance, 14*(3), 310–332.

Ghysels, E., Gourieroux, C., & Jasiak, J. (2004). Stochastic volatility duration models. *Journal of Econometrics, 119*(2), 423–433.

Harris, L., & Hasbrouck, J. (1996). Market vs. limit orders: The SuperDOT evidence on order submission strategy. *Journal of Financial and Quantitative Analysis, 31*(2), 213–231.

Hendershott, T. (2003). Electronic trading in financial markets. *IT Professional Magazine, 5*(4), 10.

Jasiak, J. (1999). Persistence in intertrade durations. Available at SSRN 162008.

Manganelli, S. (2005). Duration, volume and volatility impact of trades. *Journal of Financial Markets, 8*(4), 377–399.

Obizhaeva, A., & Wang, J. (2013). Optimal trading strategy and supply. *Journal of Fiancial Markets, 16*(1), 1–32.

O'hara, M. (1995). *Market microstructure theory* (Vol. 108). Cambridge, MA: Blackwell.

Pacurar, M. (2008). Autoregressive conditional duration models in finance: A survey of the theoretical and empirical literature. *Journal of Economic Surveys, 22*(4), 711–751.

Russell, J. R. (1999). Econometric modeling of multivariate irregularly-spaced high-frequency data. Manuscript, GSB, University of Chicago.

Simonsen, O. (2007). An Empirical Model for Durations in Stocks. *Annals of Finance, 3*(2), 241–255.

Zhang, M. Y., Russell, J. R., & Tsay, R. S. (2001). A nonlinear autoregressive conditional duration model with applications to financial transaction data. *Journal of Econometrics, 104*(1), 179–207.

Assessment of Drug Interactions with Repeated Measurements

Shouhao Zhou, Chan Shen, and J. Jack Lee

1 Introduction

Drug combination therapy has become a major treatment approach in oncology and other branches of medicine, applying a growing number of drugs approved by the FDA in recent years. Synergistic drug combinations, which are more effective than predicted from summing the effects of the individual drugs, often achieve greater efficacy at lower doses, while also reducing toxicity (Chou 1991). Although dose response assessment and drug interaction analysis play integral parts of early-stage drug discovery, determining optimal designs for in vitro studies remains elusive.

Despite thousands of papers published in the field of drug combination discovery, the procedure to characterize a two-drug interaction proposed by Chou and Talalay (1984) is still the most commonly used method. Assuming the median effect equation holds for the marginal dose-effect curves of the single agents and the combination doses at a fixed ray (i.e., $d_1/d_2 = c$, where c is a constant forming a ray in the $d_1 \times d_2$ dose plane when considering a 2-drug combination), Chou and Talalay assessed the drug interaction at the observed combinations by estimating the interaction index derived from Loewe's additivity model (Loewe and Muischnek 1926; Berenbaum 1985; Greco et al. 1995; Tallarida 2000). Comprehensive reviews of this approach are available (Chou 2006; Lee et al. 2007). To assess the uncertainty of the estimation, Lee and Kong (2009) proposed an analytic approach to construct

S. Zhou (✉) • J.J. Lee
Department of Biostatistics, The University of Texas MD Anderson Cancer Center, Houston, TX 77030, USA
e-mail: szhou@mdanderson.org; jjlee@mdanderson.org

C. Shen
Department of Health Services Research, Division of Cancer Prevention and Population Sciences, The University of Texas MD Anderson Cancer Center, Houston, TX 77030, USA
e-mail: cshen@mdanderson.org

© Springer International Publishing AG 2017
D.-G. Chen et al. (eds.), *New Advances in Statistics and Data Science*,
ICSA Book Series in Statistics, https://doi.org/10.1007/978-3-319-69416-0_16

the confidence intervals for the interaction index, which is close to what is generated using Monte Carlo techniques (Belen'kii and Schinazi 1994).

Although the interaction index can be estimated with only one observation at each combination dose, there have been new developments in the implementation of experiments for assessing drug combinations. Given the low cost of conducting in vitro studies, repeated measurements are collected to better estimate the dose response curves. For example, to investigate synergy for different ratios of the compounds in the mixture, Sanofi (2013) recommends performing the experiment 3 times sequentially with 10 concentrations in triplicate for robust estimation of synergy using a ray design. However, the estimation of the interaction index and its confidence interval was implemented by simply applying Chou and Talalay's method after averaging over the effects at each single or combination dose, leading to estimation inefficiency due to discarded data points and induced correlation (Hennessey et al. 2010).

The objective of this study is to improve the accuracy of the point and interval estimation of the interaction index in a fixed ray design by taking into account the variability between experiments and/or between replicates of the repeated measurements. The framework of Loewe's additivity for potency and the median effect model for estimating the dose response curve is introduced in Sect. 2, followed by generalization to the data with repeated measurements in the experiment. In Sect. 3, we propose a procedure to estimate the interaction index at some observed dose of the drug combination and construct its associated confidence interval. Because investigators are usually not only interested in examining synergism at the tested dose levels, but also identifying the region of the drug combination effect that shows significant synergism, in Sect. 4, we propose an additional procedure to estimate the interaction index along the drug effect on interval $(0, 1)$ and construct its associated confidence bound. Section 5 provides some simulation results showing improvement in the estimation by introducing random effects for repeated measurements. In Sect. 6, we apply our methods in an experimental study conducted at MD Anderson Cancer Center. The last section is devoted to a discussion.

2   Median Effect Model for Drug Combination Effects

In this section, we review popular method and design for assessing drug combination effects, then generalize the ideas of the median effect model in the setting of repeated measurements.

2.1 Median Effect Model

Chou and Talalay (1984) considered the estimation of the drug effect with various dose concentrations. The dose response curve was estimated with the median effect equation, which has the following form

$$E = \frac{\left(\frac{d}{D_{med}}\right)^m}{1 + \left(\frac{d}{D_{med}}\right)^m},$$
(1)

where d is the dose of a drug eliciting effect E, D_{med} is the median effective dose of the drug that achieves the effect $E = 1/2$, and m is the Hill coefficient (Hill 1910a,b), a slope parameter that depicts the shape of the curve. When E describes the proportion of cells surviving, m is negative, and the curve described by Eq. (1) falls with increasing drug concentration; when E describes the percentage of inhibition, m is positive, and the curve rises with increasing drug concentration.

A transformation of the median effect equation can be written as

$$\text{logit}(E) = \log \frac{E}{1 - E} = m \log(d) - m \log(D_{med}) = \beta_0 + \beta_1 \log(d),$$
(2)

where $\beta_0 = -m \log(D_{med})$ and $\beta_1 = m$, making a 1-to-1 mapping between the unknown parameters $\{m, D_{med}\}$ and $\{\beta_0, \beta_1\}$. For an arbitrary dose level d, suppose the observable drug effect is y. The median effect model (2) has the form

$$\text{logit}(y) = \beta_0 + \beta_1 \log(d) + \varepsilon,$$
(3)

with the model error ε following $N(0, \sigma^2)$. If there are k candidate drugs, the marginal dose-effect curve for the ith drug, $i = 1, \cdots, k$, can be estimated by $\text{logit}(\hat{y}) = \hat{\beta}_{0,i} + \hat{\beta}_{1,i} \log(d)$, or equivalently, $\hat{y} = \text{logit}^{-1}(\hat{\beta}_{0,i} + \hat{\beta}_{1,i} \log(d))$.

2.2 Ray Design

A ray design is used to assess k-drug interactions for any integer $k \geq 2$ by fixing the ratio of multiple drug concentrations in order to better estimate synergism (Tallarida 2000). In practice, the individual agents are combined in amounts that retain constant relative proportions of each drug. A simple example of a combination of 2 agents is illustrated in Fig. 1, where the different lines correspond to the different rays, each with a specific fraction (**f**) value with $\mathbf{f} = (f, 1 - f)$, and the dots represent various concentrations within a mixture. In cases of $k > 2$, $\mathbf{f} = (f_1, \cdots, f_k)$ with $0 \leq f_k \leq 1$ and $f_k = 1 - f_1 - \cdots - f_{k-1}$.

Fig. 1 Illustration of a ray design. The *x*-axis corresponds to the concentration of agent B and the *y*-axis to the concentration of agent A. Each line corresponds to a different ray with a specific relative potency *f* value with respect to Agent A, and the dots represent various concentrations within a ray

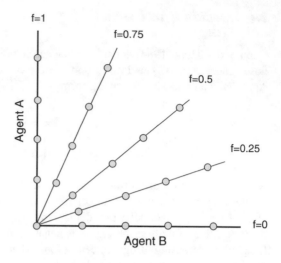

For a combination of k drugs ($k \geq 2$) at dose level $\mathbf{d} = (d_1, \cdots, d_k)$, we have $d_i = f_i A_i$ for each $i = 1, \cdots, k$ and a total dose of the combination

$$d = \sum_{i=1}^{k} d_i = \sum_{i=1}^{k} f_i A_i,$$

where A_i is the dose level of the ith single agent in a ray design (Straetemans et al. 2005). Because all dose concentrations have a constant ratio between drug combinations, a drug combination on a fixed ray can be considered as a special drug with the dose-effect curve $\text{logit}(\hat{y}) = \hat{\beta}_{0,c} + \hat{\beta}_{1,c} \log(d)$.

2.3 Loewe Additivity

In drug interaction analysis, the Loewe additivity model was considered to be the gold standard for defining drug interactions (Berenbaum 1989). For a k-drug combination with dose level $\mathbf{d} = (d_1, \cdots, d_k)$, the potency of the combination can be characterized as

$$\tau = \frac{d_1}{D_{E,1}} + \cdots + \frac{d_k}{D_{E,k}} = \sum_{i=1}^{k} \frac{d_i}{D_{E,i}}. \tag{4}$$

Here, $d_1, \cdots, d_k$ are doses of each drug in the mixture of the k drugs resulting in effect E, and $D_{E,1}, \cdots, D_{E,k}$ are the doses of the drugs that result in the effect E for each respective drug when given alone. The summation (4) is the interaction index (Tallarida 2002), which has a value that is less than the constant number of

1 for synergistic drug combinations, equal to 1 for additive drug combinations, and larger than 1 for antagonistic drug combinations. Because E is the unknown true effect of the drug combination $\mathbf{d} = (d_1, \cdots, d_k)$, and for any given effect E, the dose level of each drug given alone is unknown, Chou and Talalay proposed the following estimate of the interaction index:

$$\hat{\tau}(\mathbf{d}) = \sum_{i=1}^{k} \frac{d_i}{\hat{D}_{y,i}} \tag{5}$$

for a single observation $\mathbf{d} = (d_1, \cdots, d_k)$ on that ray resulting in observed effect y, where $\hat{D}_{y,i} = \exp\left(-\frac{\hat{\beta}_{0,i}}{\hat{\beta}_{1,i}}\right)\left(\frac{y}{1-y}\right)^{1/\hat{\beta}_{1,i}}$.

2.4 Drug Combination Effects with Repeated Measurements

Denote n_c and n_i as the number of observations when a k-drug combination is used and the ith drug is used alone, respectively, $i = 1, \cdots, k$. Conventionally, any study with repeated measurements requires at least three 96-well plates for data collection, which translates into a minimum total sample size ($n = n_c + \sum_{i=1}^{k} n_i$) of 250 after excluding the positive and negative controls, which is sufficient for the normal approximation of the confidence interval proposed in the following sections. In Sanofi's guideline (Sanofi 2013) for robust estimation of the dose response curve, cell viability at each dose level is measured 9 times, first in 3 replicates, then repeating the experiment 3 times, which requires nine 96-well plates to complete a study.

Suppose there exists some bias α_j, for instance, the random effect from the jth plate or the jth well on the 96-well plate, with observations of drug effects $y_{i,j,r}$ for the ith drug in model (3),

$$\text{logit}(y_{i,j,r}) = \beta_{0,i} + \alpha_j + \beta_{1,i} * \log(d) + \varepsilon_{i,j,r}, \tag{6}$$

where the subscript r stands for repeated measurements and α_j follows $N(0, \sigma_\alpha^2)$, $j = 1, \cdots, J$. Chou and Talalay's estimate for the potency of k-drug combinations can be generalized with repeated measurements given a certain estimator $\hat{y}$ for y,

$$\hat{\tau}(\mathbf{d}) = \sum_{i=1}^{k} \frac{d_i}{\hat{D}_{\hat{y},i}}. \tag{7}$$

The commonly used estimators for $\hat{y}$ include the average raw effect $\bar{y}$ at dose $\mathbf{d}$, and $\text{logit}^{-1}(\hat{\beta}_{0,c} + \hat{\beta}_{1,c}\log(d))$ based on the marginal dose-effect curve of the combination drug without random effects.

3 Confidence Interval Estimation at the Observed Combination

Under the assumption that the dose-effect curves follow the median effect equation, Lee and Kong (2009) investigated the characteristics of the interaction index at an observed combination $\mathbf{d}$ and its logarithmic transformation and proposed a procedure for constructing the confidence interval for the estimated interaction index without repeated measurements by approximating the variance of $\mathrm{Var}(\hat{\tau}(\mathbf{d}))$ using the delta method (Bickel and Doksum 2001).

In the experiment with repeated measurements, we use a similar approach by first estimating the variance of $\log(\hat{\tau}(\mathbf{d}))$. Because $\log(\hat{\tau}(\mathbf{d}))$ has a distribution that is more symmetric than $\hat{\tau}(\mathbf{d})$ in (7), we construct the confidence interval of $\hat{\tau}(\mathbf{d})$ with the exponential transformation for better normal approximation. Compared with the 95% confidence interval constructed directly with the estimated variance of $\hat{\tau}(\mathbf{d})$, our approach guarantees that the lower limit of the confidence interval is greater than zero all the time due to the exponential transformation. As shown in the simulation study in Sect. 5, our approach also increases the estimation accuracy in terms of the confidence coverage rate being close to the nominal rate.

Let $p_i = d_i/d$. The logarithm of the interaction index for a single observation $\mathbf{d} = (d_1, \cdots, d_k)$ can be written as

$$\log(\hat{\tau}(\mathbf{d})) = \log(d) + \log(\sum_{i=1}^{k} \frac{p_i}{\hat{D}_{\hat{y},i}}). \tag{8}$$

In Eq. (8), both quantities d and p_is are constant. For any effect y in (6), the dose estimate

$$\hat{D}_{y,i} = \exp\left(-\frac{\hat{\beta}_{0,i}}{\hat{\beta}_{1,i}}\right)\left(\frac{y}{1-y}\right)^{1/\hat{\beta}_{1,i}}$$

is a function of $\{\hat{\beta}_{0,i}, \hat{\beta}_{1,i}\}$, such that the randomness of (8) indeed only comes from the estimation of $\hat{y}$ and $2k$ parameters $\hat{\boldsymbol{\beta}} = \{\hat{\beta}_{0,1}, \hat{\beta}_{1,1}, \cdots, \hat{\beta}_{0,k}, \hat{\beta}_{1,k}\}$. Any two pairs of parameters $\{\hat{\beta}_{0,i}, \hat{\beta}_{1,i}\}$ and $\{\hat{\beta}_{0,j}, \hat{\beta}_{1,j}\}$ are independent when $i \neq j$, since different experimental subjects are used to estimate the dose response curves for drug i alone and for drug j alone, respectively. Furthermore, all those patients are different from the patients who receive the combination dose $\mathbf{d}$. Thus, the estimates $\{\hat{\beta}_{0,c}, \hat{\beta}_{1,c}\}$ for the drug combination and $\hat{y} = \mathrm{logit}^{-1}(\hat{\beta}_{0,c} + \hat{\beta}_{1,c}\log(d))$ are independent of the estimates $\{\hat{\beta}_{0,i}, \hat{\beta}_{1,i}\}$, for any drug administered alone $i = 1, \cdots, k$.

Denote $g(\hat{\boldsymbol{\beta}}, y) = \sum_{i=1}^{k} p_i/\hat{D}_{y,i}$. Let $\nabla g(\hat{\boldsymbol{\beta}}, \hat{y})$ and Σ_1 respectively be the first derivative and variance-covariance matrix of $g(\boldsymbol{\beta}, y)$ at $\{\hat{\boldsymbol{\beta}}, \hat{y}\}$. For the first derivatives, we have

$$\frac{\partial g(\hat{\boldsymbol{\beta}}, \hat{y})}{\partial \hat{\beta}_{0,i}} = \frac{p_i}{\hat{\beta}_{1,i}\hat{D}_{\hat{y},i}}, \quad \frac{\partial g(\hat{\boldsymbol{\beta}}, \hat{y})}{\partial \hat{\beta}_{1,i}} = \frac{p_i}{\hat{D}_{\hat{y},i}} \frac{\text{logit}(\hat{y}) - \hat{\beta}_{0,i}}{\hat{\beta}_{1,i}^2}$$

for $i = 1, \cdots, k$, and

$$\frac{\partial g(\hat{\boldsymbol{\beta}}, \hat{y})}{\partial \hat{y}} = -\frac{1}{\hat{y}(1 - \hat{y})} \left(\sum_{i=1}^{k} \frac{p_i}{\hat{\beta}_{1,i}\hat{D}_{\hat{y},i}} \right).$$

The variance-covariance matrix Σ_1 is a blocked diagonal matrix, with the block being a 2×2 matrix except for the last diagonal element $Var(\hat{y})$. Using the multivariate delta method, we can approximate the variance of $\log(\hat{\tau}(\mathbf{d}))$,

$$Var(\log(\hat{\tau}(\mathbf{d}))) \approx \frac{1}{g(\hat{\boldsymbol{\beta}}, \hat{y})^2} Var(g(\hat{\boldsymbol{\beta}}, \hat{y}))$$

$$\approx \frac{1}{g(\hat{\boldsymbol{\beta}}, \hat{y})^2} \cdot \nabla g(\hat{\boldsymbol{\beta}}, \hat{y})^T \cdot \Sigma_1 \cdot \nabla g(\hat{\boldsymbol{\beta}}, \hat{y})$$

$$\approx \frac{1}{g(\hat{\boldsymbol{\beta}}, \hat{y})^2} \left\{ Var(\text{logit}(\hat{y})) \left(\sum_{i=1}^{k} \frac{p_i}{\hat{\beta}_{1,i}\hat{D}_{\hat{y},i}} \right)^2 + \sum_{i=1}^{k} \frac{p_i^2}{D_{\hat{y},i}^2} Var(\log D_{\hat{y},i}) \right\}$$

$$= \frac{1}{g(\hat{\boldsymbol{\beta}}, \hat{y})^2} \left\{ Var(\text{logit}(\hat{y})) \left(\sum_{i=1}^{k} \frac{p_i}{\hat{\beta}_{1,i}\hat{D}_{y,i}} \right)^2 \right.$$

$$+ \sum_{i=1}^{k} \left(\frac{p_i}{D_{\hat{y},i}} \right)^2 \left(\frac{1}{\hat{\beta}_{1,i}^2} Var(\hat{\beta}_{0,i}) + 2 \frac{\text{logit}(\hat{y}) - \hat{\beta}_{0,i}}{\hat{\beta}_{1,i}^3} Cov(\hat{\beta}_{0,i}, \hat{\beta}_{1,i}) \right.$$

$$\left. \left. + \frac{(\text{logit}(\hat{y}) - \hat{\beta}_{0,i})^2}{\hat{\beta}_{1,i}^4} Var(\hat{\beta}_{1,i}) \right) \right\}. \tag{9}$$

A natural estimate for the term $Var(\text{logit}(\hat{y}))$ in (9) can be derived from the estimation of the variance $\hat{\sigma}^2$ for the model error in regression (6). Denote $n_{c,r}$ as the number of repeated measurements at dose level $\mathbf{d}$ for the drug combination. There is no need for additional computations and the estimator $\hat{\sigma}^2/n_{c,r}$ provides a more robust estimation than the other two estimators, such as the sample variance proposed by Lee and Kong (2009). As shown by the simulation study in the following simulation section, the model variance estimator in (6) has much smaller bias than that in (3), leading to a better estimation in $Var(\log(\hat{\tau}(\mathbf{d})))$.

Once the variance for $\log(\hat{\tau}(\mathbf{d}))$ in (9) is obtained, a $(1 - \alpha) \times 100\%$ confidence interval for $\log(\tau(\mathbf{d}))$ can be constructed as

$$\left[\log(\hat{\tau}(\mathbf{d})) - z_{\alpha/2} \sqrt{Var(\log(\hat{\tau}(\mathbf{d})))}, \log(\hat{\tau}(\mathbf{d})) + z_{\alpha/2} \sqrt{Var(\log(\hat{\tau}(\mathbf{d})))} \right],$$

where $z_{\alpha/2}$ is the $1 - \alpha/2$ percentile of the standard normal distribution. Note that the large sample approximation using a normal distribution is considered especially reasonable in our setting of repeated measurements with a larger degree of freedom than the case when repeated measurements are discarded.

Therefore, a $(1 - \alpha) \times 100\%$ confidence interval for $\tau(\mathbf{d})$ can be approximated by

$$\left[\hat{\tau}(\mathbf{d}) \exp\left(-z_{\alpha/2} \sqrt{\text{Var}(\log(\hat{\tau}(\mathbf{d})))} \right), \hat{\tau}(\mathbf{d}) \exp\left(z_{\alpha/2} \sqrt{\text{Var}(\log(\hat{\tau}(\mathbf{d})))} \right) \right]. \quad (10)$$

4 Confidence Bound for Interaction Index on a Fixed Ray

Different from (7) at a given combination dose, the interaction index (4) for a given effect E can be estimated with the statistic

$$\widehat{II}(E) = \hat{d}_E \sum_{i=1}^{k} \frac{p_i}{\hat{D}_{E,i}}, \quad (11)$$

a function of $\hat{d}_E$ and $\hat{D}_{E,i}$, denoting the projected total doses for drug effect E based on the estimated dose response curves in (6) for a drug combination on the fixed ray or drug i used alone, respectively.

To assess the variation of $\widehat{II}(E)$ with normal approximation, we first derive an estimate for the variance $\text{Var}(\log(\widehat{II}(E)))$ when $\log(\widehat{II}(E))$ is more symmetric than $\widehat{II}(E)$. Let $\nabla g(\hat{\boldsymbol{\beta}}, E)$ and Σ_2 respectively be the first derivative and variance-covariance matrix of $g(\boldsymbol{\beta}, E)$ at $\hat{\boldsymbol{\beta}}$. Using the multivariate delta method (Bickel and Doksum 2001), the variance of $\log(\widehat{II}(E))$ can be approximated by

$$\text{Var}(\log(\widehat{II}(E))) = \text{Var}(\log(\hat{d}_E)) + \text{Var}(\log(g(\hat{\boldsymbol{\beta}}, E))) \quad (12)$$

$$\approx \text{Var}(\log(\hat{d}_E)) + \frac{1}{g(\hat{\boldsymbol{\beta}}, E)^2} \text{Var}(g(\hat{\boldsymbol{\beta}}, E)) \quad (13)$$

$$\approx \text{Var}(\log(\hat{d}_E)) + \frac{1}{g(\hat{\boldsymbol{\beta}}, E)^2} \cdot \nabla g(\hat{\boldsymbol{\beta}}, E)^T \cdot \Sigma_2 \cdot \nabla g(\hat{\boldsymbol{\beta}}, E)$$

$$\approx \text{Var}(\log(\hat{d}_E)) + \frac{1}{g(\hat{\boldsymbol{\beta}}, E)^2} \sum_{i=1}^{k} \left(\frac{p_i}{\hat{D}_{E,i}} \right)^2 \text{Var}(\log(\hat{D}_{E,i})) \quad (14)$$

$$= h(\hat{\beta}_{0,c}, \hat{\beta}_{1,c}, E) + \frac{1}{g(\hat{\boldsymbol{\beta}}, E)^2} \sum_{i=1}^{k} \left(\frac{p_i}{\hat{D}_{E,i}} \right)^2 h(\hat{\beta}_{0,i}, \hat{\beta}_{1,i}, E), \quad (15)$$

where $h(\hat{\beta}_0, \hat{\beta}_1, E) = \frac{1}{\hat{\beta}_1^2} \text{Var}(\hat{\beta}_0) + 2 \frac{\text{logit}(E) - \hat{\beta}_0}{\hat{\beta}_1^3} \text{Cov}(\hat{\beta}_0, \hat{\beta}_1) + \frac{(\text{logit}(E) - \hat{\beta}_0)^2}{\hat{\beta}_{1,c}^4} \text{Var}(\hat{\beta}_1)$.

Equation (12) holds because the estimation of $(\hat{\beta}_{0,c}, \hat{\beta}_{1,c})$ for the dose combination is independent of $\hat{\boldsymbol{\beta}}$. The first approximation (13) holds because of another use of the delta method. The last approximation (14) holds because $p_1, \cdots, p_k$ are constant on the fixed ray and Σ_2 is a blocked diagonal matrix, with each block being a 2×2 matrix when the pairs $(\hat{\beta}_{0,i}, \hat{\beta}_{1,i})$ and $(\hat{\beta}_{0,j}, \hat{\beta}_{1,j})$ are independent for $i \neq j$.

Based on approximation (15), a $(1 - \alpha) \times 100\%$ confidence bound for $\log(\tau)$ as a function of drug effect $E \in (0, 1)$ can be constructed as

$$\left[\log(\widehat{II}(E)) - z_{\alpha/2}\sqrt{\mathrm{Var}(\log(\widehat{II}(E)))}, \log(\widehat{II}(E)) + z_{\alpha/2}\sqrt{\mathrm{Var}(\log(\widehat{II}(E)))} \right],$$

where $z_{\alpha/2}$ is the $1 - \alpha/2$ percentile of the standard normal distribution. Again, the normal approximation is considered reasonable in our setting of repeated measurements with a large total number of observations, $n = n_c + \sum_{i=1}^{k} n_i$, where n_c and n_i denote the number of measurements taken when the k-drug combination is used and drug i is used alone, respectively, $i = 1, \cdots, k$.

Accordingly, a $(1-\alpha) \times 100\%$ confidence bound for the interaction index of drug effect $E \in (0, 1)$ can be approximated by

$$\left[\widehat{II}(E) \exp\left(-z_{\alpha/2}\sqrt{\mathrm{Var}(\log(\widehat{II}(E)))}\right), \widehat{II}(E) \exp\left(z_{\alpha/2}\sqrt{\mathrm{Var}(\log(\widehat{II}(E)))}\right) \right].$$
(16)

5 Simulation Study

To examine whether the confidence intervals and confidence bounds proposed in the previous sections have proper characteristics, we first simulated two drugs that follow the median effect equation (6) with the same slope, $m = 2$, and median effective doses: $D_{med,1} = D_{med,2} = D_{med,c} = 1$. That setting is identical to the "sham combination" of Berenbaum (1989), giving us the additive effects at an arbitrary dose combination with a constant interaction index of 1.

We adopted a fixed ray with ratio $d_2/d_1 = 1/1$ and a constant standard deviation in the model error $\sigma = 0.25$. We used two settings of the within-group standard deviation σ_α, 0.2 and 0.4, to examine the sensitivity of the estimation of the interaction index to random effects. We generated replicates of the dose effects on three doses, 0.8, 1.6 and 3.2, for each of the single drugs, and three doses, (0.6,0.6), (1.2, 1.2) and (2.4, 2.4), for the mixture (d1, d2) at the fixed ray using the median effect model

$$\mathrm{logit}(E_{i,j}) = \beta_0 + \alpha_j + \beta_1 * \log(d_i) + e_{i,j},$$

with error term $e \sim N(0, \sigma^2)$.

Table 1 The mean, median, standard deviation (st. dev.) and root mean squared error (RMSE) for the estimation of the model error $\hat{\sigma} - \sigma$. We compared the proposed method (ZSL16) with the median effect model of Chou and Talalay (CT84) using 1000 simulations

	$\sigma = 0.2$		$\sigma = 0.4$	
	ZSL16	CT84	ZSL16	CT84
Mean	−0.001	−0.145	−0.005	−0.291
Median	−0.001	−0.153	−0.006	−0.308
St. dev.	0.035	0.042	0.066	0.084
RMSE	0.035	0.151	0.066	0.303

To illustrate the effects of proper modeling for repeated measurements, we considered $\hat{y} = \bar{y}$ in the following simulations parallel to the standard approach of Chou and Talalay (1984) using the dose effect by aggregating the effects of repeated measurements at the same dose level. As a function of the model error Var(logit($\bar{y}$)), the estimate of the 95% confidence interval for the combination indices at the observed combination dose strongly depends on the estimation accuracy of the model variance σ^2. In Table 1, we compare the standard deviation and root mean squared error (RMSE) of the estimated σ^2 obtained by the proposed method or the median effect model (Chou and Talalay 1984), using previously published R code (Lee et al. 2010). In both scenarios, our method not only estimated σ^2 without bias, but also significantly reduced the variance and RMSE of the estimate.

Because the construction of the 95% confidence interval was under $H_0 : II = 1$, we assessed the probabilities of concluding synergistic, additive, and antagonistic effects based on the 95% confidence intervals of the combination indices under H_0. In both scenarios, the probability of additive effects using our proposed method was reasonably close to 95% (Table 2). The 95% confidence intervals constructed based on the work of Lee and Kong (2009) for the method of Chou and Talalay (1984) underestimated the variance of the combination indices, leading to larger than expected probabilities of false conclusions for the synergistic or antagonistic effects.

Furthermore, we investigated scenarios in which we assumed the alternative model was true by only changing $D_{med,c}$ to a value of 1.65, which equivalently translates into $\beta_{0,c} = 0.5$. Under this setting, the drug combination was always synergistic and the true interaction index was a constant of 0.78 regardless of the actual dose level or dose effect. Although both CT84 and our method tended to overestimate the coverage probabilities of the confidence intervals in the simulation (Table 3), our method produced smaller estimation errors for the parameter coefficients (not shown) and model variance (Table 4).

Table 2 The probabilities of concluding synergistic, additive, and antagonistic effects based on the 95% confidence intervals of the combination indices under H_0. We compared the proposed method (ZSL16) with that of Chou and Talalay (1984, CT84), using 1000 simulations. The implementation of the 95% confidence interval estimation for CT84 was based on the approach of Lee and Kong (2009) with R code provided by Lee et al. (2010)

	ZSL16			CT84		
Dose	0.6	1.2	2.4	0.6	1.2	2.4
$\sigma = 0.2$						
Synergistic	0.009	0.003	0.006	0.161	0.123	0.125
Additive	0.975	0.962	0.953	0.671	0.702	0.762
Antagonistic	0.016	0.035	0.041	0.168	0.175	0.113
$\sigma = 0.4$						
Synergistic	0.015	0.006	0.008	0.163	0.124	0.125
Additive	0.958	0.923	0.921	0.674	0.699	0.752
Antagonistic	0.027	0.071	0.071	0.163	0.177	0.123

Table 3 The probabilities of concluding synergistic, additive, and antagonistic effects based on the 95% confidence intervals of the combination indices under H_1. We compared the proposed method (ZSL16) with that of Chou and Talalay (1984, CT84) using 1000 simulations. The implementation of the 95% confidence interval estimation for CT84 was based on the approach of Lee and Kong (2009) with R code provided by Lee et al. (2010)

	ZSL16			CT84		
Dose	0.6	1.2	2.4	0.6	1.2	2.4
$\sigma = 0.2$						
Synergistic	0.996	1.000	0.999	1.000	0.999	0.996
Additive	0.004	0.000	0.001	0.000	0.001	0.004
Antagonistic	0.000	0.000	0.000	0.000	0.000	0.000
$\sigma = 0.4$						
Synergistic	0.995	0.999	0.981	1.000	0.999	0.996
Additive	0.005	0.001	0.019	0.000	0.001	0.004
Antagonistic	0.000	0.000	0.000	0.000	0.000	0.000

Table 4 The mean, median, standard deviation (st. dev.) and root mean squared error (RMSE) for the estimation of model error $\hat{\sigma} - \sigma$. We compared the proposed method (ZSL16) with the median effect model of Chou and Talalay (CT84) using 1000 simulations

	$\sigma = 0.2$		$\sigma = 0.4$	
	ZSL16	CT84	ZSL16	CT84
Mean	−0.001	−0.183	−0.001	−0.183
Median	−0.001	−0.194	−0.001	−0.193
St. dev.	0.043	0.052	0.044	0.052
RMSE	0.043	0.190	0.044	0.190

6 Application

In this section, we apply our methods in an experimental study conducted for soft tissue sarcoma samples at MD Anderson Cancer Center in a nested hierarchical experimental design. Soft tissue sarcomas, which arise from connective or support- ive tissues, account for 1% of adult cancers and 15% of pediatric cancers. Among 70 different histological subtypes, 5–10% are undifferentiated pleomorphic sarcomas (UPS), which are typically large and rapidly growing tumors. Patients are still at risk for both tumor recurrence and metastasis after undergoing standard treatments of radiation therapy and chemotherapy. The objective of the experiment was to explore the combination of targeted therapies for better treatment of patients with UPS.

UPS-186, a cell line derived from a sporadic UPS sample, was used to test the effectiveness of treatment regimens in Dr. Keila Torres's lab at the MD Anderson Department of Surgical Oncology. Two novel inhibitors, AEW541 and BGT226, were investigated for their drug interaction effects in combination doses at the fixed ray with $d_2/d_1 = 3/20$. The experiment was repeated three times, each with tripli- cate doses in combination or as single agents, as recommended by Sanofi (2013).

We first estimated the dose-effect curves for AEW541 and BGT226 by a mixed- effect linear regression of logit(E) on log(d) based on cell viability when treated with the single agents. The random effects in the mixed-effect regression had a nested structure to accommodate the specific design feature. The median effect plot indicates that the data followed the median effect equation (3) reasonably well (Fig. 2a, b). Using the fitted median effect equations, we calculated the interaction indices based on (11) for the varied effects (solid lines) of drug combinations at the fixed ray with $d_2/d_1 = 3/20$ and constructed their associated point-wise 95% confidence bounds (dashed lines) based on (16) in both Fig. 2c, d. The vertical bars in Fig. 2c indicate the 95% confidence interval estimates of the interaction indices at the tested doses of drug combinations using a naive estimator of the drug effects, $\hat{y} = \bar{y}$, while the vertical bars in Fig. 2d indicate those obtained with the model-based estimator $\hat{y} = \text{logit}^{-1}(\hat{\beta}_{0,i} + \hat{\beta}_{1,i}\log(d))$. Based on the estimated 95% confidence bounds (dashed lines), we conclude that the combination doses at the fixed ray are statistically synergistic, with the effect between 0.37 and 0.45.

7 Discussion

We proposed a new approach to provide both point and interval estimates for the drug interaction index in a ray design. It was implemented under the framework of the median effect model (Chou and Talalay 1984), but using repeated measurements observed for in vitro experiments. Our approach can adjust for the presence of plate-location effects that are known to be of significant magnitude, for instance, in micro-titer experiments (Faessel et al. 1999). At some observed dose levels for a multiple drug combination, we proposed a procedure to estimate the interaction

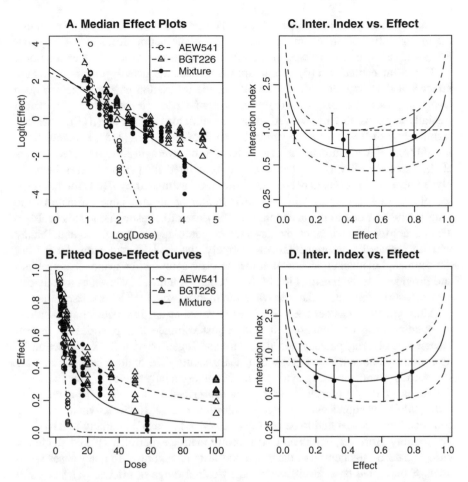

Fig. 2 Results of dose effect assessment at the fixed ray for combination doses of agents AEW541 and BGT226 to treat a cell line of undifferentiated pleomorphic sarcoma. (**a**) Median effect; (**b**) Dose-effect curves; (**c**) Interaction indices versus effects using $\hat{y} = \bar{y}$; (**d**) Interaction indices versus effects using model-based estimator $\hat{y} = \text{logit}^{-1}(\hat{\beta}_{0,i} + \hat{\beta}_{1,i} \log(d))$. In plots (**c**) and (**d**), solid curves indicate estimated interaction indices versus effects (proportion of cells surviving); dashed lines are point-wise 95% confidence bounds for the curve of interaction index versus effect based on the delta method in Sect. 4; vertical bars, from left to right, give 95% confidence interval estimates of the interaction indices based on the delta method in Sect. 3 for observed combinations respectively corresponding to the combination doses of (7.5, 50), (3, 20), (2, 13.3), (1.5, 10), (0.75, 5), (0.5, 3.3) and (0.3, 2)

index and construct its associated confidence interval. Because we can test drug combinations only at a limited number of dose levels, and investigators are interested in possible synergism at those dose levels, as well as identifying the region where the synergistic effect is significant, we proposed an additional procedure to estimate the interaction index along with the drug effect on the interval $(0, 1)$ and construct its associated confidence bound. The proposed method can help us gauge the uncertainties of the interaction indices for combination doses of two or more drugs and can also be used to provide more in-depth assessment of drug interactions.

The point estimator $\hat{\tau}(\mathbf{d})$ in our approach depends heavily on the estimated effect $\hat{y}$ at the observed dose $\mathbf{d}$. The bias in the estimation of $\hat{y}$ at a specific dose level has a larger impact on $\hat{\tau}(\mathbf{d})$ and its confidence interval than $\widehat{II}(E)$, which partially explains why the derived variance estimator (15) for $\log(\widehat{II}(E))$ could be significantly different from the variance estimator (9) for $\log(\hat{\tau}(\mathbf{d}))$ in some cases. In addition, if we estimate the drug effects $\hat{y}$ by averaging the observed effects at the same dose level, the change in the associated interaction indices between two adjacent dose levels may contradict the trend estimated by $\widehat{II}(E)$ (for example, see plot C in Fig. 1 or 2), which is an indicator of an unreliable estimate of the drug interaction due to the uncertainty in the dose effect estimation. This problem also occurs for the estimation that uses the standard approach of Chou and Talalay without repeated measurements. Alternatively, the model-based estimator $\hat{y}$ from the estimated median effect equation for the drug combination avoids that problem and provides a smooth estimation of the interaction index. However, as a trade-off, a larger estimation bias is induced when the median effect model is misspecified.

Although $\widehat{II}(E)$ has not been widely recognized or used in medical applications to examine drug combinations, it is a robust estimate that provides an overall assessment of drug potency and drug effects. Together with the construction of its confidence bound, investigators can easily identify the regions that demonstrate statistically significant drug synergism. This is especially useful in practice when the focus of drug potency is mostly circumscribed to the effect in a range of $(50\%, 90\%)$, or equivalently, the cell inhibition rate of $10–50\%$, where the drug combination is considered to be not only effective but also potentially to have limited toxicity. However, before multi-drug combination experiments are conducted in vitro, the dose-effect curve of the combined drug is unknown. In many cases when none of the tested dose levels reaches the desired range of effects, $\widehat{II}(E)$ can still provide a valuable reference for guiding whether further in vitro or in vivo studies should be conducted.

Acknowledgements The authors thank the National Institutes of Health for partial support by grant P50 CA100632. We are grateful to Dr. Yichuan Zhao and an anonymous referee for helpful comments. We also thank Dr. Keila Torres at MD Anderson Cancer Center for generously sharing their data from the in vitro experiments.

References

Belen'kii, M. S., & Schinazi, R. F. (1994). Multiple drug effect analysis with confidence interval. *Antiviral Research, 25*, 1–11.

Berenbaum, M. C. (1985). The expected effect of a combination of agents: The general solution. *Journal of Theoretical Biology, 114*, 413–431.

Berenbaum, M. C. (1989). What is synergy? *Pharmacological Reviews, 41*, 93–141.

Bickel, P. J., & Doksum, K. A. (2001). *Mathematical statistics: Basic ideas and selected topics* (pp. 306–314). Englewood Cliffs, NJ: Prentice Hall.

Chou, T. C. (1991). The median-effect principle and the combination index for quantitation of synergism and antagonism. In T. C. Chou & D. C. Rideout (Eds.), *Synergism and antagonism in chemotherapy* (pp. 61–101). San Diego: Academic.

Chou, T. C. (2006). Theoretical basis, experimental design, and computerized simulation of synergism and antagonism in drug combination studies. *Pharmacological Reviews, 58*, 621–681.

Chou, T. C., & Talalay, P. (1984). Quantitative analysis of dose effect relationships: The combined effects of multiple drugs or enzyme inhibitors. *Advances in Enzyme Regulation, 22*, 27–55.

Faessel, H. M., Levasseur, L. M., Slocum, H. K., & Greco, W. R. (1999). Parabolic growth patterns in 96-well plate cell growth experiments. *In Vitro Cellular & Developmental Biology - Animal, 35*, 270–278.

Greco, W. R., Bravo, G., & Parsons, J. C. (1995). The search of synergy: A critical review from a response surface perspective. *Pharmacological Reviews, 47*(2), 331–385.

Hennessey, V. G., Rosner, G. L., Bast, R. C., & Chen, M. Y. (2010). A Bayesian approach to dose-response assessment and synergy and its application to in vitro dose-response studies. *Biometrics, 66*, 1275–1283.

Hill, A. V. (1910). A new mathematical treatment of changes of ionic concentration in muscle and nerve under the action of electric currents, with a theory as to their mode of excitation. *Physiology, 40*, 190–224.

Hill, A. V. (1910). The possible effects of the aggregation of the molecules of haemoglobin on its dissociation curves. *Physiology, 40*, 1115–1121.

Lee, J. J., & Kong, M. (2009). Confidence intervals of interaction index for assessing multiple drug interaction. *Statistics in Biopharmaceutical Research, 1*(1), 4–17.

Lee, J. J., Kong, M., Ayers, G. D., & Lotan, R. (2007). Interaction index and different methods for determining drug interaction in combination therapy. *Journal of Biopharmaceutical Statistics, 17*, 461–480.

Lee, J. J. (2010). SYNERGY. Available at: https://biostatistics.mdanderson.org/SoftwareDownload/. Assessed 15 Sep 2016

Loewe, S., & Muischnek, H. (1926). Effect of combinations: Mathematical basis of problem. *Archiv für Experimentalle Pathologie und Pharmakologie, 114*, 313–326.

Sanofi (2013). In vitro synergy characterization: Design and methodology. Cited 14 October 2013.

Straetemans, R., O'Brien, T., Wouters, L., Van Dun, J., Janicot, M., Bijnens, L., et al. (2005). Design and analysis of drug combination experiments. *Biometrical Journal, 47*, 299–308.

Tallarida, R. J. (2000). *Drug synergism and dose-effect data analysis.* New York: Chapman and Hall.

Tallarida, R. J. (2002). The interaction index: A measure of drug synergism. *Pain, 98*, 163–168.

Statistical Indices for Risk Tracking in Longitudinal Studies

Xin Tian and Colin O. Wu

1 Introduction

Well-known regression methods for longitudinal analysis, for the most part, focus on modeling the conditional means of the response variables with various longitudinal variance-covariance structures given time and a set of covariates, which could be either time-varying or time-invariant. The conditional means and the longitudinal variance-covariance structures can be modeled either parametrically or nonparametrically. These conditional mean-based regression models have been well-established in the literature, e.g., Hart and Wehrly (1986), Shi et al. (1996), Hoover et al. (1998), Fan and Zhang (2000), James et al. (2000), Lin and Carroll (2001), Rice and Wu (2001), Diggle et al. (2002), Molenberghs and Verbeke (2005), Zhou et al. (2008), Fitzmaurice et al. (2009) and Sentürk and Müller (2010). Although the conditional mean-based models are popular in practice, they may be inadequate when the scientific objectives of the study require the evaluation of the conditional distribution functions.

Longitudinal analysis based on conditional distributions has two important objectives which may not be easily fulfilled by evaluating the conditional means. First, when the outcome variable has a non-Gaussian or skewed distribution, the temporal trends of the outcome variable and the covariate effects may be better described through the time-varying patterns of conditional distributions. The conditional mean-based regression models, on the other hand, do not lead to useful inferences on the distribution functions, when the distributions of the error terms are non-Gaussian or unknown. One aspect we should note is that the estimation of the conditional distribution functions generally requires a larger sample size than

X. Tian (✉) • C.O. Wu
Office of Biostatistics Research, National Heart, Lung, and Blood Institute, Bethesda,
MD 20892, USA
e-mail: tianx@nhlbi.nih.gov; wuc@nhlbi.nih.gov

© Springer International Publishing AG 2017
D.-G. Chen et al. (eds.), *New Advances in Statistics and Data Science*,
ICSA Book Series in Statistics, https://doi.org/10.1007/978-3-319-69416-0_17

the estimation of the conditional means. Second, unlike the conditional mean-based models, the conditional distributions and their functionals provide a natural and clinically simple approach for describing tracking of risk factors over time. Of note, the concept of tracking is originated from the need of predicting future values of risk factors from serial measurements in epidemiological studies or longitudinal clinical trials, and it has been studied by Clarke et al. (1978), Ware and Wu (1981), Foulkes and Davis (1981) and McMahan (1981) under two general definitions and various model formulations. As discussed in Foulkes and Davis (1981), the first definition of tracking is concerned with the ability to predict the future values of an outcome variable from its repeated measurements in the past, while the second definition of tracking describes the maintenance of relative ranking over time among a study population. Despite different technical definitions, tracking has important implications in longitudinal biomedical studies that aim to identify persistent disease risk factors related to the development and the occurrence of diseases later in life.

Applications of conditional distribution functions and risk factor tracking are widely available in biomedical studies. For example, Mahoney et al. (1991) described the factors affecting tracking of coronary heart disease risk factors in a pediatric study, and Wilsgaard et al. (2001) analyzed tracking of cardiovascular risk factors in an epidemiology study with an adult population. In these studies, the scientific objective is to determine whether an individual with unfavorable levels of cardiovascular risk factors, such as blood pressure, body mass index, and serum lipids, at younger ages is more likely to have unfavorable levels of the same risk factors at an older age relative to the reference population, or equivalently, the tracking properties of these cardiovascular risk factors.

In this paper, the motivating example is the National Heart, Lung, and Blood Institute Growth and Health Study (NGHS). The NGHS is a large epidemiological study of childhood growth and cardiovascular risks of 2379 girls, who were 9 or 10 years old at enrollment, with detailed anthropometric and laboratory measurements obtained at each of 10 annual visits during 1986–1997 (NGHSRG 1992). Previous publications (Daniels et al. 1998; Obarzanek et al. 2010) investigated the effects of age, race and other covariates on the cardiovascular risk factors using the conditional mean-based methods. Since obesity and hypertension of a child are defined by the conditional distributions of body mass index (BMI) and blood pressure (BP) level given the child's age, gender and height (NHBPEP 2004; Obarzanek et al. 2010), an important question on tracking is whether having the abnormal level of a risk factor, such as BMI or BP, at an early age could increase the likelihood of having the abnormal level of the same risk factor at a later age. The appropriate answer to this question may be used to justify longitudinal studies in young children and track those subjects who have abnormal risk levels from childhood to young adulthood. Motivated by the NGHS, Wu and Tian (2013a,b) and Tian and Wu (2014) proposed two statistical tracking indices, namely, the rank-tracking probability (RTP) and the rank-tracking probability ratio (RTPR), to quantify the tracking of a longitudinal risk variable over time, and investigated a number of nonparametric estimators of the RTP and RTPR under different regression models. The applications of the RTP and RTPR estimators to the NGHS data demonstrate that both BMI and BP in this population of adolescents have good tracking abilities as children with high levels of BMI or BP at a younger age are more likely to have high levels of BMI and BP at an older age. These RTPs and RTPRs are *local* statistical indices in the sense that they are functions of two specific time points, $(t, t + \delta)$, with $t > 0$ and $\delta > 0$, so that their values may change with t or δ and the clinical interpretations depend on the specific time points $(t, t + \delta)$. In many situations, however, it may be more convenient to measure tracking of risk factors by certain *global* tracking indices. For example, if the RTP (or RTPR) of a risk factor only changes with δ and stays mostly constant for $t \in [t_1, t_2]$, then it is reasonable to use the *mean-integrated* RTP (or RTPR) over the time range $[t_1, t_2]$ as a function of the *elapsed or lagging time* δ only.

Here we propose a class of mean-integrated RTP and RTPR (mRTP and mRTPR) to quantify the global tracking of time-dependent variables in a longitudinal study. In general, we may expect that a risk factor's tracking ability diminishes over the lagging time δ. Thus, we first consider the mRTP and mRTPR over a given time range $t \in [t_1, t_2]$, which, as functions of δ, can be used to quantify how the rank-based tracking of the variable changes over the elapsed time. When an overall tracking index is required, we can also quantify the global tracking of a time-dependent variable by a global mean-integrated RTP and RTPR (gRTP and gRTPR) over both time ranges for t and δ. As useful alternatives to the local RTP and RTPR for given (t, δ), these global measures of tracking indices can be easily used to compare the overall tracking of disease risk factors over short-term or long-term follow-up.

For the rest of the paper, we present in Sect. 2 the various definitions and interpretations of the local and global RTPs and RTPRs, derive in Sect. 3 the estimation and inference methods for these tracking indices, and demonstrate the applications of these tracking indices to the NGHS data in Sect. 4. Finally, we investigate in Sect. 5 the statistical properties of these tracking indices through a simulation study, and give some concluding remarks in Sect. 6.

2 Rank-Based Tracking Indices

We consider the longitudinal design commonly seen in large biomedical studies. Motivated by the NGHS study (NGHSRG 1992), we focus on the following longitudinal data structure that is mathematically tractable and simple to interpret in biomedical studies: (a) The sample has n independent subjects, and the ith subject has n_i observations at time points $\{t_{ij} \in \mathscr{T}; j = 1, \ldots, n_i\}$, where $\mathscr{T} = [T_0, T_1]$ is the time interval of interest or the study duration. The total number of observations is $N = \sum_{i=1}^{n} n_i$. (b) At any time point $t \in \mathscr{T}$, $Y(t)$ is the real-valued outcome variable. For simplicity, we assume that $Y(t)$ is non-negative and the covariate X is time-invariant and categorical, taking values $x \in \{1, \ldots, K\}$, and denote the longitudinal sample for $(Y(t), X, t)^T$ by $\mathscr{Z} = \{(Y_{ij}, X_i, t_{ij}); 1 \leq i \leq n, 1 \leq j \leq n_i\}$. In general, the methods of this paper can be easily extended to any range of $Y(t)$ on the real line with continuous and time-dependent covariates. The assumption of categorical and time-invariant covariate X is made for mathematical simplicity and practical interpretations. We review in this section the local statistical tracking indices, RTP and RTPR, defined by Wu and Tian (2013a,b) and Tian and Wu (2014), and then introduce the corresponding mean-integrated global tracking indices.

2.1 Rank-Tracking Probabilities

Given that our objective is to evaluate the conditional percentiles and ranks of the subjects' health status (e.g., Kavey et al. 2003; Thompson et al. 2007; Obarzanek et al. 2010), we define here a class of conditional probabilities to quantitatively measure a subject's percentile or *rank* and the *tracking ability* (or *tracking*) of the outcome variable $Y(t)$ at different time points. Suppose that, for a given $t \in \mathscr{T}$ and $X = x$, the subject's health status is determined by a set $A(x, t)$ for the response value $Y(t)$, we can quantify the conditional probability of a certain health status by

$$P_A(x, t) = P[Y(t) \in A(x, t) | X = x, t]. \tag{2.1}$$

The choice of $A(x, t)$ depends on the scientific objective of the study. For example, if $Y(t)$ is a subject's BMI at age t, then $A(x, t)$ can be chosen as the overweight risk set defined by the BMI values greater than the age-adjusted 85th percentile from the growth chart (Obarzanek et al. 2010); if $Y(t)$ is a subject's blood pressure, then $A(x, t)$ can be chosen as the high blood pressure risk set defined by the blood pressure levels greater than the 90th percentile conditional on age, gender and height (NHBPEP 2004). Specifically, if $A(x, t) = (y, \infty)$ for a given value y, $P_A(x, t)$ = 1- $F_t(y|x)$, where $F_t(y|x)$ is the conditional cumulative distribution function (CDF) of $Y(t)$ given $X = x$ and t, i.e.,

$$F_t(y|x) = P[Y(t) \le y | X = x, t]. \tag{2.2}$$

In practice, it is sometimes useful to allow $A(x, t)$ to change with x and t. For pediatric studies, because the health categories for children and adolescents are often defined by the conditional distributions given age, gender and other covariates (e.g., Kuczmarski et al. 2002; NHBPEP 2004), it is meaningful to evaluate the conditional CDF defined by $F_t[y(x, t)|x] = P[Y(t) \le y(x, t)|x, t]$, where $y(x, t)$ is a pre-determined risk threshold curve.

To quantify the tracking of $Y(t)$ at two time points t and $t + \delta$, with $\delta > 0$, the *rank-tracking probability* based on $A(x, t)$ at t and $t + \delta$ is defined by

$$\text{RTP}_A(x, t, t + \delta) = P[Y(t + \delta) \in A(x, t + \delta) | Y(t) \in A(x, t), X = x], \tag{2.3}$$

which is the conditional probability of $Y(t + \delta) \in A(x, t + \delta)$ given that $X = x$ and $Y(t) \in A(x, t)$. By comparing (2.1) with (2.3), we see that (2.3) measures the likelihood of $Y(t + \delta) \in A(x, t + \delta)$ at time $t + \delta$ given that, at time t, $Y(t)$ is already within $A(x, t)$, while (2.1) at time $t + \delta$ only measures the likelihood of $Y(t+\delta) \in A(x, t+\delta)$ without knowing the subject's health status at time t. Thus (2.3) takes the knowledge of $Y(t) \in A(x, t)$ into account and describes the ability to track the subject's health status determined by $Y(t) \in A(x, t)$ and $Y(t + \delta) \in A(x, t + \delta)$. When $\text{RTP}_A(x, t, t + \delta) = 1$ at a given t, it indicates *perfect tracking*, i.e., certain health status of $Y(t)$ is always maintained from t to $t + \delta$. Since $\text{RTP}_A(x, t, t+\delta)$ is a function of the two time points t and $t + \delta$, it is a local measure of tracking based on $A(x, t)$ in the sense that the value of (2.3) is time-specific. For the special case that $A(x, t)$ is the interval $A_\alpha(x, t) = (y_\alpha(x, t), \infty)$, where $y_\alpha(x, t)$ is the $(100 \times \alpha)$th percentile of $Y(t)$ given $X = x$, the quantile-based RTP of (2.3) is

$$\text{RTP}_{\alpha_1, \alpha_2}(x, t, t+\delta) = P\big[Y(t+\delta) > y_{\alpha_2}(x, t+\delta)\big|Y(t) > y_{\alpha_1}(x, t), X = x\big], \quad (2.4)$$

which is the probability that $Y(t)$ is above the $(100 \times \alpha_2)$th percentile at time $t + \delta$ given that $X = x$ and $Y(t)$ is already above the $(100 \times \alpha_1)$th percentile at time t.

2.2 Rank-Tracking Probability Ratios

A potential problem of $\text{RTP}_A(x, t, t+\delta)$, which takes values in $[0, 1]$, is that it does not provide a relative scale as compared to the conditional probability of $Y(t+\delta) \in A(x, t + \delta)$ without knowing the information of $Y(t)$. Thus, an alternative tracking index for measuring the *relative strength* of tracking ability for $Y(t)$ at time points t and $t + \delta$ is the relative value of $\text{RTP}_A(x, t, t + \delta)$ compared with the conditional probability $P\big[Y(t + \delta) \in A(x, t + \delta)\big|X = x\big]$. This relative tracking index is defined to be the *rank-tracking probability ratio*,

$$\text{RTPR}_A(x, t, t + \delta) = \frac{\text{RTP}_A(x, t, t + \delta)}{P\big[Y(t + \delta) \in A(x, t + \delta)\big|X = x\big]}. \quad (2.5)$$

If $\text{RTPR}_A(x, t, t + \delta) = 1$, then the knowledge of $Y(t) \in A(x, t)$ does not increase the chance of $Y(t+\delta) \in A(x, t+\delta)$, and this implies that $Y(t) \in A(x, t)$ does not have tracking potential for $Y(t+\delta) \in A(x, t+\delta)$. On the other hand, if $\text{RTPR}_A(x, t, t+\delta)$ is greater or less than 1, then $Y(t) \in A(x, t)$ has positive or negative tracking for $Y(t + \delta) \in A(x, t + \delta)$, respectively. The strength of the positive tracking ability can be measured by how much $\text{RTPR}_A(x, t, t + \delta)$ is greater than 1.

2.3   Mean-Integrated RTPs and RTPRs

By integrating out the time variable in RTP of (2.3) over an interval $\mathscr{T}_0 = [t_1, t_2]$, we can obtain a mean-integrated RTP (mRTP), which represents the average value of RTP over the time range $\mathscr{T}_0$ as a function of the *lagging time* δ,

$$\text{mRTP}_{A, \mathscr{T}_0}(x, \delta) = \frac{\int_{t_1}^{t_2} \text{RTP}_A(x, t, t + \delta)\, dt}{t_2 - t_1}. \tag{2.6}$$

When the $\text{RTP}_A(x, t, t + \delta)$ curve does not change significantly over $t \in \mathscr{T}_0$, it is appropriate to measure the tracking ability of $Y(t)$ within $\mathscr{T}_0$ using the simpler index, $\text{mRTP}_{A, \mathscr{T}_0}(x, \delta)$, which, for a fixed $X = x$, is a function of δ only. As δ changes, $\text{mRTP}_{A, \mathscr{T}_0}(x, \delta)$ measures the mean tracking ability of $Y(t)$ for any given lagging time δ, which is expected to decrease with δ in most biomedical studies. For the special case of quantile-based RTP of (2.4), the mRTP is denoted by

$$\text{mRTP}_{(\alpha_1, \alpha_2), \mathscr{T}_0}(x, \delta) = \frac{\int_{t_1}^{t_2} \text{RTP}_{\alpha_1, \alpha_2}(x, t, t + \delta)\, dt}{t_2 - t_1}. \tag{2.7}$$

When the RTPR curve is used for tracking of outcome $Y(t)$, the mean-integrated RTPR (mRTPR) over $t \in \mathscr{T}_0 = [t_1, t_2]$ is given by

$$\text{mRTPR}_{A, \mathscr{T}_0}(x, \delta) = \frac{\int_{t_1}^{t_2} \text{RTPR}_A(x, t, t + \delta)\, dt}{t_2 - t_1}. \tag{2.8}$$

Similar to (2.6), (2.8) is an appropriate global measure of tracking when the values of $\text{RTPR}_A(x, t, t + \delta)$ do not vary significantly over $t \in \mathscr{T}_0$, and is likely to be a decreasing function of the lagging time δ. To fully use all the observations in the design time range or during the entire study follow-up $\mathscr{T} = [T_0, T_1]$, we can let $\mathscr{T}_0 = \mathscr{T}_\delta = [T_0, T_1 - \delta]$. Thus for any $\delta > 0$, $t \in \mathscr{T}_\delta = [T_0, T_1 - \delta]$, we can estimate $\text{RTP}_A(x, t, t + \delta)$ and $\text{RTPR}_A(x, t, t + \delta)$, then obtain $\text{mRTP}_{A, \mathscr{T}_\delta}(x, \delta)$ in (2.6) and $\text{mRTPR}_{A, \mathscr{T}_\delta}(x, \delta)$ in (2.8).

Although the above tracking indices, $\text{mRTP}_{A, \mathscr{T}_0}(x, \delta)$ and $\text{mRTPR}_{A, \mathscr{T}_0}(x, \delta)$, characterize some of the global tracking features of a variable $Y(t)$, their dependence on δ makes them "partially global". For example, if we would like to compare the degrees of tracking for two disease risk factors $Y^{(1)}(t)$ and $Y^{(2)}(t)$ within the time range $t \in \mathscr{T}_0$, $\text{mRTP}_{A, \mathscr{T}_0}(x, \delta)$ and $\text{mRTPR}_{A, \mathscr{T}_0}(x, \delta)$ for $Y^{(1)}(t)$ and $Y^{(2)}(t)$ only describe the tracking abilities of $Y^{(1)}(t)$ and $Y^{(2)}(t)$ at a specifically given lagging time δ, and they do not provide an overall comparison for a range of δ values. To use certain global tracking indices that capture the time ranges for both $t \in \mathscr{T}_0$ and $\delta \in \mathscr{T}_1 = [d_1, d_2]$, we consider the global mean-integrated RTP (gRTP) and RTPR (gRTPR) defined by

$$\text{gRTP}_A(x) = \frac{\int_{d_1}^{d_2} \text{mRTP}_{A,\,\mathscr{T}_0}(x, \delta)\, d\delta}{(d_2 - d_1)} \qquad (2.9)$$

and

$$\text{gRTPR}_A(x) = \frac{\int_{d_1}^{d_2} \text{mRTPR}_{A,\,\mathscr{T}_0}(x, \delta)\, d\delta}{(d_2 - d_1)} \qquad (2.10)$$

respectively. Compared to the tracking indices defined in (2.3) through (2.8), the gRTP and gRTPR defined in (2.9) and (2.10) are the overall measures of tracking for $Y(t)$ because they are not functions of either t or δ. When the RTPs and RTPRs do not change significantly with (t, δ) for $t \in \mathscr{T}_0$ and $\delta \in \mathscr{T}_1$, the $\text{gRTP}_A(x)$ and $\text{gRTPR}_A(x)$ are appropriate global tracking indices for $Y(t)$ within the corresponding time ranges.

3 Estimation and Inference Methods

We establish a nonparametric method based on B-spline approximations for the estimation and inferences of the tracking indices defined in Sect. 2. Assuming the covariate X is discrete and time-invariant, our estimation method is based on the nonparametric mixed models of Shi et al. (1996) and Rice and Wu (2001). We briefly discuss a potential extension of the estimation method with continuous and time-varying covariates.

3.1 Nonparametric Mixed Models and Prediction

Global smoothing through basis approximations is a natural extension of the linear mixed-effects models and popular in nonparametric longitudinal analysis. For the simple case of evaluating the time trend of $Y(t)$ without covariates, Shi et al. (1996) and Rice and Wu (2001) have proposed to model $Y_i(t)$ at time t by the nonparametric mixed-effects model,

$$Y_i(t) = \mu(t) + \zeta_i(t) + \epsilon_i(t), \qquad (3.1)$$

where $\mu(t)$ is the mean curve of $Y_i(t)$, $\zeta_i(t)$ is the subject-specific deviation from $\mu(t)$ for the ith subject with $E[\zeta_i(t)] = 0$, and $\epsilon_i(t)$ is the mean zero measurement error. For the subgroup analysis conditioning on $X = x$, the model (3.1) can be applied by specifying $\mu_x(t)$, $\zeta_{i,x}(t)$ and $\epsilon_{i,x}(t)$ as the corresponding mean curve, subject-specific deviation curve and error process for $X = x$, so that, conditioning on $X = x$,

$$Y_i(t)\big|_{X=x} = \mu_x(t) + \zeta_{i,x}(t) + \epsilon_{i,x}(t). \qquad (3.2)$$

The estimation of the mean and subject-specific deviation curves can be achieved through a least squares method for the B-spline approximated model of (3.1) or (3.2). When B-splines are used for (3.1), we have the approximations

$$\mu(t) \approx b_0(t)^T \xi \quad \text{and} \quad \zeta_i(t) \approx b_1(t)^T \eta_i,$$

so that the B-spline approximated model for (3.1) is

$$Y_i(t) = b_0(t)^T \xi + b_1(t)^T \eta_i + \epsilon_i(t), \tag{3.3}$$

where, for some positive integers m_0 and m_1,

$$b_0(t) = \left(b_{01}(t), \ldots, b_{0m_0}(t)\right)^T \quad \text{and} \quad b_1(t) = \left(b_{11}(t), \ldots, b_{1m_1}(t)\right)^T$$

are the B-spline basis functions and

$$\xi = \left(\xi_1, \ldots, \xi_{m_0}\right)^T \quad \text{and} \quad \eta_i = \left(\eta_{i1}, \ldots, \eta_{im_1}\right)^T$$

are the corresponding population and subject-specific coefficients. We assume that the subject-specific coefficient vectors η_i, $i = 1, \ldots, n$, are independent and have a multivariate normal distribution with mean zero and variance-covariance matrix Φ. If we denote by Y_i the column vector consisting of the observed $Y_i(\mathbf{t_i})$ values at the time points $\mathbf{t_i} = (t_{i1}, \ldots, t_{in_i})^T$, B_{0i} and B_{1i} the corresponding $n_i \times m_0$ and $n_i \times m_1$ spline basis matrices, and ϵ_i the measurement error vector evaluated at these time points, respectively, the matrix representation of the B-spline approximation (3.3) for the observed data is

$$Y_i = B_{0i} \xi + B_{1i} \eta_i + \epsilon_i, \tag{3.4}$$

where $\epsilon_i = \left(\epsilon_i(t_{i1}), \ldots, \epsilon_i(t_{in_i})\right)^T$.

Under the assumption that ϵ_i has the mean zero normal distribution, i.e. $\epsilon_i \sim N(0, \Sigma)$, the maximum likelihood estimators (MLEs) or the restricted MLEs of $\{\xi, \Sigma, \Phi\}$ are $\{\widehat{\xi}, \widehat{\Sigma}, \widehat{\Phi}\}$, and the best linear unbiased predictors (BLUPs) of the random effects $\widehat{\eta}_i$ can be computed by the EM algorithm as described in Rice and Wu (2001) and implemented by using the statistical packages (e.g., the lme4 package in R, Bates et al. 2016). The B-spline predicted outcome trajectory curve for the ith subject at any time point t is then

$$\widehat{Y}_i(t) = b_0(t)^T \widehat{\xi} + b_1(t)^T \widehat{\eta}_i, \tag{3.5}$$

which is computed by plugging the coefficient estimates into (3.3). Estimation of the mean and subject-specific curves in (3.2) can be obtained using the same method as outlined in (3.3) through (3.5), except that the estimated coefficients in (3.5) depend on the given covariate $X = x$. In this case, the B-spline predicted outcome trajectory curve for the ith subject at any time point t is

$$\widehat{Y}_i(t)\big|_{X_i=x} = b_0(t)^T \widehat{\xi}_x + b_1(t)^T \widehat{\eta}_{i,x}. \tag{3.6}$$

In general, we allow $b_0(t)$ and $b_1(t)$ to be B-spline basis functions with possibly different m_0 and m_1. In practice, we may take $m_0 = m_1 = m$ for computational simplicity, so that $b_0(t) = b_1(t) = b(t)$. The number of terms for the B-spline bases, m_0, m_1 or m, may be chosen by the model selection criteria or cross-validation. We used B-spline basis in our computation for curve estimation and outcome trajectory prediction because of its good numerical properties and simplicity in practical implementation. Other smoothing methods, such as the Fourier basis approximations or penalized smoothing splines, may also be applied.

We note that, as an extension of model (3.1), when a set of continuous and time-dependent covariates $X(t)$ are included, Liang et al. (2003) proposed to use a class of mixed-effects varying coefficient models to predict the outcome $Y(t)$ given $X(t)$. However, this extension does not lead to useful interpretation of the global tracking indices in Sect. 2.3 and requires further methodological development than the indices provided in this paper.

3.2 Estimation of Tracking Indices

The predicted trajectory for $Y(t)$ can be used to estimate the tracking indices. Estimation of the local tracking indices, RTP and RTPR, based on this approach has been described in Tian and Wu (2014). We further extend this estimation approach to the global tracking indices defined in Sect. 2.3.

For a brief description of the local RTP and RTPR estimators, we first note that RTP of (2.3) and RTPR of (2.5) can be written as

$$\text{RTP}_A(x, t, t+\delta) = \frac{E\{1_{[Y(t+\delta)\in A(x,t+\delta)], Y(t)\in A(x,t), X=x]}\}}{E\{1_{[Y(t)\in A(x,t), X=x]}\}} \tag{3.7}$$

and

$$\text{RTPR}_A(x, t, t+\delta) = \frac{\text{RTP}_A(x, t, t+\delta)}{E\{1_{[Y(t+\delta)\in A(x,t+\delta), X=x]}\}} \tag{3.8}$$

respectively, where $1_{[\cdot]}$ is the indicator function. Let

$$\widetilde{Y}_i(t) = \widehat{Y}_i(t) + \widehat{\epsilon}_i(t) \tag{3.9}$$

be the estimated *pseudo-observation* of the ith subject at time t, where $\widehat{\epsilon}_i(t)$ is estimated measurement error. Then, by substituting the expected values of (3.7) and (3.8) with their corresponding empirical estimators, we obtain the estimators,

$$\widehat{\text{RTP}}_A(x, t, t+\delta) = \frac{\sum_{i=1}^n 1_{[\widetilde{Y}_i(t+\delta)\in A(x,t+\delta), \widetilde{Y}_i(t)\in A(x,t), X_i=x]}}{\sum_{i=1}^n 1_{[\widetilde{Y}_i(t)\in A(x,t), X_i=x]}} \tag{3.10}$$

and

$$\widehat{\text{RTPR}}_A(x, t, t+\delta) = \frac{\widehat{\text{RTP}}_A(x, t, t+\delta)}{(1/n)\sum_{i=1}^{n} 1_{[\widetilde{Y}_i(t+\delta)\in A(x, t+\delta), X_i=x]}} \qquad (3.11)$$

for RTP and RTPR, respectively. The reason for using $\widetilde{Y}_i(t)$ of (3.9) in the estimators (3.10) and (3.11) is that $\widehat{Y}_i(t)$ is the subject-specific average at t for the ith subject, while $\widetilde{Y}_i(t)$, which includes the random measurement error for the subject, is an "observation" for the subject and appropriate for estimating the distribution functions. Two remarks for the estimators (3.10) and (3.11) have been noted in Tian and Wu (2014). First, the $\widehat{\epsilon}_i(t)$ can be computed from the maximum likelihood estimator of $\epsilon_i(t)$ in (3.1) or the estimated error from the fitted model residuals. The potential bias of using $\widehat{Y}_i(t)$ instead of $\widetilde{Y}_i(t)$ in (3.10) and (3.11) has been shown by simulation. Second, in some situations, the risk threshold in set $A(\cdot)$ is not known and may be estimated through a sample splitting approach.

Based on (3.10) and (3.11), we can obtain the estimators of the global tracking indices through integration over the time ranges of interest. Replacing the RTP and RTPR in (2.6) and (2.8) with the estimators in (3.10) and (3.11), we obtain the estimators

$$\widehat{\text{mRTP}}_A(x, \delta) = \frac{\int_{t_1}^{t_2} \widehat{\text{RTP}}_A(x, t, t+\delta)\, dt}{t_2 - t_1} \qquad (3.12)$$

and

$$\widehat{\text{mRTPR}}_A(x, \delta) = \frac{\int_{t_1}^{t_2} \widehat{\text{RTPR}}_A(x, t, t+\delta)\, dt}{t_2 - t_1} \qquad (3.13)$$

for mRTP and mRTPR, respectively, where the integration in the numerators can be computed numerically. Similarly, the estimators for gRTP and gRTPR of (2.9) and (2.10) are given by

$$\widehat{\text{gRTP}}_A(x) = \frac{\int_{d_1}^{d_2} \widehat{\text{mRTP}}_A(x, \delta)\, d\delta}{(d_2 - d_1)} \qquad (3.14)$$

and

$$\widehat{\text{gRTPR}}_A(x) = \frac{\int_{d_1}^{d_2} \widehat{\text{mRTPR}}_A(x, \delta)\, d\delta}{(d_2 - d_1)} \qquad (3.15)$$

respectively, through further integration over the range of the lagging time δ.

3.3 Bootstrap Confidence Intervals

As the asymptotic distributions of the estimators in (3.12) through (3.15) are still unavailable, the *resampling-subject bootstrap* approach is used to construct the corresponding approximate bootstrap confidence intervals (Hoover et al. 1998). In this approach, we obtain B bootstrap samples by resampling the subjects with replacement one at a time, and compute the corresponding estimates within each bootstrap sample. The average and the lower and upper $[100 \times (\alpha/2)]$th percentiles of the B bootstrap estimates are used as our bootstrap estimate and the $[100 \times (1-\alpha)]\%$ bootstrap confidence interval. Alternatively, we can compute the sample standard deviations (SD) of the estimates from the bootstrap samples, and approximate the $[100 \times (1 - \alpha)]\%$ confidence interval by the *estimate* $\pm z_{\alpha/2} \times SD$ *error band*. In our numerical applications, we used $B = 500$ bootstrap samples, and the simulation results show the coverage probabilities of these bootstrap confidence intervals are reasonably good.

4 Application to the NGHS Data

The NGHS is a multi-center population-based cohort study aimed to assess the racial differences and longitudinal changes in cardiovascular risk factors for adolescent girls. A total of 1166 Caucasian and 1213 African-American girls at age 9 or 10 years enrolled in NGHS and had height, weight, blood pressure and other cardiovascular risk factors measured at annual visits through age 18–19 years. The study design was described in NGHSRG (1992). Tian and Wu (2014) studied tracking of body mass index (BMI) and systolic blood pressure (SBP) using the local rank-tracking indices. Building on this earlier work, we evaluate here the global indices discussed in Sect. 2 to track the health status of overweight/obesity and high blood pressure in these adolescent girls.

4.1 Rank-Tracking for BMI

Based on Obarzanek et al. (2010), the overweight and obesity status for girls ($\geq$ 85th percentile) was defined by using the age- and sex-adjusted percentile from the Centers for Disease Control and Prevention (CDC) growth charts. We fit separate nonparametric mixed-effects models (3.2) to the NGHS BMI data by race with cubic B-spline approximation and 4 equally-spaced knots. Then we computed the subject-specific BMI trajectories over 9–19 years of age, and estimated the mean-integrated global RTP and RTPR of BMI for both races over the age range and the lagging time interval.

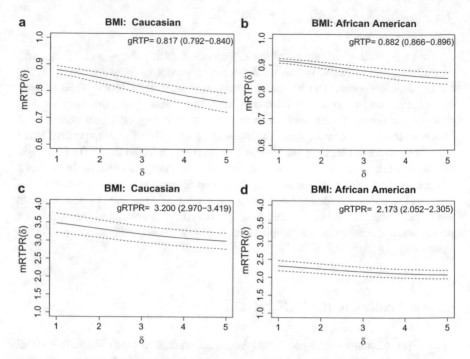

Fig. 1 The estimated BMI $mRTP_{A_{0.85}}(x, \delta)$, $mRTPR_{A_{0.85}}(x, \delta)$ and their 95% pointwise bootstrap percentile confidence intervals for Caucasian ($x = 0$) and African-American ($x = 1$) girls (**a–d**). The estimated BMI $gRTP_{A_{0.85}}(x)$ or $gRTPR_{A_{0.85}}(x)$ and its 95% bootstrap percentile confidence interval are indicated in each plot

Figure 1a, b shows the estimated $mRTP_{A_{0.85}}(x, \delta)$ curve over the range of the lagging time $\delta \in [1, 5]$ years, for Caucasian ($x = 0$) and African-American ($x = 1$) girls, respectively. Here $A_{0.85} = A_{0.85}(t)$ represents the risk set for the over-weight/obesity status, containing the set of BMI values greater than the age-adjusted 85th CDC percentile for girls' BMI at age t. At each given δ, $mRTP_{A_{0.85}}(x, \delta)$ was calculated from integrating the $RTP_{A_{0.85}}(x, t, t + \delta)$ curve over the entire time range of $[9, 19 - \delta]$ years. That is, when $\delta=2$, for each $t \in [9, 17]$, we estimated the local $RTP_{A_{0.85}}(x, t, t + 2)$, then obtained $mRTP_{A_{0.85}}(x, \delta = 2)$ by integrating $RTP_A(x, t, t + 2)$ over [9, 17] for t; when $\delta=4$, we obtained $mRTP_{A_{0.85}}(x, \delta = 4)$ by integrating $RTP_{A_{0.85}}(x, t, t + 4)$ over the time [9, 15] for t. The 95% pointwise bootstrap percentile confidence intervals for mRTP estimators were computed from $B = 500$ bootstrap replications.

For Caucasian and African-American girls at 9–19 years of age, the estimated mRTP curves show that, on average, the conditional probability of being overweight or obese were 76–88% and 85–92% for those girls who were already overweight one to 5 years earlier, respectively. As expected, the mRTP curves tended to decrease with $\delta \in [1, 5]$. Further, the global indices $gRTP_{A_{0.85}}(x)$ and their 95% bootstrap confidence intervals were estimated to be 0.817(0.792–0.840) for Caucasian girls and $0.882(0.866-0.896)$ for African-American girls by averaging over the interval for δ, respectively, which suggested that African-American girls were more likely to remain in the undesirable overweight status compared to Caucasian girls. The relative strength of the BMI tracking ability is shown by the mRTPR curves and gRTPR in Fig. 1c, d. For both racial groups, these relative global tracking indices were significantly greater than 1, indicating that the knowledge of a girl's overweight status in an earlier age increased the chance of being overweight at a later age about two to three times compared to the probability of her being overweight without the knowledge of her previous weight status. Consistent with the snapshot results based on the local RTPs and RTPRs in Tian and Wu (2014), these global tracking results indicate that there was a very high degree of positive tracking for BMI over 1–5 years for these adolescent girls.

4.2 Rank-Tracking for SBP

For children and adolescents, the blood pressure status was defined by the age-, sex- and height-specific conditional percentiles (NHBPEP 2004). We studied here the tracking of SBP by comparing it with the risk set $A_{0.75}(t) = \{y : y > q_{0.75}(t)\}$ where $q_{0.75}(t)$ was the age-adjusted 75th SBP percentile for a girl at age t with median height from the guideline table in NHBPEP (2004).

Similarly, we fit the nonparametric mixed-effects models to the NGHS SBP data by race separately, using cubic B-spline approximation with 4 equally-spaced knots selected from Bayesian information criterion (BIC). Then we estimated the mean-integrated global rank-tracking indices based on the predicted trajectories of individual SBP curves. Figure 2a, b shows the estimated $\text{mRTP}_{A_{0.75}}(x, \delta)$ curve over the range of 1–5 years, for both racial groups ($x = 0$ for Caucasians and $x = 1$ for African-Americans), respectively. The 95% pointwise bootstrap percentile confidence intervals for the estimators were obtained from $B = 500$ bootstrap samples.

For both Caucasian and African-American girls at 9–19 years of age, the estimated mRTP curves had a slight decreasing trend over the lagging time δ, indicating more recent SBP status such as SBP measured 1 or 2 years earlier might be more predictive of the current SBP status compared to the SBP status 5 years ago. On average, the conditional probability of having elevated SBP (in the upper quartiles of the population) was 30–37% for Caucasian girls and 36–43% for African-American girls given those girls who already had elevated SBP 1–5 years earlier. Further, the global indices $\text{gRTP}_{A_{0.75}}(x)$ and their 95% bootstrap confidence intervals (CIs) averaging over the lagging time were estimated to be $0.336(0.303-0.370)$ and $0.402(0.370-0.432)$, respectively. These results suggest SBP had a moderate and positive tracking ability for adolescent girls, although not as high compared to using BMI to track overweight status (Fig. 1). The relative strength of the SBP tracking ability evaluated by the mRTPR curves and gRTPR are displayed in Fig. 2c, d. Compared to the probability of a girl having elevated SBP

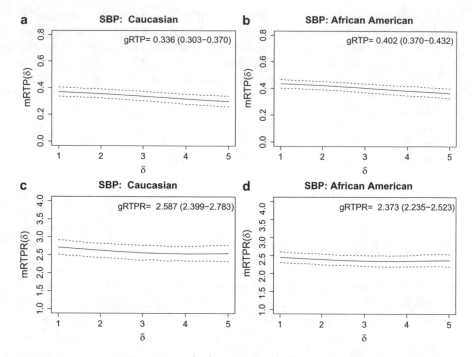

Fig. 2 The estimated SBP $\text{mRTP}_{A_{0.75}}(x, \delta)$, $\text{mRTPR}_{A_{0.75}}(x, \delta)$ and their 95% pointwise bootstrap percentile confidence intervals for Caucasian ($x = 0$) and African-American ($x = 1$) girls (**a**–**d**). The estimated SBP $\text{gRTP}_{A_{0.75}}(x)$ or $\text{gRTPR}_{A_{0.75}}(x)$ and its 95% bootstrap percentile confidence interval are indicated in each plot

without knowing the SBP status at an earlier age, knowing that a girl already had elevated SBP in an earlier age increased the likelihood of her having elevated SBP at a later age more than 2 times: the estimated gRTPR = 2.587 (95% CI 2.399–2.783) for Caucasian and gRTPR = 2.373 (95% CI 2.235–2.523) for African-American girls, respectively.

5   Simulation

To study the performance of our estimators, we consider a small simulation that mimics the NGHS SBP data structure. The simulated samples were generated based on the model (3.1), $Y_i(t) = \mu(t) + \zeta_i(t) + \epsilon_i(t)$, for $t \in [0, 10]$. Each simulated sample consisted of $n = 1000$ subjects, each with 10 random visit times. Within each sample, we generated the ith subject's jth visiting time, t_{ij}, from the uniform distribution $U[(j-1), j]$ for $j = 1, \ldots, 10$, so that, $t_{i1} \sim U[0, 1], \ldots, t_{i10} \sim U[9, 10]$. Similar to the patterns of the SBP growth curves in NGHS, we chose $\mu(t) = 100 - 0.9t + 18\sin(\pi t/25)$. The random effect of the model was $\zeta_i(t) = \gamma_{0i} + \gamma_{1i}t$, where $(\gamma_{0i}, \gamma_{1i})^T$ followed the bivariate normal distribution with zero-mean and covariance $\Gamma = (\Gamma_1, \Gamma_2)$ such that $\Gamma_1 = (9, -0.15)^T$ and $\Gamma_2 = (-0.15, 0.04)^T$, i.e., $\text{corr}(\gamma_{0i}, \gamma_{1i}) = -0.25$. The random error $\epsilon(t_{ij})$ was uncorrelated with $(\gamma_{0i}, \gamma_{1i})^T$ and had the $N(0, 4)$ distribution.

For each simulated sample, we estimated $\text{mRTP}_{A_\alpha, \mathscr{T}_0}(\delta)$ and $\text{mRTPR}_{A_\alpha, \mathscr{T}_0}(\delta)$ defined in (2.6) and (2.8), where $\delta \in [1, 5]$, $\mathscr{T}_0 = [0, 5]$, and $A_\alpha(\cdot) = (q_\alpha(t), \infty)$, with the $(100 \times \alpha)$th percentile $q_\alpha(t)$ computed from the normal distribution based on the simulation model. Using the procedures in Sect. 3, we fit a mixed-effects model (3.1) to each sample with the cubic B-spline basis approximation and equally-spaced knots selected from BIC, and computed the estimators $\widehat{\text{mRTP}}_{A_\alpha}(\delta)$ and $\widehat{\text{mRTPR}}_{A_\alpha}(\delta)$ using the predicted subject-specific curves $\widehat{Y}_i(t)$ for $t \in [0, 10]$. Furthermore, we calculated the $\widehat{\text{gRTP}}_{A_\alpha}$ and $\widehat{\text{gRTPR}}_{A_\alpha}$. The bootstrap confidence intervals for the estimators were obtained with $B = 500$ bootstrap replications.

We repeated the simulation $M = 1000$ times. Figure 3 shows the true curves of tracking indices computed based on the known simulation model, the averages of their estimates and the lower and upper 2.5% pointwise percentiles of the estimated curves $\widehat{\text{mRTP}}_{A_\alpha}(\delta)$ and $\widehat{\text{mRTPR}}_{A_\alpha}(\delta)$ with $\alpha = 75\%$ and $\delta \in [1, 5]$. These plots indicate that these average curves were reasonably close to the true curves, and the widths of the intervals bounded by the lower and upper 2.5% pointwise percentiles were relatively small. We carried out the simulations for a range of (α, δ) values. For $\alpha = 75\%$ and $\delta = 1, 2, \ldots, 5$, the averages and the square roots of the mean squared errors (MSEs) of the mRTP, gRTP, mRTPR and gRTPR estimates and the empirical coverage probabilities for the bootstrap percentile confidence intervals are summarized in Table 1. Other α and δ values are not tabled because the simulation results for the corresponding estimators were very similar to those in Table 1. We

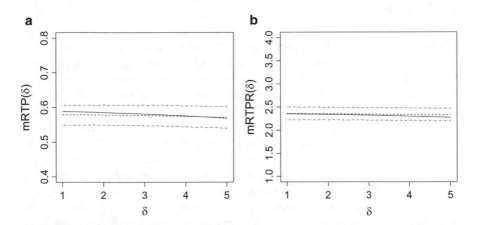

Fig. 3 The true curves (solid lines) of tracking indices, the averages of their estimates (dash lines) and the lower and upper 2.5% pointwise percentiles (dotted dash lines) of the estimated curves for (**a**) $\widehat{\text{mRTP}}_{A_{0.75}}(\delta)$ and (**b**) $\widehat{\text{mRTPR}}_{A_{0.75}}(\delta)$ at $\delta \in [1, 5]$ from 1000 simulations

Table 1 The true values of $\text{mRTP}_{A_\alpha}(\delta)$, gRTP_{A_α}, $\text{mRTPR}_{A_\alpha}(\delta)$, and gRTPR_{A_α} with $\alpha = 75\%$ under the simulation model, the averages and the square roots of the MSEs for the estimates and the empirical coverage probabilities of the 95% bootstrap confidence intervals from 1000 simulations

		True value	Average estimate	Average root MSE	Coverage probability
$\text{mRTP}(\delta)$	$\delta = 1$	0.588	0.579	0.018	0.914
	$\delta = 2$	0.585	0.578	0.017	0.922
	$\delta = 3$	0.581	0.576	0.016	0.940
	$\delta = 4$	0.575	0.574	0.016	0.954
	$\delta = 5$	0.569	0.570	0.016	0.951
gRTP		0.580	0.576	0.015	0.936
$\text{mRTPR}(\delta)$	$\delta = 1$	2.353	2.359	0.071	0.948
	$\delta = 2$	2.341	2.353	0.072	0.942
	$\delta = 3$	2.323	2.345	0.072	0.938
	$\delta = 4$	2.301	2.336	0.076	0.919
	$\delta = 5$	2.274	2.327	0.086	0.916
gRTPR		2.320	2.344	0.072	0.930

also repeated the simulation study using the sample size of $n = 200$ or $n = 500$ in each simulated sample, and the results were comparable to those in Table 1. In summary, these results show that our proposed methods for estimating the global tracking indices perform well: the averages of the estimates were close to the true curves and the coverage probabilities of the bootstrap confidence intervals were also near the nominal level of 95%.

6   Discussion

We have developed in this paper a class of global tracking indices for a time-dependent variable, and showed that these statistical indices quantitatively measure the *rank-tracking abilities* of risk factors in a longitudinal epidemiological study. These global tracking indices are constructed based on the local tracking indices, RTP and RTPR, defined in Tian and Wu (2014), which can be intuitively interpreted as the conditional probabilities of a subject's health status at a later time point given that the same subject had certain health status at an earlier time point. Compared with the commonly used serial correlations in the literature, our tracking indices give more intuitive quantitative measures of the variables' tracking abilities over time and do not depend on the assumptions for the distribution of the longitudinal variable of interest. In contrast, serial correlations may not have adequate interpretations if the relationship between the outcome variable evaluated at two time points is not linear or their joint distribution is significantly different from normality. Furthermore, the Pearson's correlation or other rank-based nonparametric correlation coefficients may not provide an adequate estimate of dependence at any two different time points using sparse observations due to missing or random study visits. However, the estimation and inference procedures of our global tracking indices are constructed under the nonparametric mixed-effects models, which use all the available data and are sufficiently flexible in many longitudinal settings. Therefore, the inherent model flexibility and the scientific interpretations enable our global track indices to be used as a convenient statistical tool to identify certain disease risk factors that track over time.

Notably, the findings from applying these global tracking indices to the NGHS study of the adolescent girls suggest that both BMI and SBP had positive tracking ability over 1–5 years with certain differences by the race groups. These results would be expected to have important implications in the design of long-term pediatric studies and in developing guidelines for the primary prevention of cardiovascular disease beginning in childhood. In general, the global rank-tracking indices may be applied to other large epidemiological studies with even longer follow-up, such as the Framingham Heart Study (with over 65 years of follow-up; Mahmood et al. 2014) and the Coronary Artery Risk Development in Young Adults (CARDIA) Study (with over 30 years of follow-up; Cutter et al. 1991). In this context, these global indices can be used to evaluate tracking of various disease risk factors and subclinical measures over a short term (such as 5–10 years) or very long term (such as over 20–30 years) period of time from early life and to determine the optimal risk threshold levels and timing for early intervention to prevent the occurrence of diseases later in life.

Further methodological and theoretical research in this topic is still warranted in at least two fronts. First, we need to develop the asymptotic properties, including the asymptotic mean squared errors and the asymptotic distributions, for the estimators of (3.12) through (3.15). These asymptotic properties can be used to establish the asymptotic inference procedures for the tracking indices. Second, estimation methods other than the ones proposed in this paper need to be developed. We present here the method of estimating the conditional probabilities from individual outcome trajectories based on the nonparametric mixed-effects models. Alternatively, various distribution-based regression approaches may be used to estimate the conditional distribution functions and the related tracking indices (Wei et al. 2006; Wu and Tian 2013b). The potential advantages and disadvantages of the alternative estimation methods may be compared with the B-spline based estimators.

References

Bates, D., Mächler, M., Bolker, B., & Walker, S. C. (2016). LME4: Fitting linear mixed-effects models using lme4. *R package version 1.1–12.*

Clarke, W. R., Schrott, H. G., Leaverton, P. E., Connor, W. E., & Lauer, R. M. (1978). Tracking of blood lipids and blood pressures in school age children: The Muscatine Study. *Circulation, 58,* 626–634.

Cutter, G. R., Burke, G. L., Dyer, A. R., Friedman, G. D., Hilner, J. E., Hughes, G. H., et al. (1991). Cardiovascular risk factors in young adults. The CARDIA baseline monograph. *Controlled Clinical Trials, 12,* 1S–77S.

Daniels, S. R., McMahon, R. P., Obarzanek, E., Waclawiw, M. A., Similo, S. L., Biro, F. M., et al. (1998). Longitudinal correlates of change in blood pressure in adolescent girls. *Hypertension, 31*, 97–103.

Diggle, P. J., Heagerty, P., Liang, K.-Y., & Zeger, S. L. (2002). *Analysis of longitudinal data* (2nd ed.) Oxford: Oxford University Press.

Fan, J., & Zhang, J. T. (2000). Functional linear models for longitudinal data. *Journal of the Royal Statistical Society, Series B, 62*, 303–322.

Fitzmaurice, G., Davidian, M., Verbeke, G., & Molenberghs, G. (Eds.). (2009). *Longitudinal data analysis*. Boca Raton, FL: Chapman & Hall/CRC.

Foulkes, M. A., & Davis, C. E. (1981). An index of tracking for longitudinal data. *Biometrics, 37*, 439–446.

Hart, J. D., & Wehrly, T. E. (1986). Kernel regression estimation using repeated measurements data. *Journal of the American Statistical Association, 81*, 1080–1088.

Hoover, D. R., Rice, J. A., Wu, C. O., Yang, L. P. (1998). Nonparametric smoothing estimates of time-varying coefficient models with longitudinal data. *Biometrika, 85*, 809–822.

James, G. M., Hastie, T. J. & Sugar, C. A. (2000). Principal component models for sparse functional data. *Biometrika, 87*, 587–602.

Kavey, R., Daniels, S. R., Lauer, R. M., Atkins, D. L., Hayman, L. L., & Taubert, K. (2003). American Heart Association guidelines for primary prevention of atheroclerotic cardiovascular disease beginning in childhood. *Circulation, 107*, 1562–1566.

Kuczmarski, R. J., Ogden, C. I., Guo, S. S., Grummer-Strawn, L. M., Flegal, K. M., & Mei, Z. (2002). 2000 CDC growth charts for the United States: Methods and development. *Vital Health Statistics Series, 11*(246), 1–190. National Center for Health Statistics.

Liang, H., Wu, H., & Carroll, R. J. (2003). The relationship between virologic and immunologic responses in AIDS clinical research using mixed-effects varying-coefficient models with measurement error. *Biostatistics, 4*, 297–312.

Lin, X., & Carroll, R. J. (2001). Semiparametric regression for clustered data using generalized estimating equations. *Journal of the American Statistical Association, 96*, 1045–1056.

Mahmood, S. S., Levy, D., Vasan, R. S., & Wang, T. J. (2014). The Framingham Heart Study and the epidemiology of cardiovascular disease: A historical perspective. *Lancet, 383*, 999–1008.

Mahoney, L. T., Lauer, R. M., Lee, J., & Clarke, W. R. (1991). Factors affecting tracking of coronary heart disease risk factors in children. The Muscatine Study. *Annals of the New York Academy of Sciences, 623*, 120–132.

McMahan, C. A. (1981). An index of tracking. *Biometrics, 37*, 447–455.

Molenberghs, G., & Verbeke, G. (2005). *Models for discrete longitudinal data*. New York, NY: Springer.

National Heart, Lung, and Blood Institute Growth and Health Research Group (NGHSRG). (1992). Obesity and cardiovascular disease risk factors in black and white girls: The NHLBI Growth and Health Study. *American Journal of Public Health, 82*, 1613–1620.

National High Blood Pressure Education Program Working Group on High Blood Pressure in Children and Adolescents (NHBPEP Working Group). (2004). The fourth report on the diagnosis, evaluation, and treatment of high blood pressure in children and adolescents. *Pediatrics, 114*, 555–576.

Obarzanek, E., Wu, C. O., Cutler, J. A., Kavey, R. W., Pearson, G. D., & Daniels, S. R. (2010). Prevalence and incidence of hypertension in adolescent girls. *The Journal of Pediatrics, 157*(3), 461–467.

Rice, J. A., & Wu, C. O. (2001). Nonparametric mixed effects models for unequally sampled noisy curves. *Biometrics, 57*, 253–259.

Shi, M., Weiss, R. E., & Taylor, J. M. G. (1996). An analysis of paediatric CD4 counts for acquired immune deficiency syndrome using flexible random curves. *Applied Statistics, 45*, 151–163.

Thompson, D. R., Obarzanek, E., Franko, D. L., Barton, B. A., Morrison, J., Biro, F. M., et al. (2007). Childhood overweight and cardiovascular disease risk factors: The National Heart, Lung, and Blood Institute Growth and Health Study. *Journal of Pediatrics, 150*, 18–25.

Tian, X., & Wu, C. O. (2014). Estimation of rank-tracking probabilities using nonparametric mixed-effects models for longitudinal data. *Statistics and Its Interface, 7*, 87–99.

Sentürk, D., & Müller, H. (2010). Functional varying coefficient models for longitudinal data. *Journal of the American Statistical Association, 105*, 1256–1264.

Ware, J. H., & Wu, M. C. (1981). Tracking: Prediction of future values from serial measurements. *Biometrics, 37*, 427–437.

Wei, Y., Pere, A., Koenker, R., & He, X. (2006). Quantile regression methods for reference growth charts. *Statistics in Medicine, 25*, 1369–1382.

Wilsgaard, T., Jacobsen, B. K., Schirmer, H., Thune, I., Løchen, M., Njølstad, I., et al. (2001). Tracking of cardiovascular risk factors. *American Journal of Epidemiology, 154*, 418–426.

Wu, C. O., & Tian, X. (2013a). Nonparametric estimation of conditional distribution functions and rank-tracking probabilities with longitudinal data. *Journal of Statistical Theory and Practice, 7*, 259–284.

Wu, C. O., & Tian, X. (2013b). Nonparametric estimation of conditional distributions and rank-tracking probabilities with time-varying transformation models in longitudinal studies. *Journal of the American Statistical Association, 108*, 971–982.

Zhou, L., Huang, J. Z., & Carroll, R. J. (2008). Joint modelling of paired sparse functional data using principal components. *Biometrika, 95*, 601–619.

Statistical Analysis of Labor Market Integration: A Mixture Regression Approach

Tapio Nummi, Janne Salonen, and Timothy E. O'Brien

1 Introduction

Integration of young people into the labor market is a complex and socially important issue which must be understood as a process in time. The majority of young people attach to the labor market quite quickly, some after their studies although some do remain unemployed (e.g. Pareliussen 2016). Moreover, different stages may not necessarily follow a straightforward progression. For example, it is quite common in the Finnish system for students to work during their studies. Meaning, one person can have several different statuses at the same time (throughout 1 year). Obtaining an overall picture of such complex and heterogeneous longitudinal data is a challenging task.

In this paper we present one possible approach to this complex data analysis problem. The approach is based on the mixture regression applied to multivariate longitudinal binary data. In applied statistics, these methods are often referred to as latent class regression models, or trajectory analysis (Nagin 2005). The idea is that data consists of unknown sub-populations with some common properties that can be revealed through longitudinal data. Recently these methods have been very popular in many fields of science, including psychology, education, sociology, marketing

T. Nummi (✉)
Faculty of Natural Sciences, University of Tampere, Tampere, Finland
e-mail: tan@uta.fi

J. Salonen
Research Department, The Finnish Centre for Pensions, Helsinki, Finland
e-mail: Janne.Salonen@etk.fi

T.E. O'Brien
Department of Mathematics and Statistics and Institute of Environmental Sustainability,
Loyola University of Chicago, Chicago, IL, USA
e-mail: teobrien@gmail.com

© Springer International Publishing AG 2017
D.-G. Chen et al. (eds.), *New Advances in Statistics and Data Science*,
ICSA Book Series in Statistics, https://doi.org/10.1007/978-3-319-69416-0_18

and health sciences (Korpela et al. 2017; Kokko et al. 2008; Jolkkonen et al. 2017; Mani and Nandkumar 2016; Nummi et al. 2014, 2017).

In this paper we present a 4-dimensional binary mixture regression model that is used to identify the sub-groups in the data gathered. We find that there are ten main groups that lead to different development paths of young men. Most people integrated into the labor market quite quickly after various intermediate stages, but in a few groups the integration is weaker or slower. In terms of society, the groups of weak attachment are of central interest, because they may later require special support or action from society. For instance, in some countries a special youth guarantee policy has been promoted (Keränen 2012; Escudero and Mourelo 2015).

2 Methods

2.1 Data

The data comes from the administrative registers of the Finnish Centre for Pensions and Statistics Finland. In the administrative registers there is a range of information pertaining to all of the pension insured (total population) people in Finland. For this study we choose the male cohort born in 1987. For other studies of the same cohort we can refer to Paananen and Gissler (2013). We follow all individuals between 2005 to 2013, when the cohort is 18–26 years of age. We take a sub-population of those who are Finnish citizens and who have lived in Finland during the specified period. The research population is 29,383 males.

Labor market attachment is measured using days when working, in education, in unemployment and on various social benefits per year. This yields the 4-dimensional response vector as follows:

- Variable 1 (Employed): Individual employed for days/year in private or public sector or self-employed.
- Variable 2 (Education): Individual in education leading to a degree and/or is receiving student financial aid.
- Variable 3 (Unemployed): Individual receives unemployment benefits, either earnings related or paid by the state.
- Variable 4 (Leave): Individual receives sickness benefits or is on vocational rehabilitation. Parental leave and the permanently disabled are included here as well.

The original data is measured as days/year. For our analysis, the data was dichotomized (Yes/No) because in this type of longitudinal data, the most important factor in the formation of an individual's career trajectory is the several different statuses of the individuals. This makes the analysis of data much simpler and more uniform.

2.2 Multivariate Binary Mixture

Our aim is to identify clusters of individuals with the same kind of mean develop-mental profiles (trajectories). Let $\mathbf{y}_i = (y_{ij1}, y_{ij2}, \ldots, y_{ijT})'$ represent the sequence of measurements on individual i for the variable j over T periods and let $f_i(\mathbf{y}_i|\mathbf{X}_i)$ denote the marginal probability distribution of $\mathbf{y}_i$ with possible time dependent covariates $\mathbf{X}_i$ that are same to all $j = 1, \ldots, s$ variables. It is assumed that $f_i(\mathbf{y}_i|\mathbf{X}_i)$ follows a mixture of K densities

$$f_i(\mathbf{y}_i|\mathbf{X}_i) = \sum_{k=1}^{K} \pi_k f_{ik}(\mathbf{y}_i|\mathbf{X}_i), \quad \sum_{k=1}^{K} \pi_k = 1 \text{ with } \pi_k > 0, \tag{1}$$

where π_k is the probability of belonging to the cluster k and $f_{ik}(\mathbf{y}_i|\mathbf{X}_i)$ is the density for the kth cluster (see e.g. McLachlan and Peel 2000). The natural choice is to use the Bernoulli distribution for the mixture components. It is assumed that s variables in $\mathbf{y}_i$, $i = 1, \ldots, N$, are independent. Also measurements given the kth cluster are assumed to be independent. This yields the density

$$f_{ik}(\mathbf{y}_i|\mathbf{X}_i) = \prod_{j=1}^{s} \prod_{t=1}^{T} p_{ijtk}^{y_{ijt}} (1 - p_{ijtk}^{1-y_{ijt}}), \tag{2}$$

where p_{ijtk} is a function of covariates $\mathbf{X}_i$. For modeling the conditional distribution of p_{ijtk} we use the logistic regression model. For the ith individual we can then write

$$p_{ijtk} = \frac{\exp(\mathbf{x}_i'\beta_{jk})}{1 + \exp(\mathbf{x}_i'\beta_{jk})}, \tag{3}$$

where $\mathbf{x}_i'$ is the tth row of $\mathbf{X}_i$, β_{jk} is the parameter vector of the jth variable in the kth cluster. For our analysis we took the second degree model

$$\mathbf{x}_i'\beta_{jk} = \beta_{0jk} + \beta_{1jk}t + \beta_{2jk}t^2 \tag{4}$$

for modeling the probabilities within the variable j and cluster k in time t. Maximum likelihood estimates can then be obtained by maximizing the log likelihood $\log \sum_{i=1}^{N} f_i$ over unknown parameters β_{jk}, $j = 1, \ldots s; k = 1, \ldots K$ (Nagin 1999; Jones et al. 2001; Nagin and Tremblay 2001; Jones and Nagin 2007, Nagin and Odgers 2010a,b). When the model parameters are estimated the posterior probability estimate provides a tool for assigning individuals to specific clusters. Individuals can then be assigned to specific clusters to which their posterior probability is the largest.

3 Analysis

Choosing the number of trajectories (clusters) K is an important issue when applying mixture modeling. The selection of K can be based on technical criteria, substantive examination, or both. We used the information criteria BIC, which is perhaps the most widely used in this context. Here we present the values of BIC for $k = 5, \ldots, 10$: -397509.4, -394554.5, -392966.5, -389504.3, -388897.6 and -383596.6. The maximum (note: SAS implementation) is obtained for $k = 10$ and is therefore our choice for the number of clusters K. Increasing K could yield to more difficult to interpret and insignificantly small clusters. The final estimated model is summarized in Tables 1 and 2 (in Appendix). The trajectory plots (Figs. 1, 2, 3, and 4) present conditional point means calculated for each of the four variables.

Table 1 Clusters k, their estimated absolute N_k and relative sizes $\hat{\pi}_k$

Group (k)	N_k	$\hat{\pi}_k$ (%)
1:	545	1.9
2:	3009	10.2
3:	1971	6.7
4:	1975	6.7
5:	5942	20.2
6:	5933	20.2
7:	1510	5.1
8:	3141	10.7
9:	4093	13.9
10:	938	3.2

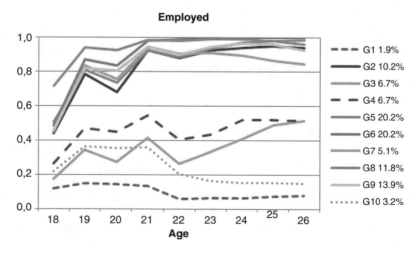

Fig. 1 Time-point means (proportions) over trajectories for the variable Employed

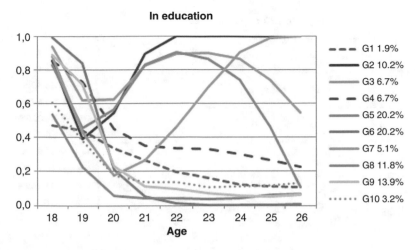

Fig. 2 Time-point means (proportions) over trajectories for the variable Education

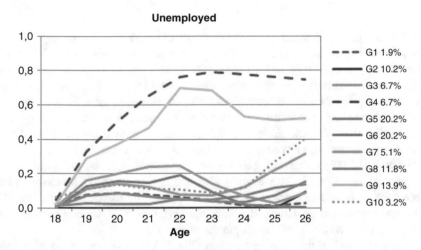

Fig. 3 Time-point means (proportions) over trajectories for the variable Unemployed

These plots are used as the main tool for the interpretation of the results obtained from the mixture regression fit. The computations were carried out by SAS proc traj procedure.

3.1 Normal Life-Course

In the trajectory plots the solid lines indicate groups (total of 88.1%) where labor market integration is good (Fig. 1). It is quite common for young people ages 18–21 to be in post-secondary or vocational education (Fig. 2). From Fig. 1 we note that

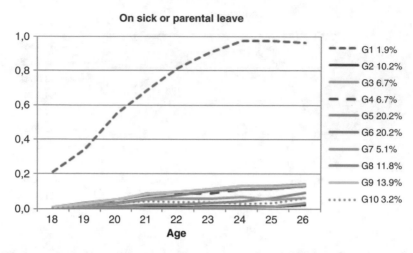

Fig. 4 Time-point means (proportions) over trajectories for the variable Leave

about 74.6% of young males are in the trajectories where the percentage of people who have employment status after 21 years of age is surprisingly high (>80%). We refer to this group of trajectories (groups 2, 5, 6, 7, 8 and 9) as the HES group (high employment status group). Trajectories 5 and 2 (30.4%) from the HES group both have high percentage of people (>50%) in education after 21 years of age (Fig. 2). This reflects the well-known fact that the majority of students in Finland work during their studies. Group 2 (10.2%) contains typical university students. Note that this group also has a high percentage of people in employment.

Group 9 (13.9%) is interesting as we can see from Fig. 3 that this group has a low percentage of people in education after the age of 21 (Fig. 2). However, the percentage of people in employment is still high and increases with age (Fig. 1). This group contains low-educated young men who work in various part-time or temporary jobs and experience unemployment periods.

In general most of the trajectory groups (Fig. 3) have low percentage of people who are unemployed, with many young men experiencing short unemployment periods. These unemployment spells are usually short throughout their normal life-course. This is also true for sickness and disability periods (Fig. 4). As the trajectories indicate, young Finnish men participate in family life (take parental leave), and this participation increases with age. However, due to short follow-up time, a more thorough analysis of parental leave is not possible as the first child is usually born after this time.

From employment and education trajectories we can see a change at age 20 (Figs. 1 and 2). This is due to the fact that the Finnish male cohort (80% of males) enters military service at this age. Service lasts less than a year, and therefore these men in the military have no status in the labor market or on education during this time.

3.2   Weak Labor Market Integration

In the figures the dotted lines indicate groups (total of 11.8%) where labor market integration is poor for longer time periods. We refer to this group of trajectories (groups 1, 3 and 10) as the LES group (low employment status group) which is our main interest and focus. These young men are experiencing difficulties in the labor market and have therefore been the target government support programs.

From Fig. 2 we can identify four groups (1, 3, 4 and 10) with low percentages in terms of employment. There is one positive indication, however, as group 3 contains higher percentage in education (Fig. 2). The LES group is not particularly active in education, as they perhaps receive some vocational education in their late teens.

Unemployment and leave trajectories (Figs. 3 and 4) explain the LES group in more detail. Group 4 (6.7%) is clearly unemployed after secondary and vocational education. The percentage of unemployment in this group is nearly 80% at the end of the follow up period.

The sickness and parental leave trajectory plot indicates that Group 1 (1.9%) has the highest percentage (Fig. 4). In fact this group is not on parental leave, but receives occupational rehabilitation or a disability pension instead. This is clearly the group with the most difficulties in the labor market. In Finland occupational rehabilitation is rather effective, so these young men may have a chance to attend school or work later in life.

As an ex-post validation of these trajectory groups we can measure or sum up the working days over the follow-up period. The length of working life is on average 5.1 years for the HES group and only 1.3 years for the LES group. The results confirm that this analysis has found clusters that also have practical importance.

4   Concluding Remarks

It is clear that our mixture regression analysis is an effective tool for the identification of different clusters of register-based data. Naturally, the central interest is on those who have difficulties with labor market integration. We think that our analysis provides new insight into this important social issue. We mainly concentrated on a descriptive analysis of results. However, it would also be interesting to analyze the identified clusters further using covariates like social class, living area, parents' education, or parents' income. The best way to proceed may be the joint modeling of clusters and mixing percentages using multinomial regression. This more subject-oriented analysis remains a topic of further research.

Acknowledgements The authors wish to thank the Finnish Centre for Pensions and Statistics Finland for providing the research data for this study. We also like to thank the referees for the comments that led to improvements of the paper.

Appendix

Table 2 Summary of the estimated model: variables, clusters, parameter estimates and their standard errors

Variable	Group	$\hat{\beta}_0$	SE($\hat{\beta}_0$)	$\hat{\beta}_1$	SE($\hat{\beta}_1$)	$\hat{\beta}_2$	SE($\hat{\beta}_2$)
1	1	2.398	4.0937	−0.3086	0.3809	0.0043	0.0088
1	2	−33.1751	1.6662	2.8697	0.1567	−0.0572	0.0036
1	3	−1.3307	1.4851	−0.082	0.1356	0.0052	0.0031
1	4	−10.4101	1.4206	0.8602	0.1308	−0.0177	0.003
1	5	−18.5665	1.4307	1.4459	0.1371	−0.0223	0.0033
1	6	−30.6046	3.7969	2.2395	0.3836	−0.0297	0.0097
1	7	−49.6895	2.1645	4.5499	0.201	−0.0993	0.0046
1	8	−64.2231	2.9188	5.9415	0.2719	−0.1288	0.0062
1	9	−48.3674	1.6773	4.3293	0.1584	−0.0912	0.0037
1	10	−10.4439	2.556	1.0078	0.2392	−0.0264	0.0055
2	1	11.1319	2.9527	−0.8535	0.2754	0.013	0.0064
2	2	399.1368	10.4145	−41.2003	1.0772	1.0621	0.0278
2	3	−20.6646	1.6869	2.0785	0.156	−0.0485	0.0036
2	4	36.9462	1.8208	−3.1096	0.1655	0.0635	0.0037
2	5	−54.0624	0.9532	5.2318	0.0885	−0.1231	0.002
2	6	165.358	4.3881	−14.2717	0.3962	0.2974	0.0089
2	7	151.7117	4.8462	−14.7589	0.4754	0.3563	0.0116
2	8	72.251	2.3522	−6.5804	0.2146	0.1428	0.0048
2	9	83.5415	2.0619	−7.2462	0.1871	0.1515	0.0042
2	10	45.0733	2.7618	−4.0274	0.2565	0.0857	0.0059
3	1	−37.1495	7.5126	3.338	0.7054	−0.0805	0.0164
3	2	−3.5307	99.786	−15.2704	54.119	0.5892	2.0791
3	3	7.1229	2.1854	−1.0465	0.1995	0.0284	0.0045
3	4	−61.0014	2.0817	5.2682	0.1901	−0.1111	0.0043
3	5	−1.4631	1.5541	−0.2562	0.1412	0.0092	0.0032
3	6	−110.2661	3.8561	10.3492	0.3723	−0.246	0.009
3	7	−54.1435	3.2046	4.9123	0.2998	−0.1141	0.007
3	8	8.3929	3.0624	−1.3156	0.2777	0.0354	0.0062
3	9	−58.2828	1.2639	5.0717	0.1153	−0.1092	0.0026
3	10	19.9764	2.9505	−2.2136	0.2699	0.0548	0.0061
4	1	−22.1081	4.2901	1.4843	0.4084	−0.0185	0.0097
4	2	−16.5855	5.8831	0.9372	0.5318	−0.0173	0.0119
4	3	6.3987	8.9441	−1.345	0.7973	0.0372	0.0176
4	4	−33.001	3.2404	2.5058	0.2873	−0.0505	0.0063
4	5	−11.5583	2.6232	0.3925	0.2318	−0.0015	0.0051

(continued)

Table 2 (continued)

Variable	Group	$\hat{\beta}_0$	SE($\hat{\beta}_0$)	$\hat{\beta}_1$	SE($\hat{\beta}_1$)	$\hat{\beta}_2$	SE($\hat{\beta}_2$)
4	6	−36.7212	2.2235	2.7618	0.1953	−0.0548	0.0043
4	7	−38.7528	4.6765	3.0266	0.4167	−0.0633	0.0092
4	8	−30.3185	2.4405	2.2794	0.2174	−0.0456	0.0048
4	9	−33.8236	2.1217	2.6022	0.1885	−0.0529	0.0042
4	10	−20.8289	6.5442	1.4166	0.591	−0.0281	0.0132

References

Escudero,V., & Mourelo, M. L. (2015). *The Youth Guarantee programme in Europe: Features, implementation and challenges*. Geneva: ILO.

Jolkkonen, A., Kurvinen, A., Virtanen, P., Lipiäinen, L., Nummi, T., Koistinen, P. (2017). Labour market attachment following major workforce downsizings: A comparison of displaced and retained workers. *Work, Employment and Society*. https://doi.org/10.1177/0950017017706305.

Jones, B. L., & Nagin, D. S. (2007). Advances in group-based trajectory modeling and an SAS procedure for estimating them. *Sociological Methods & Research, 35*(4), 542–571.

Jones, B. L., Nagin, D. S., & Roeder, K. (2001). A SAS procedure based on mixture models for estimating developmental trajectories. *Sociological Methods & Research, 29*(3), 374–393.

Keränen, K. (2012). Young people within services — best practices for the promotion of the youth guarantee. The Ministry of Employment and the Economy in Finland.

Kokko, K., Pulkkinen, L., Mesiäinen, P., Lyyra, A.-L. (2008). Trajectories based on postcomprehensive and higher education: Their correlates and antecedents. *Journal of Social Issues, 64*(1), 59–76.

Korpela, K., Nummi, T., Lipiäinen, L., De Bloom, J., Sianoja, M., Pasanen, T., & Kinnunen, U. (2017). Nature exposure predicts well-being trajectory groups among employees across two years. *Journal of Environmental Psychology*. https://doi.org/doi:10.1016/j.jenvp.2017.06.002.

Mani, D., & Nandkumar, A. (2016). The differential impacts of markets for technology on the value of technological resources: An application of group-based trajectory models. *Strategic Management Journal, 37*(1), 192–205.

McLachlan, G., & Peel, D. (2000). *Finite mixture models*. Hoboken, NJ: Wiley.

Nagin, O. S. (1999). Analyzing developmental trajectories: Semi-parametric group-based approach. *Psychological Methods, 4*, 39–177.

Nagin, D. S. (2005). *Group-based modeling of development*. Cambridge, MA: Harvard University Press.

Nagin, D. S., & Odgers, C. L. (2010a). Group-based trajectory modeling (nearly) two decades later. *Journal of Quantitative Criminology, 26*(4), 445–453.

Nagin, D. S., & Odgers, C. L. (2010b). Group-based trajectory modeling in clinical research. *Annual Review of Clinical Psychology, 6*, 109–138.

Nagin, D. S., & Tremblay, R. E. (2001). Analyzing developmental trajectories of distinct but related behaviors: A group-based method. *Psychological Methods, 6*(1), 18–34.

Nummi, T., Hakanen, T., Lipiäinen, L., Harjunmaa, U., Salo, M., Saha, M. T., & Vuovela, N. (2014). A trajectory analysis of body mass index for Finnish children. *Journal of Applied Statistics, 41*(7), 1422–1435.

Nummi, T., Virtanen, P., Leino-Arjas, P., & Hammarström, A. (2017). Trajectories of a set of ten functional somatic symptoms from adolescence to middle age. *Archives of Public Health, 75*, 11.

Paananen, R., & Gissler, M. (2013). *International Journal of Epidemiology, 41*, 941–945.

Pareliussen, J. K. (2016). Age, skills and labour market outcomes in Finland. OECD Economics Department Working Papers, No. 1321. Paris: OECD Publishing.

Bias Correction in Age-Period-Cohort Models Using Eigen Analysis

Martina Fu

1 Introduction

Age-period-cohort (APC) analysis is a popular technique that is often used in epidemiology to examine chronic disease incidence or mortality rates and in sociology to examine social event rates. It analyzes age-year-specific rates, found in $a \times p$ tables with a rows of consecutive age groups and p columns of consecutive periods, using regression models. When the time spans in each age group and period group are equal, the diagonals of the table represent birth cohorts (generations). Recognizing the importance of all the age, period, and cohort effects, biostatisticians and quantitative scientists simultaneously estimate the fixed effects of all three factors in the APC models (Mason et al. 1973; Rodgers 1982; Kupper et al. 1983; Wilmoth 1990; Glenn 2003; Smith 2008).

However, age, period, and birth cohort have a linear relationship: Period – Age = Cohort. This linear dependence among the covariates of APC regression models leads to multiple estimators and multiple trends in age, period, and cohort, resulting in parameter indetermination (Mason et al. 1973; Rodgers 1982; Smith et al. 1982; Kupper et al. 1983). This identification problem attracted much attention in the 1970s and 1980s, and several approaches have been studied to address this problem, including specifying an extra constraint on the parameters (Mason et al. 1973; Kupper et al. 1985) or identifying estimable functions (Rodgers 1982; Smith et al. 1982). In particular, the constraint method specifies a relationship among the parameters so that a unique estimator can be determined. Different constraints, however, may lead to different parameter estimates and, very often, a seemingly reasonable constraint assumed on the parameters yields an insensible

M. Fu (✉)
Research Lab of Dr. Yi Li, Department of Biostatistics, University of Michigan,
Ann Arbor, MI, USA
e-mail: Fumm95@yahoo.com

© Springer International Publishing AG 2017
D.-G. Chen et al. (eds.), *New Advances in Statistics and Data Science*,
ICSA Book Series in Statistics, https://doi.org/10.1007/978-3-319-69416-0_19

trend (Kupper et al. 1985). An estimable function approach, on the other hand, looks for characteristics of the parameters or the trend that are independent of the constraint (Rodgers 1982; Smith et al. 1982; Kupper et al. 1985). The search for an estimable function that completely determines the parameters was not successful (Kupper et al. 1985; Clayton and Schifflers 1987) and the identification problem had remained unsettled until recently.

In recent years, several new methods have been studied to address the identification problem, including the smoothing trend method (Heuer 1997), the intrinsic estimator and ridge regularization methods (Fu 2000), the smoothing cohort model (Fu 2008), the mechanism-based approach (Winship and Harding 2008), and the partial least-squares method (Tu et al. 2011). Specifically, the intrinsic estimator has the expectation of an estimable function that completely determines the parameters, yielding robust parameter estimation with finite samples and consistent estimation with diverging samples (Fu 2016). Furthermore, constrained estimators have asymptotic bias, leading to biased estimation (Fu 2016). Thus, the intrinsic estimator provides a simple method to achieve unbiased estimation among multiple estimators, and has been shown to produce meaningful data analysis results in the literature (Yang et al. 2004; Schwadel 2010; Fu 2016).

However, before the intrinsic estimator was introduced in Fu (2000), many studies used an equality constraint for technical convenience to determine a unique estimation based on subjective assumptions (Mason and Smith 1985). It is known that using a constraint introduces bias unless the constraint is satisfied by the true parameters of the model (Kupper et al. 1985), and it has been recently shown that an equality constraint almost surely introduces bias (Fu 2016). Such estimation bias needs to be corrected so that correct inferences can be made. Calculating the unbiased estimation using the intrinsic estimator method requires the original data (Fu 2016). Unfortunately, many publications only report the analysis results, either through numerical estimates or graphical plots, but do not report raw data. For example, see Jemal et al. (2001), Cayuela et al. (2004), and Chen et al. (2011). Bias correction becomes even more challenging when the original data is no longer available after the analysis has been published. In this paper, we develop a method that directly corrects the bias in the estimation. It possesses the following properties. (1) It requires no raw data and no model fitting; (2) It is easy to implement with simple calculations; and (3) It provides the standard error of the parameter estimates if the previously reported analytical results have variance or standard error estimations, regardless of the constraint used to achieve the unique parameter estimation.

This article is organized as follows. Section 2 reviews the APC model, the identification problem, and the intrinsic estimator method. Section 3 develops a bias correction method and provides algorithms for bias correction and standard error estimation. Section 4 demonstrates the bias correction method with two studies, one with the raw data and the other with only graphical plots and no raw data. Section 5 provides a discussion and conclusion. The R program is available from the author upon request, and will be posted on the internet.

2 Age-Period-Cohort Model and the Identification Problem

2.1 The Age-Period-Cohort Model

Assume the investigator is interested in analyzing data in an $a \times p$ table with a rows of consecutive age groups and p columns of consecutive periods. Y_{ij} is the rate of the ith age group in the jth period, $i = 1 \ldots a, j = 1 \ldots p$, as shown in Table 1 for cervical cancer incidence rate among U.S. females aged 15–84 from 1975 to 2009 from the Surveillance Epidemiology and End Results (SEER) database (National Cancer Institute, n.d.)). The APC accounting model or multiple classification model fits a linear model to the logarithm of the rate Y_{ij} on the fixed effect of age, period, and cohort:

$$\log \left(Y_{ij} \right) = \mu + \alpha_i + \beta_j + \gamma_k + \varepsilon_{ij}, \tag{1}$$

where μ is the intercept, α_i is the ith age group effect, β_j is the jth period effect, γ_k is the kth cohort effect with $k = a - i + j$, and ε_{ij} is the random error with mean 0 and common variance σ^2. Alternatively, if non-Gaussian response variables are considered, one may fit a generalized linear model with the same covariate structure as in model (1):

$$g \left(EY_{ij} \right) = \mu + \alpha_i + \beta_j + \gamma_k, \tag{1*}$$

where EY_{ij} is the expected value of the response, and g is a link function, such as the log link for Poisson log-linear models or the logit link for the logistic regression.

Table 1 Cervical cancer incidence rate (per 100,000) among U.S. females 1975–2009[a]

Age\period	1975–1979	1980–1984	1985–1989	1990–1994	1995–1999	2000–2004	2005–2009
15–19	0.26	0.33	0.29	0.33	0.48	0.17	0.23
20–24	2.99	2.41	2.01	2.61	1.76	1.50	1.46
25–29	8.94	7.84	7.78	7.87	7.11	6.15	4.33
30–34	14.51	12.86	11.99	11.70	11.90	10.58	9.12
35–39	18.38	15.34	16.37	15.09	14.13	11.02	12.63
40–44	19.23	16.86	16.84	15.76	15.54	13.25	12.22
45–59	21.48	17.39	17.60	16.99	16.43	12.42	11.49
50–54	21.07	18.10	17.94	16.77	14.37	11.77	10.46
55–59	24.83	18.82	16.09	16.24	14.29	12.36	10.21
60–64	25.77	20.55	18.41	18.54	15.32	13.14	10.83
65–69	27.05	21.21	19.14	18.56	14.73	13.12	12.18
70–74	27.41	20.70	18.86	14.99	13.42	11.26	11.69
75–79	26.44	20.93	18.95	15.98	14.75	11.15	9.35
80–84	27.92	20.92	17.01	18.22	12.57	12.70	7.78

[a]Obtained from the SEER cancer registry database

As in ANOVA models, parameter centralization is required separately on the fixed effects of the age, period and cohort.

$$\sum_{i=1}^{a} \alpha_i = 0, \sum_{j=1}^{p} \beta_j = 0, \sum_{k=1}^{a+p-1} \gamma_k = 0 \tag{2}$$

Alternatively, a reference level may be set for each parameter $\alpha_1 = \beta_1 = \gamma_1 = 0$. If model (1) determines a unique parameter estimate, then the temporal trends in age, period, and cohort can be obtained by plotting the age effect against age, period effect against period, and cohort effect against birth cohort.

For notational convenience, the APC model (1) can also be written in a matrix form:

$$\log(Y) = Xb + \varepsilon, \tag{3}$$

where Y is a column vector of the event rate and b is a column vector of the model parameters such that its transpose $b^T = (\mu, \alpha_1, \ldots, \alpha_{a-1}, \beta_1, \ldots, \beta_{p-1}, \gamma_1, \ldots, \gamma_{a+p-2})$. With parameter centralization (2), the parameters α_a, β_p, and γ_{a+p-1} do not appear in b. X is the design matrix and ε is a vector of independent random errors, each with mean 0 and common variance σ^2.

2.2   The Identification Problem

Because of the linear dependence: Period − Age = Cohort, models (1) and (1*) yield multiple estimators. Each one leads to a different temporal trend, which makes it difficult to estimate and interpret the parameters (Fig. 1). To determine a unique trend, an additional constraint can be set on the parameters (Smith et al. 1982; Kupper et al. 1983). Many studies choose to set an equality constraint assuming its justification based on the investigator's prior knowledge. For example, the first two age effects may be set as equal assuming that the event rates in the early ages do not vary much. Similar assumptions can be made for identical period effects or cohort effects (Fig. 1). However, seemingly reasonable constraints often lead to insensible trend estimations (Kupper et al. 1985), such as the overall decreasing age trend in the top panel of Fig. 1 based on a reasonable assumption that cervical cancer risk stays low and constant in early ages. Furthermore, different constraints may yield different temporal trends, as shown in Fig. 1, where three different temporal trends are obtained for the cervical cancer incidence rates in Table 1 with three constraints: identical first two age effects, identical first two period effects, and identical first two cohort effects. The different trend estimations clearly indicate that bias can be introduced by setting a constraint. To help address the issue, one major question may be asked about which constraints would yield unbiased parameter estimation. A logical answer is that a constraint satisfied by the true parameter values will yield unbiased estimation. However, this argument quickly leads to a paradox, because it is impossible to confirm whether a constraint is satisfied by the true parameter values

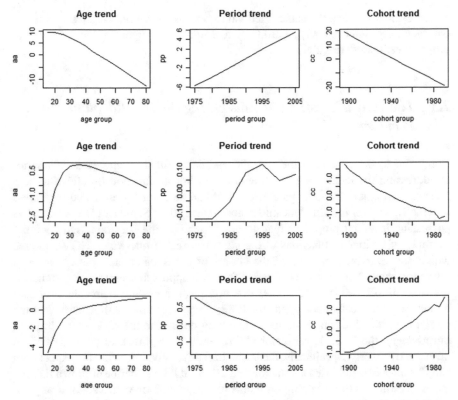

Fig. 1 Temporal trend in age, period and cohort of the cervical cancer incidence rates in Table 1 generated by equality constraints. Top panels: $\alpha_1 = \alpha_2$; Middle panels: $\beta_1 = \beta_2$; Bottom panels: $\gamma_1 = \gamma_2$

before the parameters are accurately estimated. Consequently, the identification problem cannot be resolved with the constraint approach.

To understand the mechanism of the identification problem, we study the APC model in matrix form (3). The linear dependence among age, period, and cohort induces a singular design matrix X with 1- less than its full rank (Kupper et al. 1983). This implies that there exists an eigenvector v in the null parameter space of the matrix X, corresponding to the unique eigenvalue 0, i.e. $Xv = 0$. By Kupper et al. (1983), $v^{\mathrm{T}} = (0\, A\, P\, C)$, where

$$A = \left(1 - \frac{a+1}{2}, \ldots, a - 1 - \frac{a+1}{2}\right),$$

$$P = \left(\frac{p+1}{2} - 1, \ldots, \frac{p+1}{2} - (p-1)\right), \qquad (4)$$

$$C = \left(1 - \frac{a+p}{2}, \ldots, a + p - 2 - \frac{a+p}{2}\right).$$

All estimators have the same fitted value because $X(u+tv) = Xu$, where u is a parameter estimator and t is an arbitrary real number. Different values of t lead to different estimators (Fu 2000).

2.3   The Intrinsic Estimator Addressing the Identification Problem

Compared to the constraint method, the estimable function approach is superior in addressing the identification problem. An estimable function is defined to be a linear combination of model parameters that can be uniquely estimated regardless of which estimator is used (McCulloch and Searle 2001; Seber and Lee 2003), thus possessing invariant properties that do not depend on the constraint. One popular example of estimable functions is the contrasts in the one-way ANOVA model, which are invariant regardless of the choice of either parameter centralization or reference level. Although the estimable function approach seems to be promising, it has been observed in APC studies that nonlinear trends are estimable but linear trends vary with constraint (Rodgers 1982; Kupper et al. 1985). This makes the search for estimable functions that completely determine the parameters difficult. Surprisingly, the intrinsic estimator has recently been shown to possess such an invariance property. Specifically, the intrinsic estimator has an estimable expectation and thus provides unbiased estimation (Fu 2016). It has further been shown that the intrinsic estimator of finite samples yields robust estimation with a slight change of the data by either adding or deleting one row or one column, and yields consistent estimation as the number of columns (periods) p, and thus the sample size, diverges to infinity, while the constrained estimators, particularly by the equality constraints, yield biased estimation (Fu 2016).

The intrinsic estimator was identified through a unique decomposition of the multiple parameter estimators in vector form (Fu 2000)

$$\widehat{b} = B + tB_0, \tag{5}$$

where $\widehat{b}$ is the estimate of the parameter vector b. B_0 is a normalized eigenvector of v with unit length 1. B is orthogonal to B_0 in the parameter space and is uniquely determined by the data. t is a real number that may take any value. B is named the intrinsic estimator (Fu 2000), and is a linear combination of model parameters that satisfies the projection

$$B = \widehat{b} - tB_0 = \widehat{b} - B_0B_0^T\widehat{b} = \left(I - B_0B_0^T\right)\widehat{b}, \tag{6}$$

where I is an identity matrix and the coefficients of the linear combination $B = L\widehat{b}$ satisfy $Lv = \left(I - B_0B_0^T\right)v = \left(I - B_0B_0^T\right)B_0\|v\| = 0$. This means that, geometrically, B can be obtained by projecting any given estimator $\widehat{b}$ to the vertical axis orthogonal to the eigenvector B_0, as shown in Fig. 2. B determines both linear

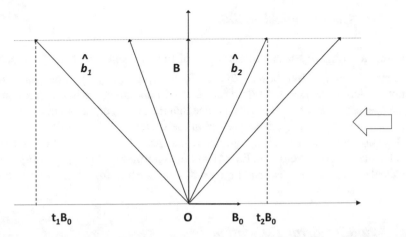

Fig. 2 Decomposition of multiple estimators by Eigen analysis. $\hat{b}_1$ and $\hat{b}_2$ are estimators with an arbitrary t value. B is the intrinsic estimator and can be obtained by projecting any estimator to the vertical axis as illustrated by the arrow. B_0 is a normalized eigenvector in the null space and is perpendicular to B

and nonlinear trends with zero bias because the bias $Lv = 0$ as defined in Kupper et al. (1985). Other estimators in Eq. (5) with $t \neq 0$ do not have an estimable expectation and thus yield nonzero bias.

3 The Bias Correction Method

For a given estimator $\widehat{b}$ (e.g. an estimator obtained by using a constraint), the unbiased estimator B can be calculated by $B = \widehat{b} - tB_0$ from (5), where $t = B_0{}^T \widehat{b}$ is an inner product between vectors $\widehat{b}$ and B_0, and B_0 can be calculated using the numbers of age groups (a) and period groups (p) as in Eq. (4), followed by a normalization

$$B_0 = \frac{v}{\|v\|}, \tag{7}$$

where $\|v\| = \sqrt{v_1^2 + \cdots + v_m^2}$ is the Euclidean norm of vector v in an m-dimensional space with $m = 2(a + p) - 3$. This provides a method of correcting the bias without fitting a model by calculating the unbiased estimation B using only the null eigenvector B_0 and the given biased estimator $\widehat{b}$. We provide an algorithm for the bias correction procedure.

3.1 Bias Correction Algorithm

1. Form an estimator $\widehat{b}$ using the estimates of the intercept, age, period and cohort effects, $\widehat{b}^T = (\mu, \alpha_1, \ldots, \alpha_{a-1}, \beta_1, \ldots, \beta_{p-1}, \gamma_1, \ldots, \gamma_{a+p-2})$. If the intercept is not available, use $\mu = 0$ because its value will not affect the bias correction for the age, period and cohort effects. Notice that the effects of the last age α_a, period β_p and cohort γ_{a+p-1} are not present in the vector $\widehat{b}$.
2. Based on the numbers of age groups a and period groups p in the estimates, calculate the eigenvector v in Eq. (4) and then normalize it to B_0 as in Eq. (7).
3. Calculate the unbiased estimator B by removing the bias from $\widehat{b}$: $B = \widehat{b} - B_0 B_0^T \widehat{b}$.

3.2 Standard Error Estimation

If the original constraint method provides standard errors for the parameter estimates of model (1) or (2), it is desirable to provide the standard errors for the parameter estimates after bias correction. For linear model (1), the parameter estimates have the variance-covariance matrix $(X_c^T X_c)^{-1} \sigma^2$, where σ^2 is the variance component and X_c is the design matrix reduced from X of model (1) by a preselected constraint on the parameters, such as $\alpha_1 = \alpha_2$, which is often provided if a constraint method is used for parameter estimation. The variance of the parameter estimates is given by the diagonal elements of the matrix $(X_c^T X_c)^{-1} \sigma^2$. Hence the variance component σ^2 can be calculated with the squares of the standard errors divided by the diagonal elements of the matrix $(X_c^T X_c)^{-1}$. Since the variance component is estimated with the residuals (r_{ij}) of the model (1) together with a specified constraint, and the residuals remain the same regardless of the constraint because all constraints yield the same fitted values, the variance component estimate $\widehat{\sigma}^2 = \frac{\sum_{ij} r_{ij}^2}{(a-2)(p-2)}$ remains the same even when different constraints may be specified based on the investigator's prior acknowledge, as shown in Fig. 3. This leads to accurate estimation of the variance of the intrinsic estimator after bias correction as follows.

Denote by V the orthonormal matrix whose column vectors are the eigenvectors of matrix $(X^T X)$ ordered by the eigenvalues in descending order. Denote by V_l and V_{-l} the last column vector of V and the submatrix excluding V_l from V, respectively. The intrinsic estimator can be computed through the principal component analysis approach (Fu 2008) with $B = VU$ and row vector $U^T = (((W^T W)^{-1} W^T R)^T, 0)$, where $W = XV_{-l}$ and R is the response vector, such as $R = \log(Y)$. Thus B has variance $Var(B) = V_{-l} (W^T W)^{-1} V_{-l}^T \sigma^2 = V_{-l} (V_{-l}^T X^T X V_{-l})^{-1} V_{-l}^T \sigma^2$. The standard error of the intrinsic estimator can therefore be calculated using the variance component σ^2 as follows.

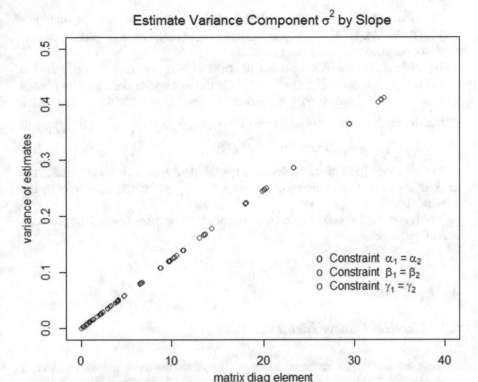

Fig. 3 Plot of variance estimate against the matrix diagonal element by different constraints. Large values of the variance (>0.5) by the equality constraint on the cohort effects are not plotted so that details can be observed for small variance close to 0 with different colors. Black dot—equality constraint on the first two age group effects $\alpha_1 = \alpha_2$; Red dot—equality constraint on the first two period effects $\beta_1 = \beta_2$; Blue dot—equality constraint on the first two cohort effects $\gamma_1 = \gamma_2$

3.3 Algorithm for Standard Error Estimation After Bias Correction

1. Form the design matrix X of model (1) and its reduced matrix X_c according to the constraint used for parameter estimation.
2. Calculate the estimate of the variance component σ^2 by dividing the squares of the standard errors by the diagonal elements of matrix $\left(X_c^T X_c\right)^{-1}$. Note that due to the use of parameter centralization (2) or reference levels, certain parameters are not present in the model. Hence, the dimension of matrix X_c is smaller than the number of parameters in model (1).
3. Calculate the orthonormal matrix V, whose column vectors are the eigenvectors of the matrix $(X^T X)$ in descending order of the eigen values. Denote by V_{-1}

the submatrix of V excluding the last column. Calculate the variance $Var(B) = V_{-l}(V_{-l}^T X^T X V_{-l})^{-1} V_{-l}^T \sigma^2$. Report the square root of the main diagonal elements as the standard errors after bias correction.

4. By the centralization (2), the standard errors of $\widehat{\alpha}_a, \widehat{\beta}_p, \widehat{\gamma}_{a+p-1}$ are calculated to be the square-root of $(1^T \Sigma 1)\sigma^2$, where 1 is the vector with elements 1 of dimension $a-1$, $p-1$, and $a+p-2$, respectively, and Σ is the variance-covariance matrix of the corresponding vectors $(\widehat{\alpha}_1,\ldots,\widehat{\alpha}_{a-1})^T$, $(\widehat{\beta}_1,\ldots,\widehat{\beta}_{p-1})^T$ and $(\widehat{\gamma}_1,\ldots,\widehat{\gamma}_{a+p-2})^T$, respectively.

For the generalized linear model (1*), the standard error estimation remains the same as above, assuming the variance component σ^2 is estimated correctly by the constraint method.

The R code for the bias correction and standard error estimation will be provided in an R package.

4 Application

4.1 Cervical Cancer Incidence Rate

To demonstrate the bias correction method, we analyze the cervical cancer incidence rates in Table 1. It has 14 age groups from 15–19 to 80–84, 7 periods from 1975–1979 to 2005–2009, and 20 cohort groups with mid birth year from 1895 to 1990. First, we use an equality constraint on the first two age effects $\alpha_1 = \alpha_2$, the first two period effects $\beta_1 = \beta_2$, or the first two cohort effects $\gamma_1 = \gamma_2$ to determine a unique trend, as shown in Table 2, with the standard errors given in parentheses. Although different constraints lead to different estimates of the age, period and cohort effects and largely different standard errors, the variance component remains the same, as shown in Fig. 3, which yields $\widehat{\sigma}^2 = 0.012$. Then we apply the bias correction method to each equality constraint estimator to obtain the corrected estimates and the standard errors, as shown in the last two columns of Table 2. Though we start with different constraint estimators, the corrected estimates and the standard errors are identical. Further examination shows that the standard errors of the bias corrected estimates are smaller than those of the constraint estimators, illustrating the efficiency of the intrinsic estimator (Fu 2016).

We also compare the novel bias correction method with the partial least-squares method, which analyzes the APC data using the maximal number of components in the partial least squares. As shown in the last column of Table 2, the partial least-squares method yields the same parameter estimates as the intrinsic estimator, but without standard errors (Tu et al. 2011). This further confirms the estimates by the bias correction method. However, the lack of standard error estimates reflects the limitation of the partial least-square method applied to APC data using the maximal

Table 2 Age, period, and cohort estimates for cervical cancer data in Table 1[a]

Constraint: $\alpha_1 = \alpha_2$		Constraint: $\beta_1 = \beta_2$		Constraint: $\gamma_1 = \gamma_2$		Bias corrected estimates (**B**)		Partial least-squares	
Age	Cohort	Age	Cohort	Age	Cohort	Age	Cohort	Age	Cohort
9.437 (0.373)	19.384 (0.603)	−2.621 (0.284)	1.761 (0.402)	−4.516 (0.922)	−1.008 (1.251)	−3.276 (0.045)	0.803 (0.105)	−3.276	0.803
9.437 (0.373)	17.238 (0.536)	−0.766 (0.241)	1.470 (0.374)	−2.369 (0.780)	−1.008 (1.251)	−1.321 (0.042)	0.613 (0.076)	−1.321	0.613
8.667 (0.285)	15.150 (0.471)	0.319 (0.198)	1.237 (0.330)	−0.993 (0.639)	−0.949 (1.066)	−0.135 (0.042)	0.481 (0.063)	−0.135	0.481
7.219 (0.224)	13.108 (0.408)	0.726 (0.156)	1.050 (0.286)	−0.294 (0.497)	−0.844 (0.924)	0.373 (0.042)	0.395 (0.056)	0.373	0.395
5.456 (0.163)	10.979 (0.345)	0.819 (0.115)	0.776 (0.243)	0.090 (0.356)	−0.827 (0.783)	0.567 (0.042)	0.222 (0.051)	0.567	0.222
3.548 (0.104)	8.977 (0.283)	0.766 (0.077)	0.629 (0.200)	0.328 (0.216)	−0.682 (0.642)	0.614 (0.043)	0.176 (0.047)	0.614	0.176
1.590 (0.054)	6.873 (0.221)	0.662 (0.048)	0.380 (0.158)	0.517 (0.083)	−0.640 (0.500)	0.612 (0.043)	0.028 (0.044)	0.612	0.028
−0.444 (0.052)	4.857 (0.160)	0.484 (0.048)	0.219 (0.118)	0.630 (0.083)	−0.510 (0.361)	0.534 (0.043)	−0.033 (0.045)	0.534	−0.033
−2.442 (0.103)	2.875 (0.102)	0.341 (0.078)	0.093 (0.081)	0.778 (0.217)	−0.344 (0.220)	0.492 (0.043)	−0.058 (0.046)	0.492	−0.058
−4.372 (0.162)	0.869 (0.055)	0.265 (0.116)	−0.058 (0.052)	0.994 (0.357)	−0.204 (0.087)	0.517 (0.042)	−0.109 (0.047)	0.517	−0.109
−6.381 (0.223)	−1.150 (0.057)	0.112 (0.157)	−0.222 (0.051)	1.132 (0.498)	−0.077 (0.082)	0.464 (0.042)	−0.172 (0.046)	0.464	−0.172
−8.496 (0.284)	−3.118 (0.107)	−0.149 (0.199)	−0.336 (0.078)	1.163 (0.639)	0.102 (0.214)	0.305 (0.042)	−0.184 (0.046)	0.305	−0.184
−10.562 (0.347)	−5.090 (0.169)	−0.359 (0.241)	−0.452 (0.115)	1.244 (0.786)	0.277 (0.354)	0.196 (0.042)	−0.200 (0.045)	0.196	−0.200
−12.657 (0.346)	−7.108 (0.225)	−0.599 (0.280)	−0.615 (0.156)	1.296 (0.913)	0.405 (0.495)	0.057 (0.044)	−0.262 (0.043)	0.057	−0.262
	−9.041 (0.286)		−0.694 (0.194)		0.618 (0.635)		−0.240 (0.046)		−0.240
Period		*Period*		*Period*		*Period*		*Period*	
−5.701 (0.189)	−10.939 (0.348)	−0.136 (0.109)	−0.736 (0.241)	0.739 (0.422)	0.866 (0.778)	0.167 (0.028)	−0.182 (0.049)	0.1672	−0.182
−3.846 (0.128)	−12.986 (0.410)	−0.136 (0.109)	−0.928 (0.284)	0.447 (0.288)	0.966 (0.919)	0.066 (0.028)	−0.273 (0.054)	0.066	−0.273
−1.911 (0.068)	−14.895 (0.473)	−0.056 (0.052)	−0.982 (0.329)	0.236 (0.144)	1.204 (1.061)	0.045 (0.028)	−0.226 (0.061)	0.045	−0.226
0.083 (0.028)	−17.134 (0.535)	0.083 (0.028)	−1.366 (0.374)	0.083 (0.028)	1.111 (1.204)	0.083 (0.028)	−0.509 (0.074)	0.083	−0.509
1.977 (0.069)	−18.849 (0.570)	0.122 (0.051)	−1.226 (0.425)	−0.169 (0.144)	1.543 (1.167)	0.022 (0.028)	−0.268 (0.117)	0.022	−0.268
3.756 (0.128)		0.046 (0.090)		−0.537 (0.284)		−0.155 (0.028)		−0.155	
5.640 (0.187)		0.075 (0.094)		−0.799 (0.426)		−0.227 (0.029)		−0.227	

[a]Age: 15–19, 20–24 ... 80–84; Period: 1975–1979, 1980–1984 ... 2005–2009; Cohort mid birth year: 1895, 1900 ... 1990

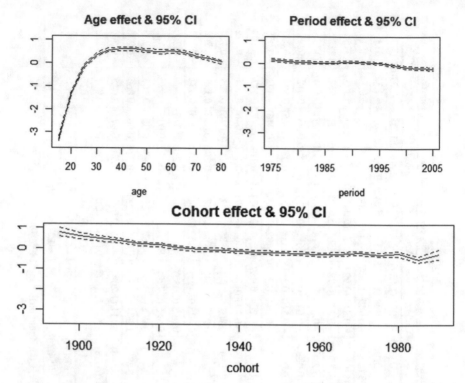

Fig. 4 Temporal trend and 95% confidence interval of cervical cancer incidence rate among U.S. females in Table 1 by the intrinsic estimator method

number of components. Notice also that the partial least-squares method cannot be used for bias correction when the original data becomes unavailable since the method requires the original data.

In order to interpret the temporal trend, we plot the corrected age, period, and cohort effects in the same scale in Fig. 4. The age trend shows that the incidence rate increased sharply from age 15 to 30, peaked around 40, and slowly decreased until age 84. The period trend shows that the incidence increased from 1975 to 1980 and then decreased slowly until 2009. The cohort trend shows that the incidence slowly decreased from the oldest cohort born in 1895 to the cohort born in 1970 and then fluctuated slightly till 1995, which may be due to unstable cohort effect estimation resulting from having few observations in the extreme cohorts. From an epidemiological point of view, the increasing-then-decreasing age trend can be well explained by the strong association between cervical cancer incidence and the human papillomavirus infection (Bosch et al. 1995; Sasieni and Adams 2000; Scheurer et al. 2005). Additionally, the decreasing period trend may be attributed to improved health care and personal hygiene while the decreasing cohort trend may be a result of educational programs about sexually transmitted diseases in younger generations.

4.2 Chronic Obstructive Pulmonary Disease Mortality

To demonstrate our method of bias correction in previously published analysis results that do not provide raw data, we apply the procedure to an age-period-cohort study of chronic obstructive pulmonary disease (COPD) mortality in Hong Kong from 1981 to 2005 (Chen et al. 2011). In this study, sex-specific mortality rates for 5 year age and period intervals among individuals 45 years and older were analyzed using an APC log-linear model with an equality constraint on two periods, 1986–1990 and 1996–2000. In the paper, the effect estimates were only plotted, and no numerical estimates were reported. We obtain the effect estimates of age, period, and cohort by reading the published figure of the temporal trend (Fig. 3 of Chen et al. 2011), centralize the effect estimates for each of age, period, and cohort, and apply the bias correction procedure since, by the large sample theory, the equality constraint almost surely yields biased estimation (Fu 2016). We compare the temporal trend of the corrected age, period and cohort effects with the reported trend for males in Fig. 5a and females in Fig. 5b.

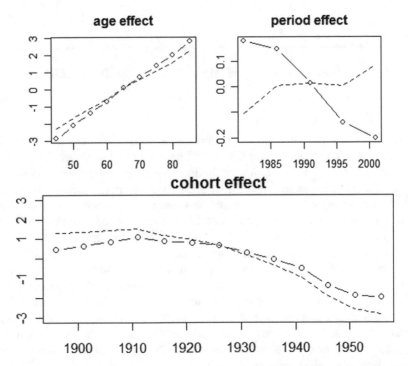

Fig. 5 (**a**) Comparison of age, period, and cohort trends before and after bias correction of COPD mortality rate in Hong Kong males. Dashed: before bias correction. Solid: after bias correction. (**b**) Comparison of age, period, and cohort trends before and after bias correction of COPD mortality rate in Hong Kong females. Dashed: before bias correction. Solid: after bias correction

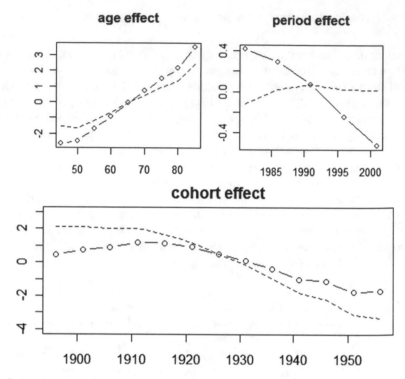

Fig. 5 (continued)

As shown in Fig. 5, the age and cohort trends remain similar before and after bias correction in both males and females. The period trend in males changes from an overall increasing pattern to a steadily decreasing one while the period trend in females changes from an increasing-then-decreasing pattern to a steadily decreasing one. It is interesting to notice that, before bias correction, the period trends between males and females were largely different, likely due to biased estimation from the equality constraint. After bias correction, they present a more or less similar pattern. This reflects the fact that both males and females lived with the same air quality, and, consequently, their period trends should have had a similar pattern, though their age trend may have been different due to the difference in the effect of aging on physiological functions between males and females. On the other hand, a closer observation reveals that the scale of the period trend is relatively small compared to that of the age and cohort trends in both males and females as shown in Fig. 6. This may imply that more effort should be focused on the age and cohort effects in order to effectively lower the mortality.

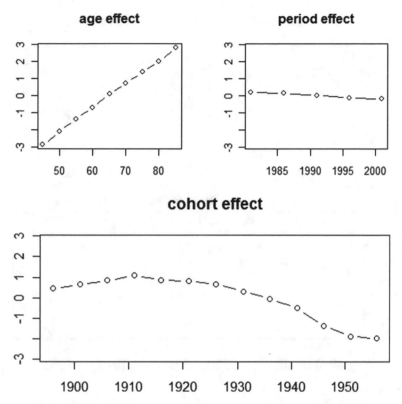

Fig. 6 (**a**) Temporal trend of COPD mortality in age, period, and cohort plotted in the same scale among Hong Kong males after bias correction. (**b**) Temporal trend of COPD mortality in age, period, and cohort plotted in the same scale among Hong Kong females after bias correction

4.3 Importance of the Variance/Standard Error Estimation

The above two examples demonstrate this powerful bias-correction method, which does not require any original data, as well as the powerful variance/standard error estimation. In the example of the cancer incidence rates, three sets of biased estimates are given, each calculated with a different equality constraint. The standard errors of the estimates also vary across the three sets. The bias correction method not only provides accurate parameter estimates through straightforward bias correction, but also provides accurate standard error estimates, even though the standard errors of the biased estimates are known to be inaccurate and vary with the estimates. As shown in Fig. 4, the accurate standard errors calculated by the correction method offers accurate 95% confidence intervals and further statistical inferences can be made about the increasing-then-decreasing age trend, the overall decreasing period, and the overall decreasing cohort trend accordingly.

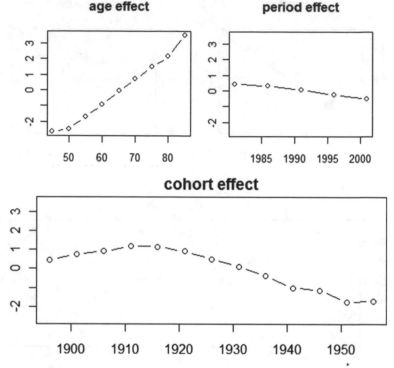

Fig. 6 (continued)

   In contrast, no standard errors were available for the biased estimates in the second, COPD study example, therefore no standard errors can be made available by the bias-correction method. The bias-correction method did yield decreasing period trend for both males and for females separately, which is much more reasonable than the increasing period trend for males and the increasing-then-decreasing period trend for females since both males and females lived in the same city and had the same air-quality. However, no statistical inferences can be made because of the lack of the standard errors for the effect estimates. Had the COPD study provided the standard error estimates, the bias-correction method would yield accurate standard error estimates no matter how inaccurate the original errors were, and meaningful statistical inference could be made to the trend estimation after bias correction.

5 Conclusion and Discussion

Age-period-cohort models have broad applications in demography, economics, marketing research, public health studies, and sociology. Although the statistical models and methods have been studied extensively in the literature, the identification problem was not settled for a long time, resulting in confusion and misinterpretation. Consequently, most studies did not analyze the age-period-cohort data correctly, and bias was frequently introduced through the constraint method by the subjective assumptions of the investigators. Although the intrinsic estimator method provides an unbiased estimation, the direct computation of the intrinsic estimator requires the original data, which may not be available in published age-period-cohort studies where bias correction is still needed. Furthermore, many studies chose not to report the original data in publications, which makes bias correction even more difficult.

Our novel bias correction method addresses this challenging issue. It requires no original data, and corrects the bias in parameter estimation obtained from using any constraint. Additionally, it is simple and easy to implement, thus making it applicable to any APC analysis that uses a constraint estimator for parameter determination. Furthermore, if the constraint method provides the standard errors of the parameter estimates for the age, period and cohort effects and the constraint used to generate the parameter estimates, our method may also yield accurate estimation of the standard errors for the parameter estimates after bias correction.

Although this bias correction method is developed based on the linear model (1), it also applies to the log-linear model (1*) and other generalized linear models because the mechanism of the identification problem remains the same and thus bias can be corrected following the same procedure. This is demonstrated in the example of the Hong Kong COPD mortality study fitted with a log-linear model, which yields much more meaningful trend after the bias correction.

It may be noted that although this uses the same mathematical formula as Eq. (14) in Yang et al. (2008), they serve very different purposes. Yang et al. (2008) used the equation to confirm the discovery of the estimable function by observing that any constraint leads to the same estimator B, which can be interpreted geometrically as estimable (independent of the constraint). Notice, however, that this is merely an interpretation, not a rigorous proof, and it was never pointed out that Eq. (14) can be used for bias correction for any given biased estimates in publications. As a matter of fact, ever since the publication of Yang et al. (2008), no bias correction has been studied yet and bias correction in APC studies has received no attention in any publication. This is because the interpretation of the estimability of B through its independence of any constraint does not constitute a rigorous proof of the estimability, therefore, no bias correction can be established yet. Currently, the same equation is being used for bias correction, especially after rigorous proof of the unbiasedness and consistency of the intrinsic estimator B as shown in Fu (2016). Only after the theoretical proof of the estimability and the consistency, could one claim the unbiasedness of the intrinsic estimator and further make bias correction through it, as demonstrated here.

References

Bosch, F. X., Manos, M. M., Muñoz, N., Sherman, M., Jansen, A. M., Peto, J., Schiffman, M. H., Moreno, V., Kurman, R., Shan, K. V., & International Biological Study on Cervical Cancer (IBSCC) Study Group. (1995). Prevalence of human papillomavirus in cervical cancer: A worldwide perspective. *JNCI: Journal of the National Cancer Institute, 87*(11), 796–802.

Cayuela, A., Rodriguer-Dominguez, S., Ruiz-Borrego, M., & Gili, M. (2004). Age-period-cohort analysis of breast cancer mortality rates in Andalucia (Spain). *Annals of Oncology, 15*, 686–688.

Chen, J., Schooling, C. M., Johnston, J. M., Hedley, A. J., & McGhee, S. M. (2011). How does socioeconomic development affect COPD mortality? An age-period-cohort analysis from a recently transitioned population in China. *PLoS One, 6*(9), e24348. https://doi.org/10.1371/journal.pone.0024348.

Clayton, D., & Schifflers, E. (1987). Models for temporal variation in cancer rates. II: Age-period-cohort models. *Statistics in Medicine, 6*, 469–481.

Fu, W. J. (2000). Ridge estimator in singular design with applications to age-period-cohort analysis of disease rates. *Communications in Statistics Theory and Method, 29*, 263–278.

Fu, W. J. (2008). Smoothing cohort model in age-period-cohort analysis with applications to homicide arrest rates and lung cancer mortality rates. *Sociological Methods and Research, 36*(3), 327–361.

Fu, W. J. (2016). Constrained estimator and consistency of a regression model on a Lexis diagram. *Journal of American Statistical Association, 111*(513), 180–199.

Glenn, N. D. (2003). Distinguishing age, period, and cohort effects. In J. T. Mortimer & M. J. Shanahan (Eds.), *Handbook of the life course*. New York: Kluwer Academic/Plenum Publisher.

Heuer, C. (1997). Modeling of time trends and interactions in vital rates using restricted regression splines. *Biometrics, 53*, 161–177.

Jemal, A., Chu, K. C., & Tarone, R. E. (2001). Recent trends in lung cancer mortality in the United States. *Journal of the National Cancer Institute, 93*(4), 277–283.

Kupper, L. L., Janis, J. M., Salama, I. A., Yoshizzwa, C. N., & Greenberg, B. G. (1983). Age-period-cohort analysis: An illustration of the problems in assessing interaction in one observation per cell data. *Communications in Statistics, 12*, 2779–2807.

Kupper, L. L., Janis, J. M., Karmous, A., & Greenberg, B. G. (1985). Statistical age-period-cohort analysis: A review and critique. *Journal of Chronic Disease, 38*, 811–830.

Mason, K. O., Mason, W. M., Winsborough, H. H., & Poole, W. K. (1973). Some methodological issues in the cohort analysis of archival data. *American Sociological Review, 38*, 242–258.

Mason, W. M., & Smith, H. L. (1985). Age-period-cohort analysis and the study of deaths from pulmonary tuberculosis. In W. M. Mason & S. Fienberg (Eds.), *Cohort analysis in social research, beyond the identification problem* (pp. 151–227). New York: Springer-Verlag.

McCulloch, C. E., & Searle, S. R. (2001). *Generalized, linear and mixed models*. New York: Wiley.

National Cancer Institute. Surveillance, epidemiology, and end results (SEER) program. https://seer.cancer.gov/statistics/summaries.html. Accessed 12 December 2016.

Rodgers, W. L. (1982). Estimable functions in age, period and cohort effects. *American Sociological Review, 47*, 774–787.

Sasieni, P. D., & Adams, J. (2000). Analysis of cervical cancer mortality and incidence data from England and Wales: Evidence of a beneficial effect of screening. *Journal of Royal Statistical Society A, 163*, 191–209.

Scheurer, M. E., Tortolero-Luna, G., Guillaud, M., Follen, M., Chen, Z., Dillon, L. M., & Adler-Storthz, K. (2005). Correlation of HPV 16 and HPV 18 E7 mRNA levels with degree of cervical dysplasia. *Cancer Epidemiology, Biomarker and Prevention, 14*(8), 1948–1952.

Schwadel, P. (2010). Age, period, and cohort effects on U.S. religious service attendance: The declining impact of sex, southern residence, and Catholic affiliation. *Sociology of Religion, 71*(1), 2–24. https://doi.org/10.1093/socrel/srq005.

Seber, G. A. F., & Lee, A. J. (2003). *Linear regression analysis*. New York: Wiley.

Smith, H. L. (2008). Advances in age–period–cohort analysis. *Sociological Methods and Research, 36*(3), 287–296.

Smith, H. L., Mason, W. M., & Fienberg, S. E. (1982). Estimable functions of age, period and cohort effects: More chimeras of the age-period-cohort accounting framework: Comment on Rodgers. *American Sociological Review, 47*(6), 787–793.

Tu, Y. K., Smith, G. D., & Gilthorpe, M. S. (2011). A new approach to age-period-cohort analysis using partial least squares regression: The trend in blood pressure in the Glasgow alumni cohort. *PLoS One, 6*(4), e19401.

Wilmoth, J. R. (1990). Variation in vital rates by age, period, and cohort. *The Sociological Review, 20*, 295–335.

Winship, C., & Harding, D. J. (2008). A mechanism-based approach to the identification of age-period-cohort models. *Sociological Methods & Research, 36*(3), 362–401.

Yang, Y., Fu, W. J., & Land, K. (2004). A methodological comparison of age-period-cohort models: The intrinsic estimator and conventional generalized linear models. *Sociological Methodology, 34*, 75–110.

Yang, Y., Schulhofer-Wohl, S., Fu, W. J., & Land, K. (2008). The intrinsic estimator for age-period-cohort analysis: What it is and how to use it. *American Journal of Sociology, 113*, 1697–1736.

Index

© Springer International Publishing AG 2017
D.-G. Chen et al. (eds.), *New Advances in Statistics and Data Science*,
ICSA Book Series in Statistics, https://doi.org/10.1007/978-3-319-69416-0

Printed in the United States
By Bookmasters